Swallowing Intervention
in Oncology

Dysphagia Series

Series Editor

John C. Rosenbek, Ph.D.

Dysphagia Assessment and Treatment Planning: A Team Approach

Rebecca Leonard, Ph.D., and Katherine Kendall, M.D.

The Neuroscientific Principles of Swallowing and Dysphagia

Arthur J. Miller, Ph.D.

Management of Adult Neurogenic Dysphagia

Maggie Lee Huckabee, M.A., and Cathy A. Pelletier, M.S.

Swallowing Intervention in Oncology

Paula A. Sullivan, M.S., and Arthur M. Guilford, Ph.D.

Manual of Dysphagia Assessment in Adults

Joseph T. Murray, M.A.

Swallowing Intervention in Oncology

Edited By

Paula A. Sullivan, M.S., CCC-SLP
Adjunct Assistant Professor
Department of Otolaryngology
University of Miami School of Medicine
Miami, Florida

and

Arthur M. Guilford, Ph.D.
Professor and Chair
Department of Communication Sciences and Disorders
College of Arts and Sciences
University of South Florida
Tampa, Florida

SINGULAR PUBLISHING GROUP, INC.
SAN DIEGO · LONDON

Singular Publishing Group, Inc.
401 West "A" Street, Suite 325
San Diego, California 92101-7904

Singular Publishing Group, Inc.
19 Compton Terrace
London N1 2UN, U.K.

Singular Publishing Group, Inc., publishes textbooks, clinical manuals, clinical reference books, journals, videos, and multimedia materials on speech-language pathology, audiology, otorhinolaryngology, special education, early childhood, aging, occupational therapy, physical therapy, rehabilitation, counseling, mental health, and voice. For your convenience, our entire catalog can be accessed on our web-site at **http//www.singpub.com**. Our mission to provide you with materials to meet the daily challenges of the everchanging health care/educational environment will remain on course if we are in touch with you. In that spirit, we welcome your feedback on our products. Please telephone (**1-800-521-8545**), fax (**1-800-774-8398**), or e-mail (**singpub@mail,cerfnet.com**) your comments and requests to us.

Typeset in 9/11 Bookman by So Cal Graphics
Printed in the United States of America by Bang Printing

Library of Congress Cataloging-in-Publication Data

Swallowing intervention in oncology / edited by Paula
  Sullivan and Arthur Guilford.
      p.   cm. — (Dysphagia series)
  Includes bibliographical references and index.
  ISBN 1-56593-751-1 (softcover : alk. paper)
  1. Deglutition disorders.   2. Cancer—Complications.   3. Cancer—
Patients—Rehabilitation.   I. Sullivan, Paula.   II. Guilford,
Arthur M.   III. Series.
  [DNLM: 1. Neoplasms—rehabilitation.   2. Deglutition Disorders—
etiology.   3. Deglutition Disorders—rehabilitation.   QZ 266S971
1998]
RC815.2.S93   1998
616.99'406—dc21
DNLM/DLC   98-29426
for Library of Congress   CIP

Contents

Foreword

A number of types of cancer and their treatments can result in changes in speech, hearing, swallowing, and subsequently nutrition. This text provides an excellent in-depth review of the types of speech, swallowing, and hearing impairments and rehabilitation needs and procedures for patients with various types and sites of tumors and their treatments. The sites of cancer that particularly affect communication and swallowing are clearly those in the head and neck, in the brain, and in the upper aerodigestive tract. Over the years, there has been increasing recognition of posttreatment morbidity—that is, the effects of the treatment on the functional abilities of the patient.

Historically, research has focused on the nature of changes in speech, swallowing, and hearing that result from various treatments to various disease sites. As the extent of posttreatment functional abnormalities has become clear, physicians and others have attempted to identify more and more effective tumor treatments, which also result in less and less functional morbidity. Unfortunately, however, even those treatments designed to eliminate or reduce morbidity, such as the organ preservation protocols being implemented and studied in many institutions using a combination of chemotherapy and radiation therapy in contrast to surgery, can result in significant functional impact.

Thus, the functional problems after treatment for cancers of the brain and upper aerodigestive tract continue despite recent treatment advances. They require expert knowledge on the part of the rehabilitation professionals involved. Unfortunately, the health care reforms of the last 5 years have made access to quality rehabilitative care difficult. Generally, a team of rehabilitation professionals is needed by these patients in order for the patient to regain optimal function posttreatment. But

health care reform has made access to rehabilitation teams experienced in the care of these patients more and more limited. Patients are often sent out into the community to look for rehabilitation resources. Third-party payers often require patients to receive their care in the community rather than at the major medical centers where rehabilitation professionals are more experienced in treating these patients. At the same time, the education of rehabilitation professionals in this area of cancer rehabilitation has diminished somewhat as graduate programs in a number of areas, particularly speech-language pathology, have reduced their coursework in such topics as laryngectomy and glossectomy and have not expanded adequately into areas such as dysphagia (i.e., the evaluation and treatment of swallowing disorders). As a result, when patients are spread throughout the community to get their rehabilitation, the patients find it difficult in many instances to identify a knowledgeable professional to care for their rehabilitation needs. These changes in health care are likely to continue and to have continuing negative impact on the functional outcomes of these patients.

More research is critically needed to expand our understanding of the continuously changing treatment effects on communication and swallowing in these patients and to identify optimal rehabilitation treatment strategies and timing of interventions for the various sites and stages of disease and treatment types.

This text can contribute significantly to the expansion of knowledge in the area of communication, swallowing, and nutritional rehabilitation in cancer patients by providing the types of in-depth knowledge needed by the professional in the major medical center and in the community in order to care for these patients effectively and efficiently. The various professionals involved in the care of the patient with communication, swallowing, and nutritional problems are well represented as chapter authors. The descriptions of the team approach and the involvement of rehabilitation professions beginning with the patient's diagnosis are thorough so that professionals who are new to the area can understand the rehabilitation process from the start. I anticipate that this text will serve as an excellent resource for a broad range of rehabilitation professionals but particularly for speech-language pathologists and audiologists who play a central role in the rehabilitation of these patients.

Jerilyn A. Logemann, Ph.D.
Ralph and Jean Sundin Professor
Department of Communication
Sciences and Disorders
Northwestern University
Evanston, Illinois

Preface

In the recent past, the word *cancer* was equated with fear, pessimism, and fatalism. Oncology rehabilitation was considered an oxymoron, as few cancer patients had any hope of long-term survival. Times are changing. Recent treatment advances have reduced mortality rates, resulting in a growing number of long-term survivors, with numbers expected to exceed 65% in the 21st century. Despite increased survival rates, cancer and its treatments often result in functional impairment to swallowing and communication, which significantly affect quality of life for both the patient and family. As new, aggressive treatment modalities continue to be developed, the potential for increased complications to the aerodigestive tract functions of swallowing, phonation, articulation, and respiration, as well as hearing and cognition, will increase. As more and more people are living longer and surviving cancer, there is a growing need for skilled, multidisciplinary health care providers to deal with the myriad issues related to cancer and its treatment. Unfortunately, many health care professionals receive little or no education in oncology rehabilitation and are ill prepared to provide services to the growing number of cancer survivors. The impact of health care reform on cancer rehabilitation, as presented in the Foreword by Dr. Jerilyn Logemann, underscores the increased need of education. Many community-based general practitioners are expected to provide "specialty" care when patients are denied access to cancer rehabilitation centers, resulting in a greater potential for patients to "fall through the cracks" during the care continuum. Thus, there is a critical need to further educate and train health care professionals in both the concept and process of cancer rehabilitation.

The motivation and inspiration to write this book came during the primary editor's 10-year tenure at H. Lee Moffitt Cancer Center and Research Institute. In the early years, the significant number of patient referrals for swallowing and communication intervention secondary to cancer or its treatment in sites other than the head and neck and brain was surprising. In subsequent years, an increased incidence of patients with functional deficits due to the late effects of therapy (e.g., fibrosis of the upper aerodigestive tract related to radiation therapy) was observed. Information to assist in these clinical endeavors was lacking. However, knowledge in the area increased due to guidance and interaction from numerous individuals and experiences. Dr. H. Worth Boyce, Jr., of the Center for Swallowing Disorders, School of Medicine, University of South Florida, emphasized and skillfully demonstrated the critical importance of the multidisciplinary team approach to dysphagia management. In his role as Cancer Center Director, Dr. John Ruckdeschel advocated for and established site-specific cancer care teams. On a daily basis, the primary editor had the opportunity to participate in and witness the positive outcomes of effective cancer care team interventions. As the Cancer Center continued to evolve and mature over time, its care teams grew in effectiveness and efficiency. Most importantly, our patients proved to be the best teachers. Again, she is grateful for another opportunity to work with an exceptional, multidisciplinary head and neck care team at the University of Miami's Sylvester Cancer Center.

In the past few years, there has been a growing interest and expansion of knowledge in the area of swallowing, communication, and nutritional rehabilitation with cancer patients. However, it has been limited primarily to the area of head and neck cancer. There is a need for increased awareness by health care specialists of the potential for posttreatment morbidity in *all* disease sites. With early intervention, treatment-related complications can be prevented or minimized.

We have endeavored to develop a clinically relevant resource that will provide interested multidisciplinary health care providers with pertinent background information related to communication, and to nutritional problems in cancer patients. More importantly, we have attempted to provide the process, or framework, through which functional outcomes are optimized—the team approach. Consequently, chapter contributors were selected to represent the broad scope of disciplines and, thus, perspectives critical in addressing the complex health care and quality-of-life issues encountered in cancer rehabilitation. These well-respected, practicing clinicians represent a variety of disciplines including medical oncology, radiation oncology, otolaryngology, gastroenterology, neurosurgery, speech-language pathology, nursing, pharmacology, psychology, psychiatry, audiology, and dietary science. Chapters 1 and 2 provide practitioners an introduction to oncology principles and management and a team-based model for integrated and comprehensive rehabilitation throughout the continuum of care. Chapters 3 and 4 discuss two primary treatment modalities, chemotherapy and radiation therapy, and their clinical applications, benefits, and impact on patient function. Malignancies in various disease sites, tumor behavior, and management issues are addressed in Chapters 5–11. Unfortunately, space would not permit representation of every specialist, population, or content area affected by cancer. Rather, subsequent chapters provide the practitioner clinically relevant information pertinent to swallowing, communication, and nutritional rehabilitation in cancer patients. Topics include but are not limited to pharmacological and psychological considerations and pediatric issues. A unique offering is the chapter dealing with legal, ethical, and clinical management issues in terminally ill patients. The book concludes with a discussion of the roles and responsibilities of providers in demonstrating the need and value of cancer rehabilitation in today's cost-driven health care environment.

We have included stories of cancer survivors told through photographs and short essays. Although unique and special, these stories do not reflect atypical outcomes. The stories of these individuals illustrate the improvements in long-term survival rates due to continued advances in surgery, radiation therapy, chemotherapy, and immunotherapy. Most importantly, these cancer survivors demonstrate the most important outcome of a combined and comprehensive approach to cancer care—improved quality of life.

As so eloquently stated by Perlman and Schulze-Delrieu in their text, *Deglutition and its Disorders*, "defining areas of current ignorance is vital to future progress and likely to spawn interdisciplinary research and clinical care." Through this collaborative effort, that is our intention and hope.

Paula A. Sullivan
Arthur M. Guilford

Acknowledgments

Indeed, I am fortunate. I have been given the opportunity to work in centers of excellence with exceptional professionals, first at H. Lee Moffitt Cancer Center and Research Institute and currently at the University of Miami's Sylvester Cancer Center, doing what brings me the greatest professional satisfaction—working with cancer survivors and their families. There can be no greater reward.

I am indebted to each chapter contributor for their unique strengths, creativity, and belief that this book will provide cancer patients an enhanced quality of life. The team effort required to see this endeavor to fruition is reflected in the commitment to this collaborative effort.

Special thanks are extended to Jay Rosenbek, series editor, and Marie Linvill, Singular Publishing Group's editor, for their expert guidance and incredible patience, understanding, and support. Their extraordinary commitments of time and effort were "above and beyond" the call of duty. I am indebted. Also, I am grateful to Dr. Andre Abitbol and Joy Gaziano for their Herculean efforts to ensure that essential and critical topics were included.

I wish to acknowledge the support and commitment to this endeavor by Dr. Jack Ruckdeschel and Dr. Albert Einstein of the H. Lee Moffitt Cancer Center and Research Institute. In addition to chapter contributions, they helped to clarify the book's aim and enlisted the support of many chapter contributors due to their belief in the need for this text. Countless other resources were provided by Moffitt Cancer Center and its staff, including the photography for the patient "Patient Profiles." I want to thank these remarkable patients who graciously and generously shared their time and cancer experiences.

To my mentor, Dr. Jeri Logemann, thank you for teaching me the critical need for clinical research and its importance to the future of dysphagia assessment and treatment, as well as providing me opportunities to participate with you in these efforts. I am honored and indebted.

To Dr. H. Worth Boyce, Jr., and Janet Jones Dawsey of the U.S.F. Center for Swallowing Disorders, special thanks for showing me the true art of medicine. You taught me that the swallow doesn't stop at the cricopharyngeus. Most importantly, you taught me that the patient as well as his or her swallowing disorder should be treated. I also owe you my appreciation of the value of a truly collaborative team.

Thank you to my parents and my family for your love and belief in me. And Dad, thank you for making me take that anatomy test. I love you all.

Most especially, I want to thank each and every one of my patients and their families for their hope, courage, and determination. You were the motivation and inspiration.

Paula A. Sullivan

Acknowledgments

When Paula and I first began planning this book, the task did not seem so daunting. However, as we began developing the project and we discovered so many areas that needed to be explored, the enormity of what was ahead became more obvious. Therefore, we certainly could not have completed this work without the strong support of Jay Rosenbek, series editor, and Marie Linvill, Singular Publishing Group Editor, and our contributing authors—without them this project would have never been completed

On a more personal level, I want to express my deep appreciation to two colleagues and former students: Paula Sullivan and Margie Wells-Friedman. It was a wonderful experience to work with and learn from them on this project. My deep appreciation to friend and mentor, Jeri Logemann, for leading the way for all of us. Also, I want to thank Diana Mullinex for jumping in and helping us on so many details. Finally, I thank my family and friends for their support and understanding during this lengthy process.

Arthur M. Guilford

Contributors

Andre A. Abitbol, M.D.
Associate Director
Radiation Oncology
Baptist Hospital of Miami
Miami, Florida

Kathryn Allen, R.D., L.D.N.
Clinical/Research Dietitian
Department of Nutrition
H. Lee Moffitt Cancer Center and Research
    Institute
Tampa, Florida

Deborah L. Borger, M.S., R.N., O.C.N.
Transplant Coordinator
Walt Disney Memorial Cancer Institute at
    Florida Hospital
Orlando, Florida

Daniel E. Buffington, Pharm.D., M.B.A.
Division of Clinical Pharmacology
University of South Florida College of
    Medicine
Tampa, Florida

Roy R. Casiano, M.D.
Associate Professor of Otolaryngology
University of Miami School of Medicine
Miami, Florida

Umesh Choudhry, M.D.
Center for Swallowing Disorders
College of Medicine
University of South Florida
Tampa, Florida

Ronald C. DeConti, M.D.
Professor of Medicine
H. Lee Moffitt Cancer Center and Research
    Institute
University of South Florida
Tampa, Florida

Albert B. Einstein, Jr., M.D.
Associate Center Director for Clinical Affairs
H. Lee Moffitt Cancer Center and Research
    Institute
University of South Florida
Tampa, Florida

Karen K. Fields, M.D.
Associate Professor
Chief, Bone Marrow Transplant Service
H. Lee Moffitt Cancer Center and Research
    Institute
University of South Florida
Tampa, Florida

Jay L. Friedland, M.D.
Assistant Professor
Department of Radiology
H. Lee Moffitt Cancer Center and Research
    Institute
University of South Florida
Tampa, Florida

Penelope Stevens Fisher, M.S., R.N., C.O.R.L.N.
Head and Neck Program
H. Lee Moffitt Cancer Center and Research
    Institute
Tampa, Florida

Joy E. Gaziano, M.A., CCC-SLP
Coordinator of Speech Pathology
    Rehabilitation Services
H. Lee Moffitt Cancer Center and Research
    Institute
University of South Florida
Tampa, Florida

Angie S. Graham, Pharm.D.
Drug Information Resident
Drug Information Analysis Service
University of California, San Francisco
San Francisco, California

John N. Greene, M.D.
Associate Professor
University of South Florida College of
    Medicine
Chief, Division of Infectious and Tropical
    Diseases
H. Lee Moffitt Cancer Center and Research
    Institute
Tampa, Florida

Annelle V. Hodges, Ph.D.
Associate Professor and Director of Audiology
Department of Otolaryngology
University of Miami School of Medicine
Miami, Florida

A. J. Jackson, II, Pharm.D.
Pharmacoeconomic Fellow
Zynr Health—Cedar-Sinai Health System
Beverly Hills, California

Paul B. Jacobsen, Ph.D.
Psychosocial Oncology Program
H. Lee Moffitt Cancer Center and Research
   Institute
Tampa, Florida

Nagi Kumar, Ph.D., R.D.
Department of Nutrition
H. Lee Moffitt Cancer Center and Research
   Institute
Tampa, Florida

Rakesh Kumar, M.D.
Chief Resident
Division of Neurosurgery
University of South Florida College of
   Medicine
Tampa, Florida

Meg Cass Kuznicki, R.N., M.S.N.
Nutritional Support Clinical Specialist
H. Lee Moffitt Cancer Center and Research
   Institute
Tampa, Florida

Alan A. Lewin, M.D.
Medical Director
Radiation Oncology
Baptist Hospital of Miami
Miami, Florida

Brenda L. Lonsbury-Martin, Ph.D.
Chandler Professor and Director of Research
Department of Otolaryngology Research Lab
University of Miami Ear Institute
Miami, Florida

Donna S. Lundy, M.A., CCC-SLP
Adjunct Assistant Professor
Department of Otolaryngology
University of Miami School of Medicine
Miami, Florida

Carole S. Mackey, M.S., R.D.
Clinical Dietician
Wesley Chapel, Florida

Jay J. Mamel, M.D.
Associate Professor of Medicine
Division of Digestive Diseases and Nutrition
University of South Florida, College of
   Medicine
Tampa, Florida

Vivek Mishra, Ph.D.
Director of Medical Physics
Baptist Hospital of Miami
Miami, Florida

Lynn C. Moscinski, M.D.
Department of Hemopathology
H. Lee Moffitt Cancer Center and Research
   Institute
University of South Florida
Tampa, Florida

S. Kirk Payne, M.D.
Associate
Department of Medicine and Program in
   Biomedical Ethics and Medical
   Humanities
University of Iowa
Iowa City, Iowa

Eva S. Quiroz, M.D.
Fellow, Infectious Diseases
University of South Florida College of Medicine
Tampa, Florida

Marion B. Ridley, M.D.
Associate Professor of Surgery
Department of Otolaryngology
College of Medicine
University of South Florida
Tampa, Florida

Maria Amelia Rodrigues, M.D.
Radiation Oncologist
Baptist Hospital of Miami
Miami, Florida

John C. Ruckdeschel, M.D.
Director and CEO
H. Lee Moffitt Cancer Center and Research
   Institute
Professor of Medicine
University of South Florida College of
   Medicine
Tampa, Florida

Ruben Saez, M.D.
Associate Medical Director of Bone Marrow
   Transplantation
Harris Methodist Fort Worth
Fort Worth, Texas

Helen M. Sharp, M.S., CCC-SLP
Doctoral Student
Department of Speech Pathology and
   Audiology
University of Iowa
Iowa City, Iowa

Paula A. Sullivan, M.S., CCC-SLP
Adjunct Assistant Professor
Department of Otolaryngology
University of Miami School of Medicine
Miami, Florida

Michael A. Weitzner, M.D.
Assistant Professor
Psychiatry Service
H. Lee Moffitt Cancer Center and Research
   Institute
University of South Florida
Tampa, Florida

Margie Wells-Friedman, M.S., CCC-SLP
Manager of Inpatient Developmental and
   Rehabilitative Services
Speech-Language Department
All Children's Hospital
St. Petersburg, Florida

Profiles of Success

Thanks to advancements in cancer treatment, long term survival rates are on the rise. However, the newer, aggressive treatments place cancer patients at greater risk for significant functional changes in swallowing and communication abilities. Clearly, with increased quantity of life must come increased quality of life. The cancer experiences of these individuals are included to demonstrate that optimal outcomes are best achieved through a collaborative and comprehensive approach to cancer care.

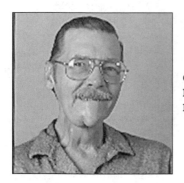

Chapter 2
Loren E.
Lowrey

Following his second surgical intervention to control advanced squamous cell cancer of the anterior floor of the mouth and mandible, efficient and effective speech rehabilitation was imperative for Loren Lowery to return to his livelihood as a radio dispatcher for his local county ambulance and fire department. His employers were concerned that unclear communication by Lowery could have life-threatening consequences. Following intensive speech and swallowing rehabilitation, Loren's cancer care team supported his efforts to return to his previous position. Loren Lowery strongly feels that speech rehabilitation was "instrumental" in his job retention as a radio dispatcher.

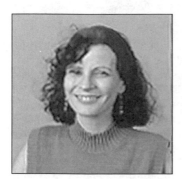

Chapter 5
Francesca
Moran Fiore

A 3-year survivor of brain cancer, Francesca Moran Fiore is grateful for "being blessed with the gift of life." Prior to her diagnosis, Francesca's life was hectic trying to manage the everyday demands of college teacher and practicing architect. She now strives to find joy in everyday activities and pursues the things she loves to do, including spending more time with her family, teaching at a Montessori school, and leading a kindergarten Sunday school class. When her cancer went into remission, Francesca made a commitment to health maintenance through proper nutrition and positive attitude.

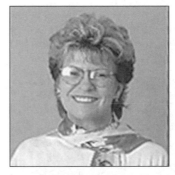

Chapter 6
Deborah
"Debby" Brown

Debby Brown required total laryngectomy for recurrent squamous cell carcinoma of the larynx. She began communicating with an artificial larynx on her 5th postoperative day, which facilitated an early discharge home. The cancer experience has not decreased Debby's activities; if anything, it has increased them. In addition to being active in her church community, Debby also assumed the office of secretary in the Chatterbox Club, a support group for laryngectomees and their families. Debby makes it a point to reach out to other laryngectomees, not only through her publication of the club's monthly newsletter, but also by serving as a visitor to newly diagnosed patients with laryngeal cancer. Prevention is important to Debby, as she is committed to increasing public awareness of head and neck cancer.

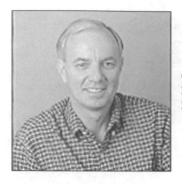

**Chapter 7
Henry "Hank"
DuFour**

Hank DuFour has a 15-year history of gastroesophageal reflux disease, with the onset at 35 years of age. In 1992, he was found to have Barrett's esophagus. Follow-up endoscopy with biopsy in March 1996 revealed changes of high-grade dysplasia with evidence of carcinoma in situ. Subsequent biopsy specimens obtained in August 1996 revealed invasive adenocarcinoma of the esophagus. Hank subsequently underwent resection, and no nodal involvement was found. Today, he is employed on a full-time basis and remains disease free. Hank has been enthusiastic in assisting his care team members in counseling patients with similar esophageal problems.

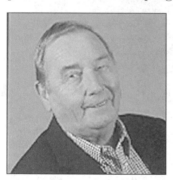

**Chapter 8
George
Forbeck**

Lung cancer was not in the retirement plans of George Forbeck, who was diagnosed with the disease in his 1st year of retirement after working 39 years as a grain trader with the Chicago Board of Trade. Cancer was not a stranger to George. His father died from cancer, as did his son, Billy Guy, at the age of 11 from neuroblastoma. George spends a part of every day working with the William Guy Forbeck Research Foundation, with the Eastern Cooperative Oncology Group Patient Recovery Committee, or one on one with other individuals with cancer. He also is committed to increasing public awareness through cancer prevention activities. Relaxing at his winter home on Hilton Head Island or in Lake Geneva, Wisconsin, during the summer months also was not in the

retirement plans of George Forbeck. "Giving back a little of what has been given to me" was one of the blessings of his cancer experience.

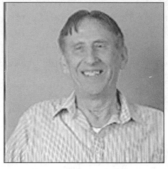

**Chapter 9
Harold
Soladay**

A positive attitude and shared partnerships with his cancer care team, family, and friends are what Harold Soladay credits for his second successful battle against cancer. Harold was recovering from prostrate cancer when he was diagnosed with acute myelogenous leukemia. His treatment of choice was an investigational chemotherapy protocol, which has provided Harold disease remission for the past 2½ years. Harold and his wife, Bernice, "live each day to the fullest" and enjoy the many things this second chance has provided.

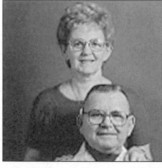

**Chapter 18
Earl and Wini
Mogk**

Earl Mogk was only 50 years of age when he underwent total laryngectomy for laryngeal carcinoma 10 years ago. Since being given a second chance at life, Earl and his wife Wini have committed their lives to helping others. He feels that cancer survivors are not fully rehabilitated until they "give it away." Currently, Earl is giving elementary, middle, and high school students a "challenge to quit" tobacco products. A couple of times a month, Earl shares his cancer experience with school groups and in the courtroom to minor offenders of Florida's new tobacco law. Earl and Wini are active members of the Nu Voice Club of Broward County and the Florida Laryngectomee Association.

A man hath no better thing under the sun, than to eat,
and to drink, and to be merry.

(Ecclesiastes 8:15)

1

Introduction to Cancer: Oncology Principles and Management

Nagi Kumar, Ph.D., R.D.

It is estimated that in the year 2000 there will be 10 million new cases of cancers diagnosed worldwide, excluding non-melanoma skin cancers (Boyle, 1997). Cancer is the second leading cause of death in the United States, and one out of every four deaths in this country is from cancer. Since 1990, there have been 4 million cancer deaths in this country (American Cancer Society, 1997). It is estimated that in the United States 1,382,400 new cases of cancer were diagnosed in the year 1997 and approximately 560,000 Americans died of the disease, which is more than 1,500 people a day. In an era when health care cost is a major concern to both the American individual and society, the National Cancer Institute (NCI) estimates overall cost for cancer at $104 billion: $35 billion for direct medical costs, $12 billion for morbidity costs, and $57 billion for mortality costs (American Cancer Society, 1997). Although the war against cancer is far from over, the past decade has witnessed remarkable progress in understanding the biology of the cancer process in addition to the development of improved screening, diagnosis, and treatment modalities. After decades of steady increases, the age-adjusted mortality due to all malignant neoplasms reached a plateau and showed a decrease of 1% from 1991 to 1994 (Bailar & Gornick, 1997).

BIOLOGY OF CANCER

The past decade has brought us closer to the sophisticated understanding of cellular biology and the regulatory abnormalities in cell behavior that has formed the basis of our understanding of the carcinogenic process. This has opened multiple avenues for novel and innovative modalities of cancer control and management, including dietary modification, biological response modification, and treatments aimed at specific regulatory abnormalities in cancer cell behavior.

The disease called *cancer* is best defined by four characteristics that describe how cancer cells act differently from their normal counterparts: (a) clonality, where cancer originates from genetic changes in a single cell that proliferates to form a clone of malignant cells; (b) autonomy, where the growth is not properly regulated by the normal biochemical and physical influences in the environment; (c) anaplasia, where the cells demonstrate a lack of normal,

1

coordinated cell differentiation; and (d) metastasis, where the cancer cells develop the capacity for discontinuous growth and dissemination to other parts of the body. The process by which a normal cell is converted into one that exhibits these four characteristic traits is termed *malignant transformation* (Mendelsohn, 1997). In general, it has been well established that the biology of cell division and differentiation is similar in both normal and cancer cells. It is now believed that three specific cellular functions tend to be inappropriately regulated in a cancer cell: proliferation, differentiation, and chromosomal and genetic organization and stability. The cancer cell differs from the normal cell in that there is a failure to regulate these functions, which results in altered phenotype and cancer (Fingert, Campis, & Pardee, 1997). More recently, observations of other alterations in cellular functions, such as signal transduction pathways that affect pathogenesis and progression and angiogenesis and tumor growth, have provided improved diagnosis and potential prevention and therapeutic opportunities.

Cell Proliferation

Normal cells reach a steady state of growth, and each organ maintains tight controls over growth rate, growth factors, and cell loss. In addition, cell proliferation is regulated by several environmental factors that control the growth of cells through the cell cycle, so several opportunities for breakdown of this control mechanism can occur in tumor cells (Cofffey & Pienta, 1987; Rollins & Stiles, 1997). It is generally believed that neoplastic cells multiply exponentially during the early phases of tumor growth. This rate of growth decreases, especially in large tumors, possibly due to decrease in growth fractions, increase in cell loss, nutritional depletion of tumor cells, or lengthening of cell cycle time (Coffey & Pienta, 1987). However, when conditions improve or when stimulated by growth factors, these same cells can reenter the division cycle. It is known that the characteristic that distinguishes most neoplasms from normal tissues is an increase in growth factors of a cell population, which initiates cell division from a nongrowing state or a quiescent state (Fingert et al., 1997).

Differentiation

Differentiation is the process by which immature cells with no apparent distinguishing cytological features acquire specialized characteristics that allow them to be recognized as belonging to a particular cell lineage; it produces differences in phenotypes, arising from differences in gene expression, without any change in genetic content (Gallagher, 1991; Rollins & Stiles, 1997). Most tumor cells show abnormalities in differentiation. A cell's ability to proliferate is intimately connected to its state of differentiation. Recent knowledge of the molecular basis for the control of differentiation provides opportunities for controlling tumor growth by manipulating the state of differentiation (Meyskens, 1990; Rowley, Aster, & Sklar, 1993). Several extracellular and intracellular factors control cellular differentiation. Normal cells respond to both stimulatory and inhibitory environmental signals that act by altering the expression of a variety of genes whose products are necessary for proliferative responses. Tumor cells, on the other hand, can escape from normal growth-controlling mechanisms by acquiring increased sensitivity to stimulatory signals or decreased sensitivity to inhibitory signals; this ability is related to an altered differentiated phenotype displayed by the tumor cell (Clement & Campisi, 1991). Analysis of differentiation by tumor cells thus provides valuable information and has logical, fundamental implications for the initial detection of cancer cells and for planning and measuring response to therapy for human cancers.

Signal Transduction and Cellular Function

The modulation of cell function is accomplished by a flow and interaction of specific signals between extracellular and intracellular macromolecules. The study of signal transduction involves the dissection of biochemical pathways involved, starting from the external stimuli leading to the specific cellular response. Recent advances in our knowledge of signal transduction and cell regulatory mechanisms appear to offer us an understanding of how normal cell function is regulated and provide the basis for understanding how abnormalities in these pathways can affect pathogenesis and progression of neoplasms.

Cancer as a Genetic Disease

Cancer is a genetic disease. It is well understood that carcinogenesis is a multistep process that results from the accumulation of genetic changes in inherited and somatic mutation of cells. The current view is that proto-oncogenes, tumor suppressor genes, and DNA repair genes are targeted by these mutations. One of the most significant advances in biomedical research has been in the identification of oncogenes, which are altered versions of the normal cellular genes called proto-oncogenes, which include any dominantly acting gene involved in the neoplastic transformation of cells. The genetic changes that occur during the carcinogenic process consist of the inactivation of tumor suppressor genes (Roulea et al., 1993; Stanbridge & Cavenee, 1989) and DNA repair genes (Hoeijmakers, 1993; Modrich, 1994) and the activation of oncogenes. More than 100 oncogenes have been identified (Levine, 1995). Tumor suppressor genes and DNA repair genes are lost or inactivated in the germ-line and their inactivation predisposes to cancer. The identification of oncogenes has led to the development of tools for molecular diagnosis and monitoring of cancer and to the development of new chemotherapeutic regimens that target specific oncogenes while sparing normal cells (Varmus, 1989). In addition, over the past decade, it has become clear that recurrent chromosomal rearrangements occur in malignant cells (Mitelman, 1994; Solomon, Barrow, & Goodard, 1991). Recent advances in identifying the genes that are believed to produce these chromo-

somal rearrangements have provided new critical diagnostic tools and further provide the opportunity to develop target therapies aimed at specific genetic defects in malignant cells.

Angiogenesis and Tumor Growth

The first observation linking angiogenesis with tumor growth was proposed in the early 1970s (Folkman, 1971), suggesting it is angiogenesis dependent. It is clear now that angiogenesis is fundamental to reproduction, development, and repair and is normally tightly regulated. However, the pathological angiogenesis that is seen in tumors is an out of control, persistent growth of blood vessels, or neovascularization, that sustains the progression of many neoplastic and nonneoplastic cells for months to years. The identification of tumor angiogenesis has pointed researchers in the direction of identifying angiogenic activity as a diagnostic tool and further into genetic angiogenic therapies and nonangiogenic or angiogenic inhibitor therapies for tumor suppression (Folkman, 1994).

CANCER ETIOLOGY

Decades of research to determine the etiology of cancer indicates that patterns of cancer incidence and death rates vary with gender, age, race, and geographic location. More recently, it has been observed that genetic alterations play a critical role in carcinogenesis. In addition, it is clear from the epidemiological evidence that variations in diet and exposure to chemical and physical agents in the external environment, such as radiation, viruses, and a variety of chemicals, contribute to the development of cancers.

Genetic Predisposition

Cancer is a genetic disease. Possibly, fewer than 1% of cancers are inherited cancer syndromes and another 5–10% are recognizable family clusters of common cancers that probably have a genetic basis (Ponder, 1994). The inherited cancer syndromes include all cancers where the genetic effect is clearly apparent (Knudsen, 1989; Mulvihill, Miller, & Fraumeni, 1977). Some examples of inherited cancer syndromes are familial polyposis, multiple endocrine neoplasia types I and II, and von Hippel-Lindau syndrome. On the other hand, familial clusters of cancers are breast and ovarian cancers and nonpolyposis colorectal cancer. Still, a hypothetical class of individuals may have a genetic predisposition without evident family clustering. Examples of these cancers include metabolic polymorphisms determining response to exogenous or endogenous carcinogens. The importance of identifying individuals with a predisposition for cancer has received significant attention in recent years. Predisposed individuals are a high-risk population that may benefit from early diagnosis and treatment. Identifying this group enables researchers to study the steps in the carcinogenic process in addition to observing if the cancer occurred from inherited, noninherited, lifestyle, or other factors. In other cases, genetic predisposition to cancer has been accompanied by abnormalities in development and control of growth in the region of cancer occurrence and elsewhere. Thus identifying individuals with a genetic predisposition to cancer has, in addition to prevention and treatment implications, a potential for researchers to gain a significant body of knowledge from observing these cases.

Despite benefits of genetic and other risk assessment, important bioethical considerations have been raised, including autonomy, privacy, justice, and equity. Identifying risk in individuals may place them in a situation with additional responsibility to deal with family psychosocial anxiety pertaining to the genetic testing of their children. Genetic counseling including psychological support may be critical. However, more recently genetic testing has been recommended only in those situations that are amenable to preventive and therapeutic intervention.

Chemical Carcinogenesis

Chemical carcinogenesis is a multistage process that begins with exposure, usually to complex mixtures of chemicals that are found in the human environment. Many cancers have been caused by occupational exposure, whereas others have been attributed to chemicals and viruses in the environment (Shields & Harris, 1990). Once an environmental agent is internalized, carcinogens are subject to competing pathways of activation and detoxification. However, some carcinogenic agents can act directly. The relative risks of individuals to chemical carcinogenesis (Harris, 1989; Weston, 1993) vary significantly depending on the metabolism of carcinogens, differences in DNA repair capacity, and response to tumor promoters. Over the past years, the sequence of events in chemical carcinogenesis has been systematically established and refined. The results of these studies have paved the way for strategies for cancer prevention and treatment.

Dietary Factors, Hormones, and the Etiology of Cancer

It has been suggested that 30–60% of all cancers in the developed world may be attributed to dietary habits (American Cancer Society, 1995). Until recently, the dietary components that received the most attention were dietary fat and fiber. Populations consuming a low-fat or high-fiber diet, such as in China, Japan, and Finland, have a lower incidence of colon, breast, endometrial, and prostate cancer than their North American and Western European counterparts consuming a high-fat, low-fiber diet (Camoriano et al, 1990). Of particular interest are the endocrine-related cancers and, specifically, breast cancer. There is increasing evidence that dietary factors, specifically fat and components of fiber, may play a role in the production, metabolism, and bioavailability of sex hormones and their impact on target tissues (Demark-Wahnefried, Winer, & Rimer, 1993; Dixon, Maritz, & Baker, 1978). Cancers of hormone-responsive organs currently account for more than 35% of all newly diagnosed male and 40% of all newly diagnosed female patients with cancer in the United States. However, it is still unclear whether the increased risk of hormonal cancer is associated with the resulting products of the different pathways of estrogen and androgenic hormone metabolism or the higher rate of production and higher concentrations of circulating hormones, which are available for metabolism. It is possible that specific components of the diet may also influence the pathways of specific sex hormone metabolism and thus their influence on target tissue.

The other group of nutrients that have consistently stimulated the interest of researchers are components in vegetables and fruits that have consistently shown a protective effect. High consumption of fruits and vegetables is associated with a reduced risk of several cancers including lung, oral, pancreas, larynx, esophagus, bladder, and stomach cancer. Although individual nutrients have been tested and it has been observed that the protective effects of these nutrients are consistent, it is in general believed that multiple nutrients that are present in vegetables and fruits are probably involved.

Ionizing and Ultraviolet Radiation and Carcinogenesis

The oncogenic effect of radiation in many tissues in humans was prevalent in the early 1900s after the discovery of the x-ray. The characteristic of ionizing radiation is its ability to penetrate cells and deposit energy within them in a random fashion, unaffected by the usual cellular barriers. The tissue effect of radiation is by apoptosis, or programmed cell death (Little, 1968; Lowe, Schmitt, Smith, Osborne, & Jacks, 1993), and radiation-induced reproductive failure. Several studies have reported induction of cancer by radiation in experimental and animal models and human studies based on epidemiological studies following exposure to high-dose radiation. Although the effects of ionizing radiation as a carcinogen have been dramatized in the

media, there is no evidence to demonstrate its carcinogenic and mutagenic effects in humans in doses below 50 cGy.

On the other hand, ultraviolet radiation carcinogenesis has received more attention in the past decade, with skin tumors accounting for more than 30% of all cancers. It has been established that the basal cell and squamous cell carcinomas of the skin are highly correlated to cumulative sunlight exposure, identified as the causative agent.

Physical Carcinogenesis

Physical carcinogenesis is a term used to define a wide range of agents that are carcinogenic because of their physical properties and physical effects. They include hard and soft materials, fibrous and nonfibrous particles, and gel materials. The mechanism of physical carcinogenesis has been regarded as a nonspecific irritative effect on cells that could cause cell proliferation, the selection of spontaneously occurring transformed clones, and finally the development of neoplasia. Physical carcinogenesis is an important public health problem, specifically in this century with a significant diffusion of particulate nonfibrous and fibrous industrial material in the workplace and in home environments and the increasing use of xenobiotic implants in plastic, orthopedic, vascular, dental, and other disciplines. The dramatic carcinogenic effects of asbestos (Maltoni et al., 1995) and the unknown effects of several alloplastic surgical components demonstrate the need for more systematic studies of the mechanism and action of physical carcinogenesis.

Viruses

Our knowledge of the mechanisms by which the retroviruses cause neoplastic transformation has increased significantly over the past decade and has contributed to the clarification of the current concept that neoplastic growth is a result of genetic alterations (Bishop, 1987) and the discovery of oncogenes that play a critical role in cell transformation. Herpes viruses such as Epstein-Barr virus, a known oncogenic virus, are associated with lymphoproliferative disease, Burkitt's lymphoma, nasopharyngeal carcinoma, and Hodgkin's disease. Other viruses that are implicated in carcinogenesis are papilloma viruses, which are associated with cervical neoplasia and cause transformation of target tissues (Kantoff et al., 1987). In addition, the association of chronic hepatitis virus infection with hepatocellular carcinoma is well established.

PRINCIPLES OF CANCER MANAGEMENT

The past decade has witnessed significant progress in surgical techniques and the use of combined modalities in cancer treatment, which has significantly affected mortality and morbidity associated with treatment of specially solid neoplasms. Integration of medical and surgical treatments in patients with cancer who have genitourinary, gastrointestinal, or biliary obstruction has reached new heights (Fainsinger, 1996). Current interdisciplinary approaches using advances in diagnosis and staging not only produce better cure rates, but in addition decrease complications of cancer treatment and improve wound healing (Ariyan, 1996; Jacquet & Sugarbaker, 1996) and especially make reconstruction and limb salvage a viable option (Upton, Kocher, & Wolfort, 1996). As most treatments in cancer are currently combined with other treatment modalities, it has become essential that the treatment is planned by a multidisciplinary team. Multidisciplinary approaches to cancer treatment have not only improved cure rates, but also have reduced the risk of disabilities and thus have improved quality of life.

Typically, the disease presents to the physician as an abnormal growth, or tumor, which causes illness by production of biochemically active molecules and by local expansion into adjacent or distant tissue sites. The symptoms of the disease depend on the location of the tumor and the specific molecular products. Developing an appropriate treatment plan for a patient with malignant disease depends on determining the extent of disease spread, the distinctive natural history, and the available therapeutic treatment options for the particular type of cancer (Mendelsohn, 1997).

Surgical Oncology

Historically, surgery was the first modality used in cancer treatment, and for the first part of this century surgery was the only cancer treatment that produced disease-free survival (Bailar & Gornick, 1997). Surgery is the treatment of choice for most confined solid neoplasms. However, more recently chemotherapy and radiation therapy combined with surgery have consistently improved management of cancers. Although surgery is the preferred treatment modality of most neoplasms, it is increasingly recognized that radiation therapy and chemotherapy complement primary surgical treatment of cancer. As accurate diagnosis is the first step to cancer therapy, the role of surgery is obtaining adequate tissue samples for pathological diagnosis. Surgery is the principal means of staging many neoplastic diseases. Twenty-five percent of patients have tumors that are confined and amenable to surgical resection alone. Surgery operates by zero-order kinetics, in that 100% of cells excised are killed. Surgery reduces tumor burden, thereby reducing the immunosuppressive effects of the tumor, increasing the efficacy of nonsurgical adjuvant therapies intended to eliminate microscopic residual disease, and decreasing the risk of recurrence. Surgery can be used as a means of cytoreduction when complete excision is not possible, and after debulking combined with additional therapy to yield significant treatment benefits. At times, surgery can be used for palliation to relieve pain and improve quality of life. Future trends indicate the use of surgical technology such as sentinel node mapping using radiolabled isotope and monitoring its path using a gamma probe (Giuliano, Kirgan, Guenther, & Morton, 1994; Krag et al., 1995). Radioimmunoguided surgery enables surgeons to localize cancer during surgery and to evaluate extent of disease (Kim, Triozzi, & Martin, 1993; Xu et al., 1994).

Radiation Oncology

Similar to surgery, radiation therapy, which is application of ionizing electromagnetic radiation to a tumor site, contributes to localized treatment of cancer, using the principle of the normal tissue and the tumor's inherent radiosensitivity. Both high-energy electromagnetic radiation produced by instruments such as linear accelerators and gamma rays produced by radioactive isotope decay, which have similar physical characteristics and biological effects, are used in radiation therapy. Radiation generates free radicals and reactive oxygen intermediates that damage cellular substituents, including DNA. The target for radiation-induced cell death is the DNA. Dose of radiation depends on cellular division, and amount of oxygen in the cells contributes to the radiosensitivity of the tumor (Little, 1994). More recently, particle beam therapy, which provides for more accurate tissue localization and uses neutrons or charged particles such as protons, has been found to cause less cytotoxicity as compared to conventional radiation therapy.

Radiation therapy is used curatively, palliatively for the management of many tumors, and for acute treatment of complications of malignant disease. More recently, combined modality treatments with radiation and chemotherapy have been used in the treatment of many types of cancers, with significantly improved therapeutic outcomes. These combined modalities have been demonstrated to be effective if chemotherapy is sufficiently active to eradicate subclinical metastases and if the primary tumor is treated effectively by surgery and/or radiation therapy or if there is spatial cooperation (Slapak & Kufe, 1994).

Antineoplastic Agents

Progress in the area of drug therapy for the treatment of cancer has resulted in the identification of several systemic chemother-

apy regimens that are curative, those that contribute significantly or are palliative, those that subsequently improve survival, and those that only contribute in a minor way to the treatment of especially solid tumors. Adjuvant therapies that are provided after surgical resections, such as in breast cancers, and neoadjuvant therapies that are provided prior to surgery, especially in head and neck and bladder carcinomas, have evolved over the recent years and provide effective conservative local therapies. Multidrug regimens that produce cure in certain cancers such as childhood leukemia and Hodgkin's disease open doors to more research in the role of drug therapy in producing sustained chemoresponsiveness. The principle of chemotherapy is based on cytokinetics, by providing cytotoxic agents during the active phase of the cell cycle, which is enhanced and uncontrolled during malignant transformation. The selection of the cytotoxic drugs, such as antimetabolites, alkylating agents, antitumor antibiotics, or glucocorticoids, is to produce the chemotherapeutic response during the various phases or all phases of these cell divisions. Recently, more cancers are treated with combination chemotherapies with excellent therapeutic outcomes, specifically, when single agents have a potential to fail. High-dose chemotherapy followed by bone marrow transplantation has been used to produce cytotoxicity followed by overcoming myelosupression (Chabner & Collins, 1993; Howell, 1997).

Tumor Immunology

Although immunostimulants and immunorestorative agents have been known to us for several decades, only recently has some light been shed on the role of biotherapeutics and its mechanism in the treatment of cancer. Immunostimulants and immunorestorative agents have been studied for the past 50 year, but their application in clinical practice has been limited because they have multiple mechanisms and their interactions are complex and unclear.

EFFECTS OF CANCER TREATMENT AND MANAGEMENT

With significant advances in the field of medical oncology in the area of diagnosis and management of cancers with aggressive treatments, although survival rates increase, patients face significant side effects of treatments and physical deficits. In addition, as prognoses for cancer patients improve, it becomes imperative that they regain normal functional status with adequate nursing, rehabilitative, psychosocial, and nutritional care that specifically outlines treatment and management of these complications.

Several complications are observed with radiation therapy, ranging from acute reactions during or immediately following therapy, such as erythema, symptoms of gastrointestinal toxicity (diarrhea, nausea, vomiting, dysphagia), and myelosupression (such as anemia, thrombocytopenia, and leukopenia; Slapak & Kufe, 1994), to long-term effects of treatment failure, such as local regrowth from cells that survive radiation therapy.

As in radiation therapy regimens, chemotherapy regimen administration is not without complications. Nausea, vomiting, stomatitis, mucositis, alopecia, and myelosupression (such as leukopenia, anemia, and thrombocytopenia) occur with most chemotherapeutic regimens. However, drug resistance is one of the central problems facing medical oncologists today. Several studies have been initiated to study the mechanisms of drug resistance of specific regimens, and chemosensitizing agents are currently being examined to overcome this obstacle while new drug development research has reached its peak.

Research in the area has provided practical means to determine emetogenic and neutropenic potential of treatment regimens and offer opportunities for developing clinical pathways to manage these side effects of treatment in a timely manner and as a part of standard treatment protocols. In addition, better understanding of the mechanism of treatments and their effects, improved patient selection criteria, better education, and management of effects of treatment with therapeutic, nutritional, and behavioral interventions have effectively complemented the use of single and multiple treatment modalities, reducing side effects of treatments and thus improving management of the cancer patient.

FUTURE DIRECTIONS OF ONCOLOGY MANAGEMENT

It is predicted, based on the increasing size of the elderly population, that a significant increase in absolute numbers of cancers will be observed in the early decades of the next century (Boyle, 1997). This has serious public health implications. In national and global terms, the greatest reduction in the burden of cancer would be from cancer prevention and standardized, multidisciplinary, early, aggressive, and effective diagnosis and management of disease. The most promising approach to the control of cancer is a national commitment to prevention and the development of economically efficient models for the management of cancer.

Greenwald defines cancer as a biomedically complex group of diseases that result partly from changes in genes that control cell growth and behavior and partly from interactions between these genetic changes and the cellular stresses that result from specific environmental and behavioral factors, including lifestyle and diet (Greenwald & McDonald, 1997), implying significant opportunities for prevention in addition to novel cancer treatments. Cancer prevention includes primary prevention, such as avoiding the known cancer-causing substances in the environment or dietary elements associated with increased risk and dietary supplementation with putative protective agents, and secondary prevention, such as early detection and removal of benign neoplasms and early detection of breast cancer by mammography (Osborne, Boyle & Lipkin, 1997). Two major programs initiated by the NCI, the Diet and Nutrition Branch and the Chemoprevention Branch, give high priority to cancer prevention. Chemoprevention is the administration of agents (nutrients/pharmaceuticals) to prevent induction or inhibit or delay the progression of cancers. The basic principles involved in identifying these nutrients and other substances for chemoprevention are that the mechanism of carcinogenesis involves mutagenesis and uncontrolled proliferation and that chemoprevention can be accomplished by interfering with these mechanisms. In addition we need to determine specific pathways involved in mutagenesis and proliferation. One of the major objectives of the NCI Chemoprevention Branch is to identify chemopreventive chemicals for human use and develop a systematic methodology, which considers the chemopreventive efficacy of the nutrient or drug, toxicity, pharmacokinetics, potential for clinical use, commercial availability, source of the agent, and cost of the agent. Over 1,500 naturally occurring and synthetic chemicals have been tested for chemopreventive activity.

The national debate on health care reform has led health care providers and payers to develop new approaches to meet the challenges of cost containment while continuing to provide quality care. The critical need for a reduction in health care costs has revolutionized the management of cancer and has established a need to standardize cancer practice via nationally accepted treatment guidelines (Kovach, 1996). Standardized guidelines for disease management must include not only the traditional clinical outcomes but also cost and quality of life of patient outcomes (Morris, 1996; Stovall, 1996). It is thus critical for institutions to examine systematic, historical research data and the economic model, which provide unequivocal evidence of the value of current modalities of treating the patient with cancer to manage costs, reduce length of stay, reduce complications, and increase response to cancer treatments.

Health care institutions must provide high-quality medical care with defined standards and guidelines for practice of credentialed professionals in this setting, contributing to early detection, proper assessment, cost-effective treatment, and prevention of cancers to improve patient outcomes while controlling health care costs. In addition, it is imperative to contribute to research and education toward innovative cancer control regimens, cancer prevention and control that significantly enhance the manageability of health care costs not only for our patient population today but also for populations to come.

REFERENCES

American Cancer Society. (1995) *Cancer facts & figures—1995* (ACS Publication No. 5008.95). Atlanta, GA: Author.

American Cancer Society. (1997). *Cancer facts & figures—1997.* Atlanta, GA: Author.

Ariyan, S. (1996). General principles of reconstruction following cancer surgery. *Surgical Oncology Clinics of North America, 5,* 741–750.

Bailar, J. C., III, & Gornick, H. L. (1997). Cancer undefeated. *New England Journal of Medicine, 336,* 1569–1574.

Bishop, J. M. (1987). The molecular genetics of cancer. *Science, 235,* 305.

Boyle, P. (1997). Global burden of cancer. *Lancet, 349* (Suppl. 2), 23–26.

Camoriano, J. K., Loprinzi, C. L., Ingle, J. N., Therneau, T. M., Krook, J. E., & Veeder, M. H. (1990). Weight change in women treated with adjuvant therapy or observed following mastectomey for node-positive breast cancer. *Journal of Clinical Oncology, 8,* 1327–1334.

Chabner, B. A., & Collins, J. M. (1993). *Cancer chemotherapy: Principles and practice of oncology.* Philadelphia: Lippincott.

Clement, A., & Campisi, J. (1991). Cell cycle regulation and growth control. In A. R. Moossa, S. C. Schimpff, & M. C. Robson (Eds.), *Comprehensive textbook of oncology* (2nd ed.). Baltimore: Williams & Wilkins.

Coffey, D. S., & Pienta, K. J. (1987). New concepts in studying the control of normal and cancer growth of the prostate. *Progressive Clinical Biological Research, 239,* 1.

Demark-Wahnefried, W., Winer, E. P., & Rimer, B. K. (1993). Why women gain weight with adjuvant chemotherapy for breast cancer. *Journal of Clinical Oncology, 11,* 1418–1429.

Dixon, J., Moritz, D., & Baker, F. (1978). Breast cancer and weight gain: An unexpected finding. *Oncology Nursing Forum, 5,* 5–7.

Fainsinger, R. L. (1996). Integrating medical and surgical treatments in gastrointestinal, genitourinary, and bilary obstruction in patients with cancer. *Hematology/Oncology Clinics of North America, 10,* 173–188.

Fingert, H. J., Campis, J., & Pardee, A. B. (1997). Cell proliferation & differentiation. In J. F. Holland, R. C. Bast, Jr., D. L. Morton, & E. Frei (Eds.), *Cancer medicine* (4th ed.). Philadelphia: Lea & Febiger.

Folkman, J. (1971). Tumor angiogenesis: Therapeutic implications. *New England Journal of Medicine, 285,* 1182–1186.

Folkman, J. (1994). Angiogenesis and breast cancer. *Journal of Clinical Oncology, 12,* 441–444.

Gallagher, R. E. (1991). Control of differentiation. In A.R. Moossa, S. C. Schimpff, & M. C. Robson (Eds.), *Comprehensive textbook of oncology* (2nd ed.). Baltimore: Williams & Wilkins.

Giuliano, A. E., Kirgan, D. M., Guenther, J. M., & Morton, D. L. (1994). Lymphatic mapping and sentinel lymphadenectomy for breast cancer. *Annals of Surgery, 220,* 391–398.

Greenwald, P., & McDonald, S. S. (1997). Cancer prevention: The roles of diet and chemoprevention. *Cancer Control, 4,* 118–127.

Harris, C. C. (1989). Interindividual variation among humans in carcinogen metabolism, DNA adduct formation and DNA repair. *Carcinogenesis, 10,* 1563.

Hoeijmakers, J. H. U. (1993). Nucleotide excisional repair II: From yeast to mammals. *Trends in Genetics, 9,* 211.

Howell, S. B. (1997). Regional chemotherapy. In J. F. Holland, R. C. Bast, Jr., D. L. Morton, & E. Frei (Eds.), *Cancer medicine* (4th ed.). Philadelphia: Lea & Febiger.

Jacquet, P., & Sugarbaker, P. H. (1996). Effects of postoperative intraperitonial chemotherapy on peritonial wound healing and adhesion formation. *Cancer Treatment Research, 82,* 327–335.

Kantoff, P. W., Gillio, A. P., McLachlin, J. R., Bordignon, C., Eglitis, M. A., Kernan, N. A., Moen, R. C., Kohn, D. B., Yu, S. F., Karson, E., et al. (1987). Expression of human adenosine deaminase in non-human primates after retrovirus-mediated gene transfer. *Journal of Experimental Medicine, 66,* 219.

Kim, J. A., Triozzi, P. L., & Martin, E. W., Jr. (1993). Radioimmunoguided surgery for colorectal cancer. *Oncology , 7,* 55.

Knudsen, A. G. (1989). Heriditary cancers: Clues to mechanisms of carcinogenesis. *British Journal of Cancer, 59,* 661.

Kovach, J. S. (1996). Need for standardization of cancer practice via nationally accepted treatment guidelines. *Oncology (Huntington), 10*(Suppl. 11), 41–43.

Krag, D. N., Meijer, S. J., Weaver, D. L., Loggie, B. W., Harlow, S. P., Tanabe, K. K., et al. (1995). Minimal-access surgery for staging of malignant melanoma. *Archives of Surgery, 130,* 654.

Levine, A. J. (1995). The genetic origins of neoplasia. *JAMA, 273,* 592.

Little, J. B. (1968). Cellular effects of ionizing radiation. *New England Journal of Medicine, 278,* 369–376.

Little, J. B. (1994). Failla Memorial Lecture changing views on cellular radiosensitivity. *Radiology Research, 140,* 299.

Lowe, S. W., Schmitt, E. M., Smith, S. W., Osborne, B. A., & Jacks, T. (1993). P53 is required for radiation-induced apoptosis in mouse thymocytes. *Nature, 362,* 847.

Maltoni, C., Pinto, C., Carnucci, R., Valenti, D., Lodi, P., & Amaducci, E. (1995). Mesotheliomas following exposure to asbestos used in railroads: 130 Italian cases. *Medicina del Lavaro (Milano), 86,* 461.

Mendelsohn, J. (1997). Principles of neoplasia. In K. J. Isselbacker, et al. (Eds.), *Harrison's principles of internal medicine* (13th ed.). New York: McGraw-Hill.

Meyskens, F. L., Jr. (1990). Coming of age: The chemoprevention of cancer. *New England Journal of Medicine, 323,* 825.

Mitelman, F. (Ed.). (1994). *Catalog of chromosome aberrations in cancer* (5th ed.). New York: Wiley-Liss.

Modrich, P. (1994). Mismatch repair, genetic stability, and cancer. *Science, 266,* 1959.

Morris, M. (1996). Implementation of guidelines and paths in oncology. *Oncology (Huntington), 10* (Suppl. 11), 123–129.

Mulvihill, J. J., Miller, R. W., & Fraumeni, J. F. (1977). Genetics of human cancer progress. In *Cancer research and therapy.* New York: Raven.

Osborne, M., Boyle, P., & Lipkin, M. (1997). Cancer prevention. *Lancet, 349*(Suppl. 2), 27–30.

Ponder, B. A. J. (1994). Genetics of malignant disease. *British Medical Bulletin,* 50.

Rollins, B. J., & Stiles, C. D. (1997). Molecular Biology. In J. F. Holland, R. C. Bast, Jr., D. L. Morton, & E. Frei (Eds.), *Cancer medicine* (4th ed.). Philadelphia: Lea & Febiger.

Roulea, G. A., Merel, P., Lutchman, M., Sanson, M., Zucman, J., Marineau, C., et al. (1993). Alteration in a new gene encoding a putative membrane-organizing protein causes neurofibromatosis type 2. *Nature, 365,* 515.

Rowley, J. D., Aster, J. C., & Sklar, J. (1993). The clinical application of new DNA diagnostic technology on the management of cancer patients. *JAMA, 270,* 2331–2337.

Shields, P. G., & Harris, C. C. (1990). Environmental causes of cancer. *Medical Clinics of North America, 74,* 263.

Slapak, C. A., & Kufe, D. W. (1994). Principles of cancer therapy. In K. J. Isselbacker, et al. (Eds.),

Harrison's principles of internal medicine (13th ed.). New York: McGraw-Hill.

Solomon, E., Borrow, J., & Goodard, A. D. (1991). Chromosome abberations and cancer. *Science, 254,* 1153–1160.

Stanbridge, E. J., & Cavenee, W. K. (1989). Heritable cancer and tumor supressor genes: A tentative connection. In R. A. Weinberg (Ed.), *Oncogenes and the molecular origins of cancer.* Cold Spring Harbor, NY: Cold Spring Harbor Press.

Stovall, E. L. (1996). Pratice guidelines: Patients' perspective. *Oncology (Huntington), 10*(Suppl. 11), 255–260.

Upton, J., Kocher, M. S., & Wolfort, F. G. (1996). Reconstruction following resection of malignan-cies of the upper extremity. *Surgical Oncology Clinics of North America, 5,* 847–892.

Varmus, H. (1989). A historical overview of oncogenes. In R. A. Weinberg (Ed.), *Oncogenes and the molecular origins of cancer.* Cold Spring Harbor, NY: Cold Spring Harbor Press.

Weston, A. (1993). Physical methods for the detection of carcinogen-DNA adducts in humans. *Mutation Research, 288,* 19–29.

Xu, G., Zhang, M., Liu, B., Li, Z., Lin, B., Xu, X., Jin, M., Li, J., Wu, J., & Dong, Z. (1994). Radioimmunoguided surgery in gastric cancer using 131–I labeled monoclonal antibody 3H11. *Semininars in Surgical Oncology, 10,* 88–94.

2

The Care Team
in Oncology

Paula A. Sullivan, M.S., CCC-SLP, and
Penelope Stevens Fisher, M.S., R.N., C.O.R.L.N.

The management of cancer and its treatment sequelae requires a comprehensive approach to rehabilitation that is provided by a skilled and seasoned multidisciplinary team of health care providers. This chapter discusses (a) health care implications related to cancer and its treatment, particularly swallowing, nutrition, and communication problems; (b) etiologies of swallowing and communication problems in cancer; (c) cancer care team organization and requisite skills; (d) outcomes of care team clinical interventions; and (e) essential components of an effective oncology care team.

HEALTH CARE
IMPLICATIONS OF CANCER

Cancer is a group of diseases characterized by uncontrolled growth and spread of abnormal cells. If the spread is not controlled, it can result in death (American Cancer Society, 1997). Cancer is the second leading cause of death in the United States and accounts for one out of every five deaths each year. About 75 million American now living, or approximately one in three, will eventually have cancer.

When the baby boom generation starts turning 65 in the next decade, they will give America its largest generation of senior citizens. The occurrence of cancer increases as individuals age, with most cases occurring in middle-aged or older adults (American Cancer Society, 1997). Continuing the aging trend of the present century, the number of elderly with cancer will escalate. Although the incidence of cancer has increased in the past 20 years, more people are surviving cancer than several decades ago. In the 21st century, the percentage of long-term cancer survivors (i.e., surviving longer than 5 years) is expected to exceed 65% (Welch-McCaffrey et al., 1989). With more and more people living longer and surviving cancer, addressing quality of life must become a top priority. The lengthening of the life span will bring increased management challenges for health care providers dealing with elderly cancer patients for two reasons: (a) older patients have greater difficulty in tolerating treatments because of concomitant health problems, and (b) consent of the patient and family is difficult to obtain (Hirano & Mori, 1998).

The changing racial and ethnic patterns in the United States also will bring new health care implications and challenges for practitioners. Although cancer is common in Americans of all racial and ethnic groups, the incidence rate varies from group to group. For example, cancer rates are highest among African-Americans as compared to a 16% lower rate in white males. Whites represent an increasingly smaller proportion of the total population. Hispanics and blacks are two particularly fast-growing population groups. It has been demonstrated that ethnicity affects individual and family roles in terminal illness (Blackhall, Murphy, & Frank, 1995). In France, Spain, Eastern Europe, and Japan, physicians rarely tell patients with cancer their diagnosis or prognosis, usually informing the family instead. In contrast, physicians in the United States often inform patients about their illness and involve them in decision making. However, this viewpoint is not held by some ethnic groups. For example, Blackhall and colleagues reported that only 47% of Korean-Americans believe that a patient should receive clinical information and make health care decisions. This study also showed a disparity between older Americans of varying ethnicity as compared to their younger counterparts. Practitioners must be aware that some of the differences in cancer incidence rates and risk factor and screening prevalence among ethnic and racial groups may be due to factors associated with social class, such as inaccessibility to health care, rather than race or ethnicity.

The societal burden of cancer is staggering, with overall cancer costs estimated at $104 billion (American Cancer Society, 1997). We can put no price tag on the human costs of cancer. Health care reform debate highlights the cost of treating cancer in a new way. Because disease and disorder prevention typically cost less than treatment, prevention of cancer and its complications will become a greater focus of managed care.

SWALLOWING AND COMMUNICATION IN CANCER

Increasing age also results in increased prevalence of diseases that can cause oropharyngeal dysphagia and communication problems, such as neurological disease and cancer. Prevalence of dysphagic symptoms in the elderly range from 16 to 22% (Bloem et al., 1990; Kjellen & Tibbling, 1981; Lindgren & Janzon, 1991). The incidence and prevalence of dysphagia in cancer patients are unknown. Some data are available for specific malignancy sites. Deglutition disorders will result in virtually all patients undergoing treatment for malignancies of the head and neck. Dysphagia is the primary symptom in approximately 90% of patients with esophageal cancer (Moses, 1991). Although the advent of new and aggressive treatment regimens has improved cancer cure or control and provided organ preservation, it has resulted in a greater number of acute and long-term impairments to swallow function. Considering the aging trend of the American people, the potential for deglutition and communication problems related to cancer and its management in the early decades of the next century is significant.

The Causes of Swallowing and Communication Problems in Cancer

The potential effects of cancer and its treatment on swallowing and communication are multifactorial and can result in a vast array of deficits. These impairments vary in severity, complexity, and frequency of occurrence and can occur at any point in the continuum of cancer care. Numerous types of cancer in various sites of the body can result in swallowing and communication deficits. However, malignancies in the brain, head and neck, and upper aerodigestive tract most commonly affect swallowing and communication. Subsequent chapters detail the various types and sites of cancers, treatment methods, and associated changes to swallowing and communication.

Deglutition and communication problems also commonly result from any of the prime treatment modalities: surgery, radiation therapy, and chemotherapy. The combination of two or more treatment methods increases the likelihood that speech and swallowing structure and/or organ and function will be impaired. Table 2–1 provides a listing of tumor effects, therapy-

TABLE 2–1. Potential Effects of Cancer on Swallowing, Communication, and Nutrition

Effects of Disease Process	Effects of Treatment Modalities (Surgery, Radiation, Chemotherapy)	Other Contributing Factors
Loss or alteration of structure(s)	Scar formation, fibrosis, fistula formation	Anorexia
Compression		Cachexia
Loss or disturbance of motility and sphincteric function	Aspiration	Learned food aversion
Incoordination of peristaltic and sphincteric functions	Altered mastication	Psychological and emotional factors
	Trismus	Social risk factors
	Early satiety	
Deinnervation of motor and/or sensory nerve supply	Gastric stasis	Cultural, religious, and ethnic influences
Changes in the peripheral and/or central nervous systems	Dumping syndrome	Medications
	Achlorhydria	Age
	Dehydration	Other comorbidity
	Edema in upper alimentary tract	
	Xerostomia	
	Mucositis	
	Stomatitis	
	Esophagitis	
	Pharyngitis	
	Malabsorption	
	Diarrhea	
	Constipation	
	Dysgeusia/ageusia/hypogeusia	
	Dysosmia	
	Odynophagia	
	Reflux	
	Nausea	
	Vomiting	
	Appetite loss	
	Neurocentral/neurosensory/ neuromotor	

related toxicities, and other contributing factors to swallowing, communication, and nutritional problems in cancer.

Finally, cancer patients are at high risk for developing swallowing, communication and nutritional problems at some point throughout the continuum of care, as the upper aerodigestive tract is a common site for the development of numerous complications in patients receiving one or more cancer treatment modalities. It is well known that the presence of coexisting swallowing and communication problems is common. For example, a patient who develops airway compromise due to tumor often has accompanying swallowing, breathing, and phonatory dysfunction.

THE CANCER CARE TEAM

Cancer is a complex disease that has physical, psychological, economic, legal, vocational, social, spiritual, and ethical implications to both the individual and society as a whole. It must be managed by a highly skilled group of health care professionals including medical oncologists, radiation oncologists, surgeons, radiologists, neurologists, dentists, gastroenterologists, pharmacists, speech-language pathologists, dietitians, social workers, nurses, psychologists, psychiatrists, physical therapists, occupational therapists, child life specialists, clergy, and cancer survivor volunteers. This team-based approach results in a more comprehensive approach to the assessment and management of cancer and its disorders. Ravich, Wilson, Jones, and Donner (1989) have suggested that a team approach may result in diagnosis and treatment of conditions that were previously missed. In addition, a team-based approach will provide continuity throughout the patient's cancer care continuum, which includes screening and prevention, diagnosis, staging, treatment, supportive care, rehabilitation, palliative care, home care, and hospice care. With input from a variety of perspectives, cancer treatments will be integrated with rehabilitation, and quality-of-life issues, such as preservation of function and avoidance of treatment-related complications, will rank in importance with cancer survival and effectiveness of treatment.

In addition to their discipline-based expertise, care team members will require additional education to effectively handle the unique array of challenges provided by the cancer patient. Each team member must possess a thorough understanding of neoplastic disease and its behavior and management in various anatomic sites. Knowledge of the effects of treatments and reconstructive procedures also is essential. In addition, cancer care team members must be aware of the potential for development of nutrition, swallowing, and communication problems in this high-risk population. Intervention by such a highly skilled multidisciplinary cancer care team is essential to developing a plan of treatment, reducing morbidity and mortality, and providing optimal outcomes, for both the patient and the team. It has been well documented that early intervention in cancer patients results in fewer complications and hospitalizations, improved wound healing, improved ability to tolerate and complete cancer treatments, and higher response rates (Daly, Weintraub, Shou, Rosato, & Lucia, 1995; Goodwin & Byers, 1993; Nayel, el-Ghoneimy, & el-Haddad, 1992).

Care teams will take on different forms depending on the setting, needs, and resources of the setting. This is illustrated by the three distinct roles served by speech-language pathologists at H. Lee Moffitt Cancer Center and Research Institute (MCC) at the University of South Florida in Tampa, Florida. Clinicians are primary team members on the University of South Florida, School of Medicine, Center for Swallowing Disorders' dysphagia team. They also serve as consultants, on an as-needed basis, to MCC's Nutrition Support Team. In addition, swallowing and communication interventions are provided in their roles as members of numerous disease site-specific cancer care teams including head and neck and neuro-oncology.

Outcomes of Care Team Intervention

An outcome is defined as the result of a clinical intervention. A clinical intervention results in several short- and long-term outcomes and reflects multiple perspectives including those of the patient, family, care team and its members, and payers. Outcomes can include clinically derived, functional, social, patient-defined, administrative, and financial measures (Frattali, 1998). Care teams composed of members with varying perspectives must identify critical components of intervention arrived at through consensus. Selected measurement tools must be appropriate for a team's particular setting and patient population. Whether standardized or "homegrown" tools are used, measures of outcomes must evaluate the components of clinical intervention determined by the team to be the most important to outcome.

Rehabilitation provided through a coordinated, multidisciplinary team effort facilitates optimal outcomes for both the patient and the team. Measures of success for the patient include regaining function, independence, and self-confidence. For the health care provider, success is measured by the patient's improvement and satisfaction, meeting clinical practice guidelines developed for quality outcomes, cost consciousness, and evaluation of the health care provider's degree of obtaining personal best practices. Most cancer care teams have defined missions that provide the framework and guide care processes. Improved cancer control or cure is the primary goal of all oncology care teams. Preventing a decline or improving health status, optimizing the quality of life, and achieving a functional outcome for patients are other common goals.

The need for focus on the structure, process, and outcome of rehabilitation in cancer care was emphasized in the 1989 position statement by the Oncology Nursing Society (ONS). The society defines cancer rehabilitation as an active, ongoing process that assists individuals, within their environments, to achieve optimal functioning within the limits imposed by the cancer or its treatment. A schematic of the ONS definition of cancer rehabilitation is represented in Figure 2–1.

Realistic and functional outcome measures must be established by the cancer care team following comprehensive medical and functional assessment of the patient by team members. Ongoing assessment is an integral part of the rehabilitation process and must rely on effective and frequent team communication and collaboration.

Most cancer rehabilitation interventions are aimed at promoting physical, psychosocial, and economic independence. Baseline and ongoing assessment of these functional abilities must be performed by members of the multidisciplinary team. Some useful cancer-specific assessment tools have been developed including the Functional Assessment of Cancer Therapy (FACT; Cella et al., 1993). The Performance Status Scale for Head and Neck Cancer (PSS-HN; List et al., 1996) is a simple, clinician-rated assessment scale of eating and communication that provides ratings of normalcy of diet, understandability of speech, and public eating.

In oncology rehabilitation, the principles of treatment are applied to the problems the patient demonstrates rather than the disease itself. The patient's cancer experience can be placed in a rehabilitation context using Dietz's (1981) goals-classification system, which allows meaningful goal setting by both the patient and the team. Using this simple system, specific patient goals can be individualized and modified according to the problems the patient

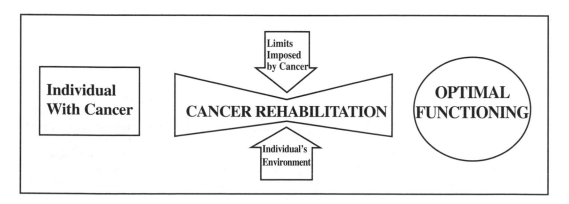

Figure 2–1. A diagram of the Oncology Nursing Society's definition of cancer rehabilitation. *Source:* From "Cancer Rehabilitation: An Overview," by P. G. Watson, 1992, *Seminars in Oncology Nursing, 8,* pp. 167–173. Reprinted with permission.

demonstrates as a result of his or her cancer or treatment modality. These oncology goals are classified as prevention, restoration, support, and palliation. *Prevention* is a general goal to reduce or prevent cancer-related disabilities. The goal of *restoration* is to return the individual to premorbid status with minimal residual disability. *Support* is provided during ongoing cancer treatment with emphasis on reducing cancer-related disability through rehabilitation interventions. Finally, *palliation* is a comfort goal for patients with active disease, with emphasis on reducing complications, maintaining patient independence, and providing emotional support.

In order to achieve optimum outcomes, patients must became stakeholders and participate in all decision making related to the rehabilitation process. Depending on the desires of the patient, the family or other care providers should be included in the team composition. Although choice of treatment depends on numerous factors, patient and family preferences regarding potential outcomes must be considered. When provided with choices of treatment for their disease, patients will often choose the treatment they perceive will provide them a better quality of life. The cancer care team must be aware of the patient's perception of the impact the disease and its treatment will have on their quality of life, as quality of life means different things to different individuals. An ongoing study by List et al. (1998) examined the value patients place on certain outcomes. These priorities include cancer cure, appearance, speech, energy, returning to activities, dry mouth, swallowing, and pain. Unexpectedly, speech was relatively low on the priority list and swallowing was ranked a middle priority. These early findings caution against making assumptions about patients' preferences when discussing treatment options and outcomes. Seckler, Meier, Mulvihil, and Paris (1991) report that surrogates provide more accurate predictions of patients' preferences than do clinicians. This underscores the importance of determining the preferences of patients and their care providers when establishing outcomes.

Considering the significant economic and social burdens of cancer and its complications, prevention should be an integral role and responsibility of cancer care teams. Primary prevention efforts may be directed toward educating the community about the risks of cigars in response to the rising sales and use of the product as well as its glamorization in the media. Secondary prevention efforts may focus on the early detection of oral cancer through screening of high-risk individuals. Cancer care team members need to be vigilant in monitoring for hearing change in patients undergoing chemotherapeutic protocols to prevent further damage or initiate early rehabilitative measures if damage is unavoidable. Although new and aggressive cancer treatments are resulting in increased survival rates, patients are incurring significant treatment toxicities. Complications may be acute, such as mucositis, and temporarily interfere with oral intake or result in permanent dysfunction of the swallowing mechanism. Prevention of and early intervention against these complications will result in improved patient outcomes.

Outcomes of Nutrition, Swallowing, and Communication Intervention

There is little doubt that the abilities to swallow and communicate are probably two of the most important determinants of quality of life. Problems with these essential and basic human needs at any point during the patient's cancer care can be frustrating and critical for numerous reasons. Communication problems may interfere with the patient's ability to express needs or desires to families or care providers or understand essential information related to care. In addition, deglutition problems may deny patients the social, cultural, religious, and personal pleasures associated with eating. Therefore, swallowing, nutrition, and communication intervention must be primary goals of oncology care teams.

Nutrition problems probably are the most common problems in cancer patients, occurring in 30–90% of hospitalized patients (Nixon et al., 1980). The negative effects malnutrition has on health and clinical outcome are well documented in Chapter 13. The assessment and implementation of an aggressive nutritional intervention plan often is the first line of treatment planning by the team's nutritional specialists to reduce morbidity and mortality and prevent delay or interruptions in cancer therapy. All members of the patient's care team should be vigilant in carefully monitoring and preventing a decline in the patient's nutrition and hydration throughout all phases of cancer treatment.

Patients presenting with dysphagia, whether temporary, fluctuating, or permanent, should be considered at high nutritional risk. Often patients' undergoing cancer treatment are unable to sustain oral intake due to treatment effects such as nausea or vomiting. Following determination of nutrition and hydration needs by the nutritional specialist, the patient's ability to tolerate and safely and efficiently handle an optimum diet should be assessed. The speech-language pathologist and dietitian must determine whether or not the patient can sustain adequate nutrition and hydration through oral intake alone. If this is not feasible, other or combined nutritional approaches must be used. Maintaining or improving nutrition and hydration must be the primary focus of all dysphagia intervention.

Traditional dysphagia outcomes, such as improving swallow physiology, may not always be realistic or feasible goals. Functional, realistic, and individualized goals must be continually redefined and modified as the patient progresses through one or more levels of care. The needs of family members and other care providers also must be considered in goal setting. For example, an outcome of the diagnostic phase of care may be the identification of the physiological factors that contribute to the patient's swallowing dysfunction and determination of the optimum food types. Tube feedings and nutritional support may be the primary focuses of care for the patient experiencing severe odynophagia associated with therapy-induced mucositis

during ongoing cancer treatment. The rehabilitative phase of care may be devoted to maximizing range of motion of oral and pharyngeal structures for swallowing and speech in the postoperative head and neck patient. For patients undergoing palliative treatment, quality-of-life issues may become the primary considerations. The goal of intervention may be to allow continued oral feeding while minimizing the risk of complications. Another frequent goal is to reduce the time spent with meals or tube feeding to provide patients and their care providers increased remaining quality of time. Other nontraditional nutrition, swallowing, and communication intervention outcomes in oncology are identified in Table 2–2. Frequent collaboration and communication among care team members will facilitate efficient and accurate formulation and modification of clinical interventions based on the patient's changing medical and disease status, treatment regimen, needs, abilities, and desires.

Measuring the Effect of Care Team Intervention

The marketplace realities of managed care and cost containment have compelled cancer providers to reevaluate their priorities and operations. Oncology care provided at major medical centers has long been perceived by payers as high quality but not necessarily cost-effective. Although a multidisciplinary team approach to care is more efficient due to the strengthened approach to problem solving, the increased use of manpower often is considered redundant and expensive. Due to these perceptions, managed care has limited patients' access to skilled care teams. It is the responsibility of teams to prove that these perceptions are misperceptions. For cancer care teams to survive and prosper in the current health care market, they must demonstrate measurable value of their services, including functional outcomes, cost (i.e., cost effective care, cost/benefit of care), and patient-defined satisfaction. Strategies for clinical service delivery reform are detailed in Chapter 21.

TABLE 2–2. Common Nutrition, Swallowing, and Communication Outcomes of Cancer Care Teams

Prevention
Screening and early identification
Pretreatment documentation of disease process
Documentation of response to surgery, radiation therapy, chemotherapy, or combined modality therapy
Reducing or preventing complications of cancer treatment
Improving health status
Maintaining or improving nutrition and hydration
Weight gain
Increased salivary flow
Maintaining or restoring highest level of functioning
Improved efficiency of feeding process by patient or family
Education regarding treatment effects
Developing cancer-related clinical guidelines and pathways
Coordinating seamless care throughout the cancer care continuum
Determining cost benefit of intervention
Ensuring adequate function with minimal intervention
Education about anticipated decline in function
Monitoring changes in swallowing function/disease progression
Accommodating decline in swallow function while minimizing risk of complications
Assessing patient's decision-making capacity
Identifying an appropriate surrogate decision maker

ESTABLISHING THE CANCER CARE TEAM

Ideally, the management of cancer and its disorders is best handled in institutions with the resources and expertise to provide a comprehensive approach to care. However, success of a team is not determined by geographic locale, size, or composition but rather by commitment to a common vision. Regular meetings led by a knowledgeable leader to plan strategies and monitor outcomes are essential. Other critical components of a well-seasoned care team include effectiveness, efficiency, competency, coordination and management, collaboration, consensus, and vision.

Effectiveness

Effectiveness is highest in a rehabilitation team when measurable outcome results are obtained from common team goals. Basic concepts of developing and advancing team effectiveness are shown in Table 2–3. Teams with shared values and clear purposes excel. Successful management of dysphagia can be based on such goals as

identification of patients at risk for aspiration, prevention of aspiration, and prevention of malnutrition (Groher & Asher, 1992). Team effectiveness can be measured by patient satisfaction and improvement, minimal variance from clinical practice guidelines, and resources accountability.

Patient satisfaction is often difficult to assess due to preexisting expectations of rehabilitation. Best practices include estab-

TABLE 2–3. Characteristics of an Effective Team

1. Interactive goals/objectives
2. Resource optimizing
3. Conflict management
4. Interactive leadership
5. Activity control
6. Feedback mechanism
7. Shared problem solving/decision making
8. Mutual assistance
9. Experimentation
10. Self-evaluation
11. Long-term commitment
12. Mutual respect
13. Collaborative practice

Source: Adapted from Quality Learning Inc. Workshop on Team Building, Lakeland, Florida, 1984.

lishing a mutual contractual outcome agreement (written or verbal) between the patient and clinician, periodic evaluation (i.e., physical examination, videofluroscopy, and subjective complaints analysis), and benchmarks for identification of improvement.

Clinical practice guidelines are one system that provides an organized approach to unifying team clinical practices. During interactive collaborative committee meetings, multidisciplinary clinicians develop guidelines for care and management of a specific diagnosis. The research-based practice is listed in an algorithm for patient flow from diagnosis through follow-up care. Critical pathways are developed for institutionalized patients, and the clinical practice can be evaluated by standards for cost, resources, and outcome. Variances can be monitored to ensure continuous quality improvement.

Resources needed to fulfill the clinical practice guideline can be systematically analyzed. Cost of staffing, supplies, tests, medications, and the physical plant can be correlated to the practice. Expenditures are recognized by the care team stimulating awareness and increasing the team's fiscal accountability. Additionally, the use of clinical guidelines has demonstrated lower hospital days, controlled costs, and consensus group practice, which enhances marketability for managed care contracts.

Efficiency

Efficiency for best practices of care can be best provided by a specialized mulitdisciplinary team with very diverse capabilities. Health care practitioners with a high level of experience in oncology or dysphagia will have increased efficiency in care performance. Care team efficiency is driven by that identified expertise and sharing of common interests in swallowing rehabilitation. When the right person does the right job, efficiency and productivity are high. Efficiency is further improved when team clinical practice guidelines are followed, time frames are in place, and objectives are monitored for outcomes. Teams with highly competent members continue to grow in efficiency.

Competency

Competency is the basis for best practices in obtaining positive rehabilitative outcomes for patients. Individual team members provide the competent, professional performance for the team to excel. Entry into practice is usually achieved after completion of quality basic education and successful performance on a knowledge-based examination managed by a state board of licensing and/or professional regulatory board. Competency is enhanced through experience and advanced education. The team environment serves as a medium for mentorship and ongoing continuing education. Methods to ensure continued professional competencies have been explored. The National Council of State Boards of Nursing identified six methods: continuing education, peer review, patient review, periodic refresher courses, competency exams, and minimal practice requirements (Cunningham, 1992). Additionally, progressive personal professional development and specialty certification build individual team members' competency, which ultimately increases the skill mix and effectiveness of the team.

Coordination and Management

A team requires continuous attention to its administration. Although each member brings diverse education, experience, and expertise, a coordinated concept of care with a universal goal must exist to realize a cohesive effort for the rehabilitation of the patient. The team design requires leadership, coordination, and management. Historically, the physician maintains overall leadership, but the work environment, complexity of patient care, objectives, and goal of the health care system direct the leadership (Yukl, 1991). The leader is often the catalyst for motivating accomplishments, enhancing involvement and cooperation, and providing vision. The leader leads others and manages self through a context of commitment, complexity, and credibility (Bennis & Nanus, 1985). Coordination is the cohesive force that keeps the team informed and patient moving toward mutual goals. On the head and neck cancer care team, otorhinolaryngology nurses often fill this role and provide skills in coordinating the treatment plan, team liaison efforts, time management, continuous quality improvement, and cost-effectiveness (Fisher, 1994).

The management of the rehabilitation team is divided into clinical care and financial accounting. Clinical management is directed by the appropriate specialist needed at that point in time to assist the patient in achieving the expected outcome. The physician remains in a leadership role for mentoring and is available for guidance and care orders. A financially solvent team manages cost-effectiveness, uses human and material resources appropriately, and gains solid revenues.

Collaboration

To have successful interdisciplinary interventions in a highly specialized care team, collaboration is paramount. Each discipline has specific practice skills to provide care for the cancer patient. Although shared values and clear purpose may drive the outcome, it is collaboration that permits the process. The environment needed to progress includes trusting relationships, mutual respect, understanding of each clinician's role, developing comfort with blending of territories, and team members' individual maturity (Kopser, Horn, & Carpenter, 1994). The environment must also be open to change and dynamic in its effort to team build and educate the members. Collaborative effort is enhanced by mutual goals. Goal setting requires the subspecialties' input and coordination for the blending into a set of mutually agreed-on outcomes for best practices and positive patient outcomes. When mutual goals are established, ownership, communications, and cohesiveness increase. Enhanced by this team-building effort, goals can be broken into manageable objectives for health care practitioners and patients. The objective outlines the expected behavior in an action statement noting the criterion for acceptable performance and what aid may be needed to accomplish the outcome.

It has been said that communication is the most important skill in life (Covey, 1989). A well-organized communication system is the vehicle for the rehabilitation team to function and grow collaboratively. Components of the communication system include formal and informal lines of communication, adoption of a conflict resolution model (Table 2–4), agreement for a problem-solving map (Figure 2–2), and mechanisms for intrateam consultation for clinical expertise support and patient care. The multifocused process of building an integrative, collaborative care team requires consensus.

Consensus

Consensus develops the strength of the rehabilitation team. As the leader provides the setting for each discipline to contribute clinical best practices, the evolution of a mutual philosophy takes form. Linked by the common value of rehabilitating the patient with a swallowing disorder, ownership is high and the philosophy is adapted. The team continually needs a forum to enhance consensus and change clinical care approaches and practices to remain on the leading edge of health care. Forums for consensus enhancement include team teaching rounds, patient care conferences, ongoing continuing education opportunities, and knowledge of and participation in research (Table 2–5). The leadership of the team provides the direction and vision for growth and accomplishment.

TABLE 2–4. Desire Conflict Resolution Model

Define the problem
Evaluate possible solution
Select an action plan
Implement the plan
Reevaluate the situation
End or start over

Source: Pat Crumbly in: Team Building. H. Lee Moffitt Cancer Center and Research Institute, Tampa, Florida, 1987.

TABLE 2–5. Team-Building Opportunities for Consensus and Education

Forum	Purpose	People Involved
Weekly teaching rounds	Review of patient care; evaluation of patient's progress	All team members and students
Weekly patient care conference	Presentation of cases for treatment planning goal achievements	All team members and students
Weekly research conference	Active and proposed protocol review; patient accrual and progress report	Physicians, research team, clinical manager, psychosocial worker, fiscal manager
Weekly discharge planning rounds	Review of patient's care in preparation for discharge	Inpatient and outpatient nursing, speech, psychosocial, dietitian, clinical nurse specialist, clinical manager
Bimonthly leadership/management meeting	Planning, problem solving, evaluation	Physician leader, clinical manager, fiscal manager

Source: Adapted from Head and Neck Oncology Program. H. Lee Moffitt Cancer Center and Research Institute, Tampa, Florida, 1991.

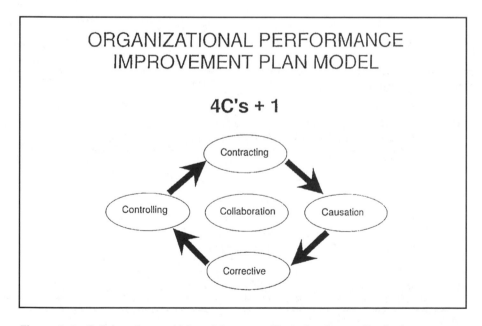

Figure 2–2. Collaboration problem-solving map. (From Continuous Quality Improvement Program. H. Lee Moffitt Cancer Center and Research Institute, Tampa, Florida, 1994.)

Vision

Vision is the ability to look to the future and see what will provide the best prac-

tices for patients, clinicians, the organization, and health care. Vision is created by the dynamic leader who is able to get by the business of the day and proactively chart the course beyond tomorrow. Leaders are motivated to this end by the dynamics, expertise, and collaborative accomplishments of the team, the changes in specialty care, and the conclusions of research. Leaders direct the team toward new goals with cooperative creativity using documented elements of organizational principles (Table 2–6). Together leaders and managers translate vision into realities. Realities for the highly specialized rehabilitation team require considerable attention to the development of a strategic plan. Embracing and using a strategic plan supports the care team's growth to excellence during the journey to greatness (Table 2–7). A care team's greatness will continue to mature in the environment of effectiveness, efficiency, competency, coordination and management, collaboration, consensus, *and* leadership as long as the horizon is explored for continuous quality improvement in best practices.

SUMMARY

Numerous cancers and their treatments can result in significant disruptions to swallowing, communication, and nutrition. These complications can occur at any time during the cancer care continuum and result in temporary or chronic functional impairments that will affect quality of life for the patient and family. Many of these complications can be reduced or prevented and patients can be assisted to regain optimum function through the rehabilitative efforts of a skilled, multidisciplinary care team. A primary responsibility of care teams is in the area of outcomes research to demonstrate the value of treatments, identify optimum clinical interventions and determine the effect of interventions on quality of life. Future improvements in cancer rehabilitation are dependent on outcomes research. Clearly, quality of life must improve with increased quantity of life.

REFERENCES

American Cancer Society (1997). *Cancer facts & figures—1997*. Atlanta, GA: Author.

Bennis, W., & Nanus, B. (1985). *Leaders: The strategies for taking charge*. New York: Harper & Row.

Blackhall, L. J., Murphy, S. T., & Frank, G. (1995). Ethnicity and attitudes toward patient autonomy. *JAMA, 274*, 820–825.

TABLE 2–6. Elements of Organizational Principles

Element	Description
Mission	Stating the business of the team
Vision	Stating the future state of the team
Values	Listing principles to be observed to meet the vision or listing principles to be served by meeting the vision
Policy	Stating the commitment to the patient through guidelines

TABLE 2–7. Process of Developing a Strategic Plan

Element	Description
Values	Reviewing and clarifying what is important
Purpose	Identifying what is done
Vision	Recognizing what the team sees
Strategic goals	Mutually agreeing on the direction to reach the desired future
Action planning	Listing specific steps that are measurable, time limited, and assigned

Source: Ulschak, Snow-Antle and Associates, 235 West Brandon Boulevard, Brandon, Florida 33511.

Bloem, B. R., Lagaay, A. M., van Beek, W., Haan, J., Roos, R. A. C., & Wintzen, A. R. (1990). Prevalence of subjective dysphagia in community residents aged over 87. *British Medical Journal, 300,* 721–722.

Cella, D. F., Tulsky, D. S., Gray, G., Sarafian, B., Linn, E., Bonomi, A., et al. (1993). The Functional Assessment of Cancer Therapy Scale: Development and validation of the general measures. *Journal of Clinical Oncology, 11,* 570–579.

Covey, S. R. (1989). *The seven habits of highly effective people.* New York: Simon & Schuster.

Cunningham, M. (1992). *Professional issues in cancer care in Core Curriculum for Oncology Nursing.* Philadelphia: W. B. Saunders.

Daly, J. M., Weintraub, F. N., Shou, J., Rosato, E. F., & Lucia, M. (1995). Enteral nutrition during multimodality therapy in upper gastrointestinal cancer patients. *Annals of Surgery, 221,* 327–338.

Dietz, J. H. (1981). *Rehabilitation oncology.* New York: John Wiley.

Fisher, P. S. (1994). Nurses and the head and neck cancer team. *Cancer Control, 1,* 40–43.

Frattali, C. M. (1998). Outcomes assessment in speech-language pathology. In A. F. Johnson & B. H. Jacobson (Eds.), *Medical speech-language pathology: A practitioner's guide* (pp. 685–709). New York: Thieme.

Goodwin, W. J., Jr., & Byers, P. M. (1993). Nutritional management of the head and neck cancer patient. *Medical Clinics of North America, 77,* 597–610.

Groher, M. E., & Asher, I. E. (1992). Establishing a swallowing program. In M. E. Groher (Ed.), *Dysphagia: diagnosis and management* (2nd ed., pp. 313–325). Newton, MA: Butterworth-Heinemann.

Hirano, M., & Mori, K. (1998). Management of cancer in the elderly: Therapeutic dilemmas. *Otolaryngology—Head and Neck Surgery, 118,* 110–114.

Kjellen, G., & Tibbling, L. (1981). Manometric oesophageal function, acid perfusion test and symptomatology in a 55-year-old general population. *Clinical Physiology, 1,* 405–415.

Kopser, K. G., Horn, P. B., & Carpenter, A. D. (1994). Successful collaboration within an integrative practice model. *Clinical Nurse Specialist, 8,* 330–333.

Lindgren, S., & Janzon, L. (1991). Prevalence of swallowing complaints and clinical findings among 50–79-year-old men and women in an urban population. *Dysphagia, 6,* 187–192.

List, M. A., Butler, P., Vokes, E. E., Kies, M., Ganzenko, N., Lundy, D., Sullivan, P., & Goodwin, W. J. (1998). *Head and neck cancer patients: How do patients prioritize treatment outcomes?* Presentation at the American Society of Clinical Oncology meeting.

List, M. A., D'Antonio, L. L., Cella, D. F., Siston, A., Mumby, P., Haraf, D., et al. (1996). The Performance Status Scale for Head and Neck Cancer and the Functional Assessment of Cancer Therapy—Head and Neck Scale. *Cancer, 77,* 2294–2301.

Moses, F. M. (1991). Squamous cell carcinoma of the esophagus. *Gastroenterology Clinics of North America, 20,* 703–716.

Nayel, H., el-Ghoneimy, E., & el-Haddad, S. (1992). Impact of nutritional supplementation on treatment delay and morbidity in patients with head and neck tumors treated with irradiation. *Nutrition, 8,* 13–18.

Nixon, D. W., Heymsfield, S. B., Cohen, A., et al. (1980). Protein-calorie under nutrition in hospitalized cancer patients. *American Journal of Medicine, 68,* 683–690.

Ravich, W. J., Wilson, R. S., Jones, B., & Donner, M. (1989). Psychogenic dysphagia and globus: Reevaluation of 23 patients. *Dysphagia, 4,* 35–38.

Seckler, A. B., Meier, D. E., Mulvihill, M., & Paris, B. E. (1991). Substituted judgement: How accurate are proxy predictions? *Annals of Internal Medicine, 115,* 92–98.

Welch-McCaffrey, D., Hoffman, B., Leigh, S., et al. (1989). Surviving adult cancers, part 2: Psychosocial implications. *Annals of Internal Medicine, 111,* 517–524.

Yukl, G. A. (1991). *Leadership in organizations.* Englewood Cliffs, NJ: Prentice Hall.

3

Chemotherapy

Ronald C. DeConti, M.D.

Any involvement in the care of patients with neoplastic disease requires a basic understanding of the roles of drug therapy in patient management because of the widespread use of these therapies and the multiple potential adverse effects associated with their use. This chapter outlines the origins of therapeutic agents, their clinical applications and benefits, and the organ systems that can be affected by them. Unfortunately, although these drugs have had, in some cases and in some diseases, dramatic life-saving and/or life-prolonging effects, these benefits are rarely achieved without some toxicity to normal tissues. A basic knowledge of these effects assists health care professionals in better supporting the needs of their patients.

ORIGINS

Although the search for effective anticancer treatments is not new, the modern use of drugs as antineoplastics is commonly dated to research on mustard gases conducted during World War II, which led to the demonstration of nitrogen mustard as an effective treatment for lymphoma. That finding fostered interest and promoted the subsequent development of a vast array of alkylating agents, whose mechanism of action was subsequently shown to be cross-linking of DNA strands. Somewhat later in the 1940s, growing understanding of cell-growth requirements and recognition of the value of antifols in the therapy of leukemia led to the development of methotrexate. As basic understandings of biochemistry and biochemical pharmacology increased, the recognition and definition of the steps leading to the synthesis of RNA and DNA made possible the development of specific enzyme inhibitors and fostered the rational development of potential antineoplastic agents directed at key sites of metabolic inhibition. The use of in vitro and subsequent animal-screening programs led to the identification and evaluation of thousands of compounds from many sources, among them natural products and antibiotics. Although no single drug has been universally effective in controlling cancer, a large number of compounds have each demonstrated an ability to be at least partially effective in reducing the size of a specific neoplasm. With evidence for progressively successful medical therapies, the role of the medical specialist in cancer care increased, leading to the development of the subspecialty of medical oncology in internal medicine. Today more than 6,000 board-certified medical oncologists, together with 4,000 hematologists, practice in the United States, and this specialty is widely recognized around the world.

CLASSIFICATION OF DRUGS

Antineoplastic agents are classified in a number of ways as shown in Tables 3–1 through 3–5. The alkylating agents are thus grouped because they share a common mechanism of biological activity though they may differ in individual toxicities, relative rates of activations and, in some cases, even relative efficacy for one neoplastic condition or another (Table 3–1). In the clinically most widely used group, the nitrogen mustards, a variety of drugs have been synthesized to modulate the rates of alkylation, permitting the development of compounds, that vary from the highly volatile (mechlorethamine) to drugs that are activated somewhat more slowly as a result of their metabolic release (e.g., cyclophosphamide and ifosfamide) as well as to permit oral formulations of the drug, for example, chlorambucil and cyclophosphamide. These agents are frequently cross-resistant with one another. Interest in the development of the nitrosoureas was stimu-

TABLE 3–1. Common Alkylating Agents and Their Major Indication

Type	Agent	Common Use
Nitrogen mustards	Mechlorethamine	Hodgkin's disease
		Lymphoma
	Cyclofosphamide	Lymphoma
		Breast cancer
		Lung cancer
	Chlorambucil	Chronic lymphocytic leukemia
	Ifosfamide	Sarcoma
	Malphalan	Breast cancer
	Estramustine	Malignant melanoma
		Prostrate cancer
Nitrosoureas	Carmustine	Glioblastoma multiforme
		Malignant melanoma
	Lomustine	Lymphoma
	Streptozocin	Islet cell carcinoma
		Carcinoid
Platinum compounds	Cisplatin	Lung cancer
		Head and neck cancer
		Ovarian cancer
	Carboplatin	Lung cancer
		Head and neck cancer
		Ovarian cancer
Ethylenimine derivatives	Thiotepa	Breast cancer
		Ovarian cancer
	Hexamethylmelamine	Breast cancer
		Ovarian cancer
Triazines	Dacarbazine	Malignant melanoma
		Sarcoma
	Tenazolamide	Malignant melanoma
		Glioblastoma multiforme
Alkylsulfonates	Busulfan	Chronic granulocytic leukemia
Miscellaneous	Procarbazine	Hodgkin's disease

TABLE 3–2. Antimetabolites

Type	Agent	Common Use
Folic acid inhibitors	Methotrexate	Acute lymphocytic leukemia
	Trimetrexate	Breast cancer
		Choriocarcinoma
		Squamous cell carcinoma of the head and neck
Pyrimidine antagonists	5-Fluorouracil	Breast cancer
	5-Floxuridine	Gastric cancer
		Colorectal cancer
		Head and neck cancer
	Cytarabine	Acute granulocytic leukemia
	5-Azacitidine	Acute granulocytic leukemia
Purine antagonists	6-Mercaptopurine	Acute lymphocytic leukemia
	6-Thioguanine	Acute myelocytic leukemia
	Deoxycoformycin	Hairy cell leukemia
		Chronic lymphocytic leukemia
	Fludarabine	Chronic lymphocytic leukemia
	Cladribine	
Substituted urea	Hydroxyurea	Acute granulocytic leukemia
		Chronic granulocytic leukemia

lated by an appreciation of their lipid solubility and their putative ability to cross the bloodbrain barrier. Their pattern of hematologic toxicity is distinctly different from that of the nitrogen mustards, with later onset and more prolonged nadirs of leukopenia and thrombocytopenia. Alkylating agents are, to varying degrees, cell-cycle nonspecific in contrast to antimetabolites. Their mechanism of action relies on cross-linking DNA, creating single and double DNA strand breaks, which result in ineffective DNA repair, ineffective cell division, and subsequent cell death. They have frequently been the subject of dose intensity studies in efforts to improve outcomes and are commonly employed in bone marrow transplantation purgative regimens (Frei, Teicher, Holden, Cathcart, & Wang, 1988).

Antimetabolites are characterized by their ability to block a defined metabolic or enzymatic process by virtue of their functional or biochemical structural similarity to the natural metabolite. They block the synthesis of DNA and/or RNA and lead to cell death. Antimetabolic agents are generally highly cell-cycle specific and depend on active DNA and RNA synthesis to induce lethality. Once DNA inhibition has been achieved, efficacy has seemed to depend more on the duration of inhibition: scheduling rather than dosage has been the key to the successful use of this group of compounds. Antimetabolites are of three types: folic acid inhibitors, pyrimidine, and purine antagonists (Table 3–2). Methotrexate and its congeners inhibit the enzyme dihydrofolate reductase. This inhibition blocks the production of tetrahydrofolate, a coenzyme necessary for the synthesis of thymidine. The pyrimidine analogs inhibit specific critical enzyme pathways in de novo pyrimidine biosynthesis. Purine analogs block purine biosynthesis and inhibit DNA synthesis.

Natural products are classified by their source as opposed to their specific function (Table 3–3). The vinca alkaloids derived from the periwinkle plant function as mitotic inhibitors and are thus highly cell-cycle specific. The taxanes derived from the yew tree stabilize microtubular protein, producing metaphase arrest. Podo-

TABLE 3–3. Natural Products

Type	Agent	Common Use
Mitotic inhibitors	Vinblastine	Hodgkin's disease
		Testicular carcinoma
	Vincristine	Lymphoma
	Vindesine	Lung cancer
	Vinorelbine	Breast cancer
		Lung cancer
Microtubule stabilizers	Paclitaxel	Ovarian carcinoma
		Lung carcinoma
		Head and neck cancer
		Bladder carcinoma
	Docetaxel	Breast cancer
Podophyllotoxins	Etoposide	Lung cancer
		Melanoma
	Teniposide	Acute lymphocytic leukemia
		Neuroblastoma
Antibiotics	Bleomycin	Lymphoma
		Testicular cancer
	Dactinomycin	Choriocarcinoma
		Sarcoma
	Daunorubicin	Acute lymphocytic leukemia
		Acute granulocytic leukemia
	Doxorubicin	Breast cancer
		Lymphoma
	Idarubicin	Acute granulocytic leukemia
	Plicamycin	Hypercalcemia
		Testicular cancer
	Mitomycin-C	Gastric cancer
		Bowel cancer
		Lung cancer
	Mitoxantrone	Breast cancer
		Lymphoma
Enzymes	Asparaginase	Acute lymphocytic leukemia

phyllotoxin derivatives from the mayapple root inhibit topoisomerase II, thereby inhibiting DNA replication and arresting cells in late S and early G2 phases of the cell cycle. The antibiotics are derived from fermentation from *Streptomyces* species. They intercalate DNA and RNA and prevent messenger transformation and signaling, resulting in cell death. A single enzyme product completes this group of drugs. Asparaginase acts by reducing the availability of preformed asparagine to dependent cells and acts as an antimetabolite.

Hormones and hormone antagonists are named for their physiological function or the physiological blockade they produce and have their action by affecting hormonally sensitive tumors in neoplasms developing in hormonally sensitive normal tissues (Table 3–4). These agents are particularly useful in the management of breast and prostate cancers. The corticosteroids are directly cytotoxic to lymphocytes and are a valuable adjunct to many leukemia and lymphoma therapies.

More recently, the explosion in understanding of the molecular bases for cell growth, its regulation, and the neoplastic process has fostered the recognition of growth modifiers, immune recognition

TABLE 3–4. Hormones and Antagonists

Type	Agent	Common Use
Estrogens	Diethylstilbestrol	Breast cancer
		Prostate cancer
Estrogen antagonists	Tamoxifen	Breast cancer
	Anastrozole	
Androgens	Fluoxymesterone	Breast cancer
Androgen antagonists	Flutamide	Prostate cancer
	Bicalutamide	
Neutral steroids	Dexamethasone	Lymphoma
		Leukemia
	Prednisone	Glioblastoma
		Myeloma
Adrenal toxins	Mitotane	Adrenocortical cancer
Adrenal synthesis inhibitors	Aminogluthethimide	Prostate cancer
		Breast cancer
Thyroid stimulating hormone release inhibitors	Thyroid hormones	Thyroid cancer
Hypothalamic hormone inhibitors	Leuprolide	Prostate cancer
	Goserelin	
Progestational agents	Megestrol acetate	Breast cancer
	Medroxyprogesterone acetate	Prostate cancer

TABLE 3–5. Biological Modifiers

Type	Agent	Common Use
Interferons	Interferons alpha 2b	Hairy cell leukemia
		AIDS-related Kaposi sarcoma
		Chronic granulocytic leukemia
		Mycoses fungoides
		Malignant melanoma
		Renal cell carcinoma
Interleukins-2	Interleukin-2	Malignant melanoma
		Renal cell carcinoma

enhancers, and natural cytotoxic killer cells as additional strategies to eliminate or eradicate neoplasms. Clinically useful biological modifiers include interferon and interleukin-2 as agents whose antineoplastic activity is mediated by the stimulation or inhibition of normal immune mechanisms. These agents promote activation of natural immune recognition cells of the body and have their actions indirectly, by stimulating normal body macrophages and lymphocytes as enhanced killer cells to destroy neoplastic cells, rather than by direct cytotoxicity. Their uses are shown in Table 3–5. Many other lines of inquiry are under investigation including other cytokines, hematopoietic growth factors, transforming growth and differentiating factors, monoclonal antibodies, antiangiogenesis agents, tumor vaccines, gene therapy, and immunotoxins. These techniques offer the hope of other approaches to control or regulate tumor expression but are not yet clinically widely useful.

Two unique examples of novel mechanisms of tumor control are noteworthy. The all-trans isomer of retinoic acid has been shown capable of inducing cell differentiation in progranulocytic leukemia, achieving clinical remissions without the dramatic cell lysis syndrome characteristic of cytotoxic treatment, with fewer bleeding and infectious complications. Used together with Idarubicin, sustained longterm remissions and possible cures are achieved in 70% of patients (Mandelli et al., 1997).

Malt lymphoma of the stomach is now believed to be the result of chronic overstimulation of locoregional lymphocytes by infection with *Helicobacter pylori*. Treatment with conventional antibiotics frequently results in regressions and probable cures (Isaacson & Spencer, 1996).

SIDE EFFECTS OF ANTINEOPLASTIC THERAPY

Common Side Effects

Inasmuch as many antineoplastics are somewhat nonspecific in their cell-killing abilities, both normal and neoplastic tissues can be affected. The normal tissues of the body that are most rapidly replicating, or in which cell renewal is high or frequent, are those most commonly affected by cancer drug therapy. These tissue renewal systems include the bone marrow, the lining of the gut, and, to a lesser extent, the squamous epithelium of the skin. The most frequent, dose-limiting toxicity of current antineoplastic agents is myelosuppression, with the potential for marked reductions in white cell count and platelet cell count leading to the susceptibility to infection and bleeding. White cell and platelet nadirs commonly occur 7 to 10 days after drug therapy. These may be noted later with the nitrosoureas and occasionally with mitomycin C. Risk of infection is increased with the use of drugs, which also damage the gut lining, increasing the opportunity for bacterial entry and subsequent sepsis. Erythema followed by ulceration is most evident in the oral cavity as mucositis with areas of erythema followed by ulceration. For some drugs, similar though generally much less evident lesions can be seen in the lower bowel lining and may be responsible for symptoms of abdominal cramping and diarrhea, which also occur in the week after treatment. The initial nausea and vomiting seen with some agents is a hypothalamic effect rather than the result of local gastrointestinal toxicity. Rash may occur as an allergic phenomenon to some drugs, but when it occurs with desquamation it is usually a manifestation of drug overdosage. Hair loss commonly develops 3 to 6 weeks following therapy, usually persists during the course of therapy, and requires several months for significant regrowth.

A number of strategies to ameliorate the side effects of chemotherapy have been implemented. Nausea and vomiting, formerly a major limitation and major clinical impediment to patient acceptance of antineoplastic drug treatment, has been dramatically improved by the 5 HT3 antagonists (serotonin receptor blockers), which have been highly successful in controlling this complication. The development of growth factors effective in promoting restoration of hematopoietic elements has been quite useful in ameliorating or preventing some effects on the hematopoietic system. Epogen has reduced the risk or severity of anemia associated with chronic drug treatment (especially with cisplatin) and decreased transfusion requirements. Granulocyte colony-stimulating factor (G-CSF) has been effective in reducing the infectious transfusion complications associated with high dosages of drug known to frequently produce a prolonged period of granulocytopenia and high risk of infection. By promoting earlier white cell recovery, fewer severe infections have been seen with these high-risk regimens. Table 3–6 outlines some helpful interventions in patient management of these usual complications.

Specific Organ Effects

Specific organ-system toxicities related to individual agents are well-known to practicing oncologists and may produce many symptoms (Table 3–7). The skin may be affected in a variety of ways. Hyperpigmentation and acneiform eruptions are common with actinomycin D. Bleomycin frequently produces itching and hyperpigmentation, particularly in scratch lines. Some patients acquire sun sensitivity while receiving 5-fluorouracil (5-FU) and all patients need to be cautioned about sun exposure to prevent this complication. When 5-FU is administered by continuous intravenous infusion, its toxicity pattern changes from that affecting predominately the bone marrow and the gut; it spares those organs and appears to affect the skin, particularly on the hands and feet, which become erythematous, swollen, and tender, with the subsequent development of fissures and ulcerations. Weakness, predominately characterized by a proximal myopathy, may be associated with prolonged use of steroids, the vinca alkaloids, and interferon. Long-lasting peripheral neuropathy, predominantly sensory, develops with cisplatin, taxol, and the vinca alkaloids; with continued use and lack of recognition this may progress to severe muscle weakness. Tinnitus and high-tone hearing loss may limit therapy with cisplatin. High doses of cytarabine and ifosfamide may sometimes produce mental confusion and occasionally leads to transient coma. Chronic exposure to the anthracyclines may affect car-

TABLE 3–6. Common Toxicities of Antineoplastic Agents

Toxicity	Organ System Risk	Intervention
Myelosuppression	Anemia	Blood product tranfusion
		Use of growth factors
	Infection	Monitor serial blood counts
		Institute antibiotics
		Modify subsequent doses
		Delay interval treatments
Nausea/vomiting	Dehydration	Monitor for occurrence and severity
		Prevent and treat with antimetics
Mucositis	Pain	Preventive hygiene
	Infection	Mouth care
	Dehydration	Alterations in diet
		Antifungals
		Anti-inflammatories
		Mucosal protectors
Diarrhea	Dehydration	Imodium
		Intravenous fluid support, if necessary
Rash	Pain	Soothing lotions
	Itch	Benadryl
		Antihistamines
Hair loss	Social	Reassurances
	Cosmetic	Hats, hairpieces

TABLE 3–7. Important Organ System Toxicities Associated With Particular Drugs

Organ System	Toxicity	Causative Agent
Skin	Hyperpigmentation	Bleomycin
		Actinomycin
	Acneiform eruption	Actinomycin
		Steroids
	Sun sensitivity	5-FU
		5-FUDR
	Hand-foot syndrome	5-FU
		5-FUDR
Neuromuscular		
Central	Confusion	Ifosfamide
	Coma	High-dose cytarabine
		Methotrexate
Peripheral	Neuropathy	Cisplatin
		Taxol
		Vinca alkaloids
Myopathy	Myopathy	Steroids
		Vinblastine
		Interferon
Cardiac	Impaired cardiac contractility	Adriamycin
		Daunomycin
		Novatrone
Renal	Reduced glomerular filtration	Cisplatin
		Mitomycin C
		Methotrexate
	Renal tubular acidosis	Cisplatin
	Hemolytic uremic syndrome	Mitomycin C
Hepatic	Cirrhosis	Methotrexate
	Hepatic occlusive disease	Ifosfamide
	Chemical hepatitis	Interferon
		GMP
	Cholangitis	Intrahepatic 5-FUDR
Endocrine	Hypothyroidism	Interferon
	Hypoadrenalism	Steroids
	Sterility	Alkylating agents
Pulmonary	Interstitial pneumonitis	Busulfan
		Bleomycin
		Nitrosureas
		Mitomycin C
		Methotrexate

diac contractility, so the total dose of these agents is limited to avoid this complication. In older individuals, cardiac ejection fractions are frequently monitored to provide a safety guide to the use of these agents. A number of drugs affect renal function, cisplatin perhaps being the major cause of azotemia, so careful attention to prehydration and glomerular filtration rate prior to the initiation of this treatment is of great importance in avoiding renal failure. Chronic cisplatin administration may result in renal tubular acidosis and a potassium-losing syndrome. Elevated liver function tests occur occasionally with many drugs; a sometimes severe chemical hepatitis occurs with androgens, 6 mercaptopurine, and interferon. Chronic low-dose methotrexate may lead to cirrhosis. Intrahepatic arterial 5-fluorouracil deoxyribonucleoside (5-FUDR) is frequently limited by ascending cholangitis. Hepatic occlusive disease is a dangerous complication associated with high-dose ifosfamide in bone marrow transplantation. Cough, fever, and shortness of breath may signal rales and an interstitial pneumonitis. This is best known to occur with continued bleomycin administration but is clearly recognized with other agents as well.

PRINCIPLES OF DRUG THERAPY

Proportional Cell Kill

The early applications of drugs carried out in L1210 and related animal leukemia models demonstrated an important principle, that of proportional cell kill. This principle is that no matter what the tumor-cell number might be, a given dose of drug kills a constant fraction of those cells. This led to an understanding of the log cell-kill concept, such that a single dose of drug could be evaluated for its log cell kill, and one could calculate the theoretical number of doses of drug necessary to eradicate the tumor, allowing for partial tumor regrowth between treatments. Animal models displayed this feature quite uniformly. In general, the models were those of leukemia where the cell inoculum was evenly distributed, usually in the peritoneal cavity of the mouse. In that situation, even a single cell retained the potential to eradicate the host with time, and prolongation in survival could be directly related to the degree of tumor-cell kill. Figure 3–1 portrays such a theoretical construct. Two examples are shown. Each treatment achieves a 2-3 log tumor-cell kill with 2-1 log tumor-cell regrowth in the interval between treat-

ments. Tumor eradication and cure are achieved more quickly with fewer treatments with 3 log kill than with 2. Resistance to treatment may be acquired at any point: early with relapse after a short partial response or later after a longer period of apparent complete clinical remission. This model was most important in planning scheduling of drugs, demonstrated the influence of schedule on cell kill, and clarified the need for additional therapy after achieving clinical remission. Unfortunately, this concept depends on the assumption that all tumor cells have the capacity to divide, that they are equally sensitive to drugs, and are independent of local host factors. Similarly, the model assumed that cell sensitivity remained unchanged.

Tumor Cell Heterogeneity

In humans, none of the aforementioned assumptions is completely true. Solid tumor models demonstrate more variability, with widely different fractions of tumor cells capable of proliferation, marked variations within a given tumor of the fraction of resting and dividing cells, and marked differences in cell-cycle time as well as spontaneous death rates.

Tumor Growth Kinetics

Overall net tumor growth is determined by the growth fraction minus the fraction of cells dying spontaneously. In general, small foci of tumors demonstrate rapid growth as a result of a high growth fraction, with a greater percentage of cells synthesizing DNA prior to replication and a higher mitotic rate. As the tumor enlarges, rates of DNA synthesis and subsequent mitosis fall, slowing growth and producing a Gompertzian growth curve. Within a single tumor focus, the center of an enlarging lesion is frequently relatively anoxic, contains more nonviable or nonreproductive cells, and contains fewer actively dividing cells. Cell division is more likely to be active at the periphery.

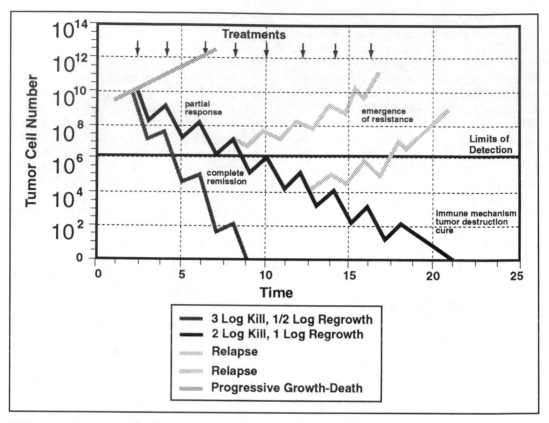

Figure 3–1. Two examples of the proportional cell-kill concept, demonstrating the relationship of achievement of cure to sensitivity to drug, number of treatments required, as well as failure with emergence of drug resistance.

Tumor cell heterogeneity is more likely to be demonstrated. These features of tumor biology are particularly pertinent to the successful application of antineoplastic agents, whose selection for a particular tumor depends on an understanding of their mechanisms of action and their relative selectivity for tumor cells at various stages of cell growth.

Cell Cycle Selectivity

The agents that have their maximal effect on cells in a particular stage of cell division are considered cell-cycle-specific agents and have their maximal effect on cells in that phase of their cycling. Thus, antimetabolites are most effective against cell populations with a high fraction of cells synthesizing DNA and mitotic

inhibitors are most effective in damaging or destroying cells in the process of mitosis. In contrast, non-cell-cycle-specific agents exert cell-killing effects independent of that feature. This concept of considering cell-cycle specificity in relationship to selection of agents is frequently relative in attempting maximal cell kill and in attempting to determine whether time of exposure to an antineoplastic or magnitude of dose is of greater importance. Dose intensity is more rational for non-cell-cycle-specific agents, whereas, for cell-cycle specific agents, once maximal inhibition is achieved, further escalation of dose serves little purpose. Rather, prolongation of exposure, attempting to inhibit later cells as they proceed to synthesize DNA, is a strategy more likely to lead to success. These principles have been applied in attempting to design the most rational approaches to the use of these agents and frequently have been responsible for improved therapeutic outcomes.

Combination Chemotherapy

For many cancers, combinations of antineoplastic agents have yielded superior response rates to those achieved with single agents alone. Both the frequency and quality of responses have been shown to improve with these combinations when compared in Phase II and Phase III trials with single-agent therapies. The curability of germ-cell carcinoma of the testes is a clear example of this, as are the strides that have been made in the management of leukemias, lymphomas, and breast cancer. Rational combinations are developed using individually active agents, attempting to augment tumor-cell kill through different mechanisms of action, and frequently employ agents with different cell-cycle killing characteristics. Some combinations seek to avoid additive toxicity, pairing agents with different toxicity patterns to produce additive or synergistic antineoplastic effects without major additive toxicities to the patient. In addition to preventing the emergence of resistance of clones and increasing cytotoxicity to both resting and dividing cells, combinations frequently have enhanced biochemical effects by blockading different biosynthetic pathways or inhibiting sequential steps in a single pathway. Some combinations achieve benefit by increasing intracellular concentration of a drug or its active metabolite or by decreasing efflux of an active agent. Some combinations can be used to achieve rescue of the host from the toxic effects of the antineoplastic agent. Leucovorin allows high-dose methotrexate to be administered over a prolonged period of time, with potential rapid reversal of blockade when leucovorin is given. The toxic effects of the metabolites of Cytoxan or ifosfamide on the bladder mucosa are preventable by concomitant or sequential administration of the uro-protector mesna,

and the availability of this agent has permitted high-dose intensity studies of this agent. These have proved particularly useful in sarcoma therapy and in bone-marrow ablative studies in bone-marrow transplantation.

In general, individually active agents are chosen unless there is a clear biochemical or pharmacological purpose for an inactive drug as described above. One must be cautious in dosing to avoid the additive toxicities when a common organ system is affected (i.e., the bone marrow). Some high-dose programs employ G-CSF in an attempt to ameliorate this toxicity. All combination studies have the potential risk that moderate reductions in the dose of each agent may abrogate any benefit achieved by the combination. Despite these provisos, marked progress has been achieved in cancer drug therapy by the recognition of the value of combination chemotherapy. As new drugs are discovered, each is explored for synergy, additive effects, or toxicity reduction. Multiple drug combinations are frequently used. Details of the use of some will be described in subsequent chapters.

Steps in Drug Evaluation

Initial human studies (Phase I) with each new agent are carried out to define the toxicity profile of the drug which is usually administered in several dose schedules as suggested by animal or in vitro studies. The biochemical pharmacological features of the agent are defined with studies of absorption, activation, metabolism, and excretion. Pharmacodynamic and pharmacokinetic features are frequently explored and dose-limiting toxicity is defined for each schedule. Phase II studies attempt to define response rates and/or efficacy in reducing the size of known evaluable or measurable metastatic lesions in 5–10 different specific neoplasms. Multiple schedules may be investigated. Objective responses are quantitated; a complete response is the disappearance of all known disease; a partial response is defined as a 50% reduction in size of the product of cross-sectioned diameters of all measurable lesions that persists for a month or more. Phase III studies of active agents compare the relative effectiveness of the new drug to that of established drugs to evaluate relative response rates, frequency of complete regressions, durations of response, toxicity incidence and severity, and effects on survival and quality of life. New drugs are then employed in combination with other known effective agents in hopes of achieving superior results. Sequentially improved treatment plans are so derived. From Phase II and III drug studies come the building blocks for integrated multimodality treatments that seek to apply surgery, radiation, and chemotherapy to improve the management of apparently localized neoplasms with poor outcomes, either because of the low probability that patients can be rendered disease-free or because of the high likelihood that relapse will ensue.

Factors Prognostic for Response

The likelihood of response to a particular treatment is a product of both treatment and host factors. Dose, dose intensity, schedule, pharmacodynamic, and pharmacokinetic features of treatment will achieve different response rates depending on host and tumor characteristics. Age, sex, performance status, prior treatment, and baseline hematologic, hepatic, and renal function variables may significantly affect outcome. Tumor variables such as histology, degree of differentiation, mitotic rate, and presence or absence of tumor-specific antigens, together with the number, size, or location of the metastatic sites, will likely affect outcome. In poorly responding tumors, younger patients with high performance status, no prior treatment, and a few small nonvisceral lesions are clearly more likely to respond than older, previously treated individuals with bulky visceral organ involvement. As treatment improves, benefitting a greater portion of those treated, benefit is likely to extend to some poorly

performing individuals with more advanced disease. Thus, drug therapy of Stage IV lung cancer patients is more apt to benefit Performance Status 1 patients, whereas the side effects of treatment are likely to be more severe and response rates are likely to be lower in more poorly functioning individuals (Ruckdeschel et al., 1986).

ACHIEVEMENTS OF CHEMOTHERAPY IN ADVANCED DISEASE

Curable Neoplasms

As additional agents have become available and our understanding of their dosage, scheduling, and use in combination with other agents has improved, our ability to control a growing number of advanced neoplastic conditions has increased. Table 3–8 outlines these achievements. The 1960s was a decade of substantial progress in both childhood and adult neoplasms, and the curative potential of drug treatments was documented. Several advanced pediatric neoplasms were demonstrated to be sensitive to the then-available agents, and their curative potential was quickly appreciated. Progressive incremental improvements in the management of childhood acute lymphocytic leukemia have led to such success that, today, the majority of children affected are cured of this disease, and progress in improving survival in the leukemias of adults has followed. Alterations in scheduling demonstrated the effectiveness of methotrexate in curing gestational trophoblastic disease without severe toxicity. The growing appreciation of the value of combination chemotherapy spurred progress in Hodgkin's disease, the non-Hodgkin's lymphomas, and breast cancer. In the 1970s, the development of platinum provided a third effective agent, which, added to a combination of vinblastine and bleomycin, now results in the cure of the majority of young men with germ cell carcinoma of the testes. More recently, strides in bone marrow trans-

TABLE 3–8. Achievements of Chemotherapy in Advanced Disease

Curative Potential	Major Improvements in Symptom Control and/or Survival	Palliative
Neuroblastoma	Breast carcinoma	Melanoma
Wilm's tumor	Prostate carcinoma	Renal cell carcinoma
Ewing's sarcoma	Ovarian carcinoma	Pancreas
Rhabdomyosarcoma	Hairy cell leukemia	Non-small cell carcinoma of the lung
Osteogenic sarcoma	Chronic lymphocytic leukemia	Squamous cell carcinoma of the head and neck
Acute lymphcytic leukemia	Mycosis fungoides	Transitional cell cancer of the bladder
Acute myelocytic leukemia	Low-grade indolent non-Hodgkin's lymphoma	Gastric cancer
Chronic myelocytic leukemia	Squamous cell carcinoma of the larynx	Colon cancer
Multiple myeloma	Nasopharyngeal carcinoma	Glioblastoma multiforme
Burkitt's lymphoma		
Hodgkin's disease		
High-grade or aggressive non-Hodgkin's lymphoma		
Germ cell carcinoma of the testes		
Gestational trophoblastic disease		
Small cell carcinoma of the lung		

plantation technology have demonstrated increased salvage of patients with relapsed leukemia and lymphoma. Intensive therapy has resulted in the eradication of Philadelphia chromosome positive cell lines in chronic granulocytic leukemia and abnormal immunoglobulin clones in select patients with multiple myeloma, adding these diseases to the curable list.

Diseases in Which Drug Treatment Produces Major Benefit

Major improvements in symptom control, quality of life, and/or long-term survival have been made in many other more advanced diseases, the most common of which are breast carcinoma and prostate carcinoma. In each of these, the availability of hormones and hormone antagonists or suppressors has contributed enormously to successful management. The vast majority of patients with metastatic prostate cancer respond to hormonal management with decreasing bone pain, fall in elevated prostate-specific antigen, and gain in performance status. Combination chemotherapy has been successful in inducing high-quality remissions in more than 50% of patients with advanced breast cancer. Platinum and taxol have extended survival for women with Stage III or IV ovarian carcinoma. The ability to manage symptoms, control tumor mass, and alleviate complications has been shown with a variety of agents for chronic lymphocytic leukemia and low-grade lymphoma. In carcinomas of the head and neck, the combination of cisplatin/5-FU as induction treatment has clearly improved quality of life and demonstrated the ability to preserve the potential for voice in Stage III and IV squamous cell carcinoma of the larynx. Deoxycoformicin has vastly simplified management of patients with hairy cell leukemia, producing a high rate of complete remission and possible cures. Nasopharyngeal carcinoma appears to be a particularly sensitive head and neck cancer, which responds well to a variety of available agents.

Limited Palliative Therapy

For an unfortunately large number of advanced neoplasms, the use of drugs remains limited to palliation. Gastrointestinal carcinomas probably represent the largest numerical group of these tumors in the United States; antineoplastic agents such as 5-FU produce objective partial responses in 20-25% of patients. Complete responses are uncommon and duration of response is limited to 4–6 months for most patients. Approximately 15% of patients with metastatic malignant melanoma and renal cell carcinoma respond to biological modifier treatments with interleukin-2 or interferon. Most responses are of limited duration, though markedly prolonged complete regressions lasting several years are achieved in 2–3% of patients.

MULTIMODALITY CANCER THERAPY

Of perhaps greater overall significance is the marked contribution drugs have made as a component of multimodality treatment plans (Table 3–9). Using information derived from the responsiveness of neoplastic disease to chemotherapy in the advanced disease setting, treatment has been applied in three ways, attempting to integrate chemotherapy into combined multimodality treatment strategies for less advanced disease.

Neoadjuvant Use

Drugs have been evaluated as initial neoadjuvant or induction treatments prior to another definitive modality, for example, radiation or surgery. For advanced localized Stage III breast cancers adherent to the chest wall, drug treatment has made possible, or easier, surgical resections with tumor-negative margins. Drugs given prior to surgery or radiation have higher response rates than in the relapsed disease situation. Cisplatin and 5-FU, for example, produce partial responses in 40–50% of patients with recurrent disease, with complete regressions in 5–8% (Roland et al., 1986), whereas induction therapy responses are seen in 80–90%, with complete remissions reaching 20–25% (Weaver et al., 1982). Although this achievement did not lead to an overall improved survival in randomized trials, it provided the impetus for the Veterans Affairs laryngeal salvage trial (Department of Veterans Affairs Laryngeal Cancer Study Group, 1991) and the subsequent demonstration of voice preservation discussed in Chapter 6. Neoadjuvant drug use in osteogenic sarcoma uses the information gained at resection to evaluate the cytotoxic results of therapy and plan further postsurgical treatment choices. Patients who show at least 90% tumor destruction have significantly improved survival. Cure rates of 50-80% may be achieved and limb-sparing resections are facilitated (Benjamin et al., 1984). This approach to therapy may also prove valuable in the management of soft tissue sarcoma.

Drug Usage Perioperatively Continues to Be Studied

Portal vein infusions at the time of colon cancer resections may prevent hepatic

TABLE 3–9. Combined Modality Treatment With Drugs

	Concomitant With		
Neoadjuvant	*Surgery*	*Radiation Therapy*	*Postsurgical Adjuvants*
Extensive localized Stage III or inflammatory breast carcinoma	Limb perfusion malignant melanoma	Rectal cancer	Breast cancer
Carcinoma of the larynx	Portal vein infusion	Nasopharyngeal cancer	Stage III malignant melanoma
Osteogenic sarcoma		Squamous cell carcinoma of the head and neck	Colon cancer
		Anal carcinoma	Ewing's sarcoma
		Lung cancer	
		Stage III localized prostate cancer	

metastases and improve survival (Piedbois et al., 1995). Isolated limb perfusion with melphalan achieves a high rate of complete regression and delays or prevents regional recurrence in regionally metastatic malignant melanoma (Reintgen, Cruse, Wells, Saba, & Slingluff, 1992).

Drugs With Radiation Therapy

Intensive efforts are underway to use drugs as radiation sensitizers either concomitantly with radiation or interdigitated with radiation therapy in many tumor sites. These have demonstrated improvements in survival in Stage III rectal cancers, where fewer local relapses and evidence of distant disease progression have been seen with a resultant improvement in survival. The North Central Cancer Treatment Group (NCCTG) study showed a relative risk reduction of 40% for local relapse and 37% for distant relapse, and improvements in disease-free survival of 30% and in overall survival of 29% (Krook et al., 1991). Altogether three trials have demonstrated the value of 5-FU in addition to radiation, and the National Institutes of Health (NIH) consensus panel of 1990 and 1991 recommended chemoradiation

therapy as standard treatment for high-risk (B2 and C) lesions. Continuous infusion therapy achieved a 10% improvement over bolus 5-FU (O'Connell et al., 1994). In head and neck cancer, many studies have suggested improved responses with combined chemotherapy and radiation therapy, but survival gains have sometimes not reached statistical significance. The data of Merlano et al. (1996), using an alternating radiotherapy and chemotherapy approach in unresectable disease, provide strong evidence supporting this approach. Combined treatment was associated with complete response more often than radiotherapy alone (43% compared to 22%; $p = .037$), and overall survival at 5 years was better (24% compared to 10%; $p = .01$). Figure 3–2 depicts the overall survival comparisons. Recently, cisplatin together with radiation therapy has been shown to improve both local control and relapse-free survival compared to radiation alone in nasopharyngeal carcinoma (Al-Sarraf et al., 1996; Dimery et al., 1993).

The use of mitomycin C and 5-FU with radiation therapy induces a high rate of complete sustained remissions and may avoid the need for abdominal perineal resection in carcinoma of the anus.

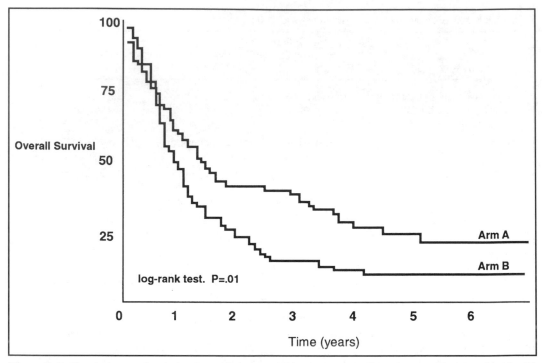

Figure 3–2. Survival according to treatment in unresectable squamous cell carcinoma of head and neck. (A) Combined chemoradiation. (B) Radiation therapy alone. *Source:* Adapted from "Five-year update of a randomized trial of alternating radiotherapy and chemotherapy compared with radiotherapy alone in treatments of unresected squamous cell carcinoma of the head and neck," by M. Merlano, M. Benasso, R. Corvo, R. Rosso, V. Vitale, F. Blengio, G. Numicao, G. Margarino, L. Bonelli, and L. Santi, 1996, *Journal of the National Cancer Institute, 88*, pp. 583-589.

Drugs as Postsurgical Adjuvants

Postsurgical adjuvant treatments have also been extensively explored and are of great value in three important neoplasms. The anti-estrogen tamoxifen is of great value in improving disease-free and overall survival for both premenopausal and postmenopausal women with estrogen receptor–positive resectable breast cancer. Chemotherapy and tamoxifen have shown additive benefit. The Oxford meeting reviewed a meta-analysis updating more than 250 trials evaluating outcomes of therapy at 15 years (*Adjuvant therapy of breast cancer tamoxifen update*, 1995; Early Breast Cancer Trialists Collaborative Group, 1992; Horton, 1996). The use of tamoxifen reduced the cancer-related risk of mortality by 14% for estrogen receptor–positive premenopausal women and 27%

for postmenopausal women. Chemotherapy reduced mortality risk by 27% for women less than 50 years of age compared to 11% for older women. Tamoxifen adds to improvement with chemotherapy in all estrogen receptor–positive patients.

High-dose adjuvant interferon given for resected high-risk malignant melanoma has been shown to produce a 42% improvement in the fraction of patients who are continuously free of disease compared to observation (Kirkwood et al., 1996). Relapse-free survival is shown in Figure 3–3. The combinations of 5-FU and leucovorin or 5-FU and levamisole have been shown to reduce risk of recurrence when given as postsurgical adjuvants for Stage B2 or C colon cancers. A large intergroup trial that enrolled 1,269 patients demonstrated an absolute reduction in risk of relapse of 15% (representing a relative

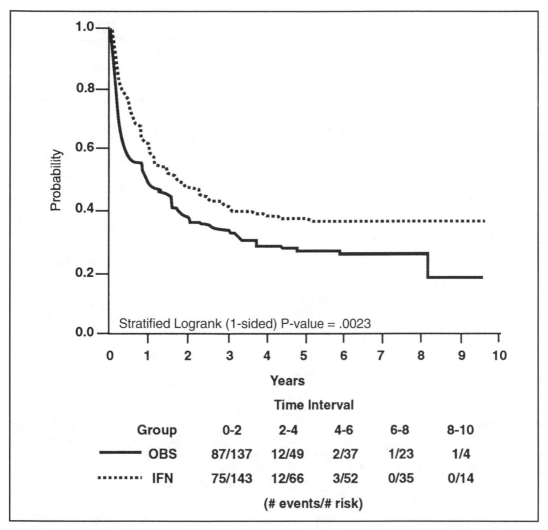

Time Interval					
Group	0-2	2-4	4-6	6-8	8-10
—— OBS	87/137	12/49	2/37	1/23	1/4
·········· IFN	75/143	12/66	3/52	0/35	0/14
(# events/# risk)					

Stratified Logrank (1-sided) P-value = .0023

Figure 3–3. Relapse-free survival of eligible patients. *Source*: Adapted from "Interferon alfa-2b adjuvant therapy of high-risk resected cutaneous melanoma: The Eastern Cooperative Oncology Group trial EST 1684," by J. M. Kirkwood, M. H. Strawderman, M. C. Ernstoff, T. J. Smith, E. C. Borden, and R. H. Blum, 1996, *Journal of Clinical Oncology, 14*, pp. 7-17.

risk reduction of 41%) and improvement in overall survival (Moertel et al., 1995). Although this study alone did not reach statistical significance for the B2 group of patients, an analysis of four separate trials has suggested the benefit for B2 patients is similar (Mamounas et al., 1996).

Applications of drugs as adjuvants to the management of other disease sites are the subject of intensive study. In gen-eral, the most active agent or combination of agents is selected for study and integrated in the above-mentioned three strategies in an attempt to improve outcome. In the disease sites illustrated, two of which are relatively poorly responsive to drugs in the advanced disease situation, therapy was successful in preventing, delaying, or eliminating the growth of micrometastatic disease, achieving substantial clinical benefit. These achievements provide a stimulus for further progress.

OVERVIEW OF IMPACT OF CHEMOTHERAPY ON SWALLOWING AND COMMUNICATION DISORDERS

This chapter summarizes broadly the contemporary use of antineoplastic drug treatment in the management of malignancy. Subsequent chapters amplify and detail its uses in specific disease sites, many of which are particularly appropriate to health care professionals interested in swallowing and communication disorders. Many of these sites of disease significantly compromise swallowing and/or communication, and, unfortunately, further definitive therapy with surgery and radiation therapy may also produce additional impediments. Chemotherapy produces similar, usually transitory, effects as well.

Dysphagia

Inhibition of mucosal cell proliferation by antineoplastics leads to cell loss, inflammation, and ulceration of the oral mucosa, resulting in clinically apparent stomatitis, pharyngitis, and esophagitis. Pain limits swallowing, resulting in dehydration, weakness, and weight loss. The breakdown of mucosal barriers makes the patient vulnerable to local infections (i.e., candidiasis and/or herpes) and provides a portal of entry for systemic bacterial infections. Restoration of mucosal integrity usually is achieved in a few days aided by anti-inflammatory, antifungal, and local anesthetic agents. In contrast to radiation therapy, recovery is not followed by fibrosis and the potential for stricture.

Hearing Loss

Some drugs, particularly cisplatin given in high doses, may produce transient to intermittent ringing in the ears. Repetitive treatments lead to eighth nerve hearing loss, which may occasionally be severe and long lasting. Pretreatment audiograms may be done to evaluate the potential for this complication in individuals whose hearing appears compromised prior to therapy. Prevention may be achieved by administering the drug in divided doses over several days to limit peak drug concentrations. Alternatively, carboplatin may be substituted for cisplatin. Its potential for neurotoxicity is markedly less.

Voice

Quality is only rarely affected by drugs. Severe edema of the vocal folds or supraglottic larynx may occur as an allergic reaction and is usually effectively treated with steroids.

Cognitive Changes

Cognitive changes are much more commonly produced by sedatives and antiemetics given in association with the administration of chemotherapy drugs than by the drugs themselves. Usually these are easily recognized, are short in duration, and require little or no intervention. Steroids may produce hyperexcitability, sleeplessness, flights of ideas, mania, and, rarely, delusions. Steroid psychosis is possible with continued use. The metabolites of ifosfamide may occasionally produce confusion, decrease in mental acuity, and slurred speech progressing to semicoma. These effects are reversible in a few hours with cessation of drug therapy and may be prevented by avoiding peak concentrations of drug. More chronic in nature may be the effects of interferon on the nervous system, producing fatigue, lethargy, mental dullness, apathy, and symptoms of depression. These changes are more likely in older individuals on a long-term adjuvant therapy. Dose reductions, antidepressants, or stimulants may be used to ameliorate these difficulties. Hopefully, the myriad ways in which chemotherapy drugs affect swallowing and communication disorders are apparent. Health care professionals acquainted with not only the benefits of therapy, but also the impact of drug toxicity on swallowing and communication difficulties, are in a better position to provide the ideal care of our patients.

REFERENCES

Adjuvant therapy of breast cancer tamoxifen update. (1995). Bethesda, MD: National Cancer Institute.

Al-Sarraf, M., LeBlanc, M., Giri, P. G. S., Fu, K., Cooper, J., Vuoung, T., Forastiere, A., Adams, G., Sakr, W., Schuller, D., & Ensley, J. (1996). Superiority of chemo-radiotherapy (CT-RT) vs radiotherapy (RT) in patients (pts) with locally advanced nasopharyngeal cancer (NPC). Preliminary results of intergroup (0099) (SWOG 8892, RTOG 8817, ECOG 2388) randomized study. *Proceedings of the American Society of Clinical Oncology,* abstract 882, 313.

Benjamin, R. S., Chawla, S. P., Murray, J. A., Carrasco, C. H., Raymond, A. K., Wallace, S., Ayala, A., Papdopoulos, N. E. J., & Plager, C. (1984). Preoperative chemotherapy for osteogenic sarcoma—A treatment approach facilitating limb salvage with major prognostic implications. In S. E. Jones & S. E. Salmon (Eds.), *Adjuvant Therapy of Cancer IV* (pp. 601-610). New York: Grune & Stratton.

Department of Veterans Affairs Laryngeal Cancer Study Group. (1991). Induction chemotherapy plus radiation compared with surgery plus radiation in patients with advanced laryngeal cancer. *New England Journal of Medicine, 324,* 1685-1690.

Dimery, I. W., Peters, L. J., Goepfert, H., Morrison, W. H., Byers, R. M., Guillory, C., McCarthy, K., Weber, R. S., & Hong, W. K. (1993). Effectiveness of combined induction chemotherapy and radiotherapy in advanced nasopharyngeal carcinoma. *Journal of Clinical Oncology, 11,* 1919-1928.

Early Breast Cancer Trialists Collaborative Group. (1992). Systemic treatment of early breast cancer by hormonal cytoxic, or immune therapy: 133 randomized trials involving 31,000 women. *Lancet, 339,* 1-15.

Frie, E., Teicher, B. A., Holden, S. A., Cathcart, K. N., & Wang, Y. Y. (1988). Preclinical studies and clinical correlation of the effect of alkylating dose. *Cancer Research, 48,* 6417-6423.

Horton, J. (1996). Special report: 1995 Oxford breast cancer overview—Preliminary outcomes. Cancer *Control Journal, 5,* 78-79.

Isaacson, P. G., & Spencer, J. (1996). Gastric lymphoma and helicobacter pylori. In V. T. DeVita, S. Hellman, & S. A. Rosenberg (Eds.), *Important advances in oncology.* Philadelphia: Lippincott-Raven.

Kirkwood, J. M., Strawderman, M. H., Ernstoff, M. C., Smith, T. J., Borden, E. C., & Blum, R. H. (1996). Interferon alfa-2b adjuvant therapy of high-risk resected cutaneous melanoma: The Eastern Cooperative Oncology Group trial EST 1684. *Journal of Clinical Oncology, 14,* 7-17.

Krook, J. E., Moertel, C. G., Gunderson, L. L., et al. (1991). Effective surgical adjuvant therapy for high-risk rectal carcinoma. *New England Journal of Medicine, 324,* 709-715.

Mamounas, E. P., Rochette, H., Jones, J., Wickerman, D. L., Fisher, B., & Wolmark, N. (1996). Comparative efficacy of adjuvant chemotherapy in patients with Dukes B vs. Dukes C colon cancer: Results from four NSABP adjuvant studies (C01, C02, C03, C04). *Proceedings of the American Society of Clinical Oncology, 15,* 205.

Mandelli, F., Diverio, D., Avvisati, G., Luciano, A., Barbui, T., Bernasconi, C., Broccia, G., Cerri, R., Falda, M., Fioritoni, G., Leoni, F., Liso, V., Petti, M., Rodeghiero, F., Saglio, G., Vegna, M., Visani, G., Jehm, U., Willemze, R., Muus, P., Pelicci, G., Bionid, A., & LoCoco, F. (1997). Molecular remission in PM1/RAR alpha-positive acute promyelocytic leukemia by combined all-trans retinoic acid and idarucibin (AIDA) therapy. *Blood, 90,* 1014-1021.

Merlano, M., Benasso, M., Corvo, R., Rosso, R., Vitale, V., Blengio, F., Numicao, G., Margarino, G., Bonelli, L., & Santi, L. (1996). Five-year update of a randomized trial of alternating radiotherapy and chemotherapy compared with radiotherapy alone in treatment of unresected squamous cell carcinoma of the head and neck. *Journal of the National Cancer Institute, 88,* 583-589.

Moertel, C. G., Fleming, T. R., MacDonald, J. S., Haller, D. G., Laurie, J. A., Tangen, C. M., Ungerleider, J. S., Emerson, W. A., Torrey, D. C., & Glick, J. H. (1995). 5-FU plus levamisole as effective adjuvant therapy after resection of stage III colon carcinoma: A final report. *Annals of Internal Medicine, 122,* 321-326.

O'Connell, M. J., Martenson, J. A., Wieand, H. S., Krook, J. E., MacDonald, J. S., Haller, D. G., Mayer, R. J., Gunderson, L. L., & Rich, T. A. (1994). Improving adjuvant therapy for rectal cancer by combining protracted-infusion 5-FU with radiation therapy after curative surgery. *New England Journal of Medicine, 331,* 502-507.

Piedbois, P., Buyse, M., Gray, R., Clark, M., Wolmark, N., Metzger, U., Fielding, L. P., Gray, B., Taylor, I., Wereldsma, J., Ryan, J., Marsoni, S., & Gruenagel,

H. H. (1995). Portal vein infusion is an effective adjuvant treatment for patients with colorectal cancer. *Proceedings of the American Society of Clinical Oncology, 14,* 192.

Reintgen, D. S., Cruse, C. W., Wells, K. E., Saba, H. I., & Slingluff, C. L. (1992). Isolate limb perfusion for recurrent melanoma of the extremity. *Annals of Plastic Surgery, 28,* 50-54.

Roland, K. M., Taylor, S. G., O'Donnell, M. R., Spiers, A., Stott, P. B., DeConti, R. C., Milner, L., & Marsh, J. C. (1986). Cisplatin-5-FU infusion chemotherapy in advanced recurrent cancer of the head and neck: An Eastern Cooperative Oncology Group Pilot Study. *Cancer Treatment Reports, 70,* 361-464.

Ruckdeschel, J. C., Finkelstein, D. M., Ettinger, D. S., Creech, R. A., Mason, R. C., Joss, B. A., & Vogel, S. (1986). A randomized trial of the four most active regimens for metastatic non-small cell lung cancer. *Journal of Clincal Oncology, 4,* 14-22.

Weaver, A., Flemming, S., Kish, J., Vandenberg, H., Jacob, J., Crissman, J., & Al-Sarraf, M. (1982). Cis-platinum and 5-fluorouracil as induction therapy for advanced head and neck cancer. *American Journal of Surgery, 144,* 445-448.

4

Radiation Therapy in Oncologic Management With Special Emphasis on Head and Neck Carcinoma

Andre A. Abitbol, M.D., Jay L. Friedland, M.S., M.D., Alan A. Lewin, M.D., Maria-Amelia Rodrigues, M.D., and Vivek Mishra, Ph.D.

Radiation therapy, one of the three main therapeutic oncologic modalities, is currently used in approximately 40–60% of all cancer patients. Radiation therapy may be used either as part of a curative plan (frequently combined with surgery and/or chemotherapy) or for palliation of disturbing symptoms (in the setting of incurable disease). Since the discoveries of x-rays by Roentgen in 1895 and radium by the Curies in 1895, the modality has evolved technologically. Radiation therapy can be broadly divided into external irradiation and internal radiation (brachytherapy). The utility of early external radiation therapy equipment was limited by the low energies of the radiation, resulting in high skin doses and inadequate dose delivery at depth. Newer linear accelerators, using a spinoff of World War II technology (i.e., the klystron unit in radars), have significant skin sparing and depth dose distribution. Additionally, the manual handling of radium sources, with its radiation exposure to personnel, has been replaced by afterloading techniques and remote afterloading techniques (com-

puter based). Newer techniques emerging in the therapeutic arena include intraoperative radiation therapy, conformal three-dimensional radiotherapy, and radiosurgery of cerebral lesions. These share the commonality of a reduction in exposure of normal surrounding tissues and delivery of focused radiation therapy, and therefore a physical dose advantage. Capitalizing on the differential radioresponsiveness of normal and malignant cells, modulating agents— including radiosensitizers (including certain chemotherapeutic drugs), radioprotectors (to protect normal tissues), hyperthermia, and regimens of altered fractionation— give a biological advantage. Hyperfractionation, frequently using two doses of radiation per day (giving a higher total dose), or accelerated fractionation (giving a shorter treatment course of radiation using multiple doses daily and/or an intensified course with short duration) are currently areas of investigation (Fowler, 1992; Peters, Ang, & Thames, 1988; Schwade et al., 1992; Van den Bogaert, Horiot, & van der Schueren, 1989; Withers, 1985). These experimental ap-

47

proaches using altered fractionation have the potential advantage of increased tumor control but the disadvantage of increased acute reaction (mucositis, as an example). Additionally, there has been a gradual shift in the surgical management of several cancers, with greater emphasis placed on organ preservation (i.e., breast, larynx, anal canal, rectum, and bladder). Germane to this concept is the frequent use of multimodality therapy combining radiation with surgery and chemotherapy. A noteworthy example of a model of integrated multidisciplinary therapy is anal carcinoma. The combination of radiation therapy, constant infusion 5 (a well-known radiosensitizer), and mitomycin C (a bioreductive drug that selectively kills metabolically deprived radioresistant cells) now results in a greater survival and local control rate, with a sphincter preservation rate of over 71% (Flam et al., 1995). Understanding the evolution of these research avenues helps one to appreciate the clinical applications of today's treatment. A synopsis of the basic principles of radiation physics and radiobiology follows.

RADIATION PHYSICS

Ionizing Radiation

A basic review of terminology and definitions is provided. Ionization is the process of absorption of radiation on biological matter. The radiation affects the orbital electrons of atoms and ejects the electron with sufficient energy. The source of the radiation may be electromagnetic or particulate. Electromagnetic radiations include x-rays and gamma rays, both of which are similar in action. X-rays are produced in an electric machine (i.e., x-ray or linear accelerator) by accelerating electrons and energizing them across an electric field (Johns & Cunningham, 1969). The energized electrons then hit a target (i.e., tungsten), converting the kinetic energy to x-rays. Gamma rays are produced within a nucleus by the unstable nucleus' decay into a more stable form. Gamma rays used in clinical practice are derived from iso-

topes such as cesium (used frequently in gynecologic work) and iridium, which is used as a low dose rate isotope (for implantation of oral tongue cancer) or a high dose rate isotope (increasingly used in gynecologic and bronchial cancers). Particulate forms of radiation include experimental types such as neutrons, alpha particles, protons, negative pi-mesons, and charged ions. A routinely used form of particulate radiation is an electron beam produced by a linear accelerator. The electron beam is captured and is used prior to hitting a target to produce x-rays. The electron beam has different depth dose characteristics than x-rays. By choosing a variety of energies from 6 meV to 18 meV, the clinician has available a facile way of treating superficial tumors of various depths.

RADIATION BIOLOGY

Absorption of Radiation in Mammalian Cells

Radiation is absorbed directly or indirectly in mammalian cells. Directly ionizing radiation interacts directly with critical targets within the absorbing atoms to produce chemical and biological transformations. This type of interaction is predominant with high linear energy transfer (LET) radiation, typical of some particulate radiations that interact by direct action. Indirect ionizing radiation first interacts with atoms or molecules in the cells (i.e., water) to produce free radicals that diffuse in the cells to reach the critical target (Figure 4–1). A free radical contains an unpaired electron and has a short life (10^{-10}s). It is estimated that two thirds of biological injuries from x-rays are due to indirect action (Hall, 1994). The indirect action of sparsely ionizing radiation (or low LET radiation) is amenable to modulation with chemical sensitizers and radioprotectors, whereas high LET radiation (predominantly direct action) is highly unresponsive to modulation by these agents. Although the deposition of radiation is instantaneous, its biological manifestation is delayed. If the end

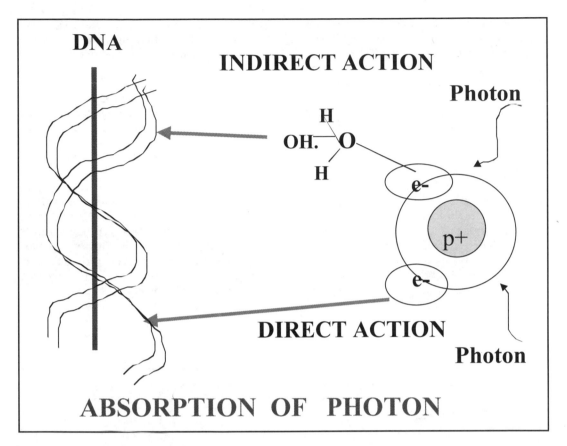

Figure 4–1. Action of radiation.

event is cell death, the cell may continue to divide for hours or days. If, however, the event is carcinogenesis, the latency period may be delayed for 5 to 15 or more years.

Biological Target

There is putative evidence to implicate DNA as the target molecule of radiation (Eric, 1994). Radiation damage to DNA, a double helix structure, may result in a base damage, single strand break, or double strand breaks. Single strand breaks that occur far from each other are of little significance because these breaks are repaired using the opposite strand as a template. If breaks occur in close proximity repair is not possible. Radiation injury is then irreversible, resulting in cell death, mutation, or oncogenesis.

Mammalian Cell Killing

A fundamental appreciation of radiobiology requires the use of a cell survival curve (Elkind & Sutton, 1960). This curve correlates the effect of radiation dose on the reproductive integrity of mammalian cells. Although a traditional end point of cell death (i.e., response) may be used, a more appropriate definition may be clonogenicity. Clonogenicity describes the ability of a cell to proliferate indefinitely. Cells exposed to radiation may undergo apoptosis (programmed cell death) or mitotic cell death. Apoptosis occurs after irradiation by activation of the oncogene p53. Cells undergoing mitosis after radiation die on the second or third attempt to replicate due to unrepaired DNA damage. These cells are no longer clonogenic.

Mammalian cell survival curves vary according to the type of ionizing radiation. For densely ionizing (high LET) radiation, the curve is a straight line from the origin, indicative of exponential cell killing (Figure 4–2). A typical cell survival curve of x-ray (low LET, or sparsely ionizing) will have an initial broad shoulder followed by a straight line at higher doses (on log-linear paper). This shoulder is indicative of repair of sublethal damage, which occurs at low doses. The killing of individual cells has a major impact on both normal tissue cells and tumor cells in clinical radiotherapy.

Dose survival curves for various normal mammalian cells indicate a wide variability in sensitivity, manifested primarily by a variation of the broad shoulder width. It is useful to categorize mammalian cell radiosensitivity according to the type of normal proliferation (Rubin & Casaret, 1968). Cells that are actively dividing or proliferating (i.e., active self-renewal) are referred to as early responding. Such cells as in the skin, mucosal surfaces, germinal, and intestinal crypt are highly sensitive to ionizing radiation. It is important to recognize that cells with active self-renewal tissues will express a radiation injury because of the short life span of their mature cells and the short time to maturity of their stem cells. An example of this cell-killing effect seen routinely in clinical practice is the acute mucositis of patients with head and neck cancer. Cells that are rarely dividing, typically highly differentiated, have low sensitivity (so-called late responding), i.e., nerve, muscle. Intermediate cells that may divide on demand (not regularly), such as following hepatic injury, have an intermediate sensitivity.

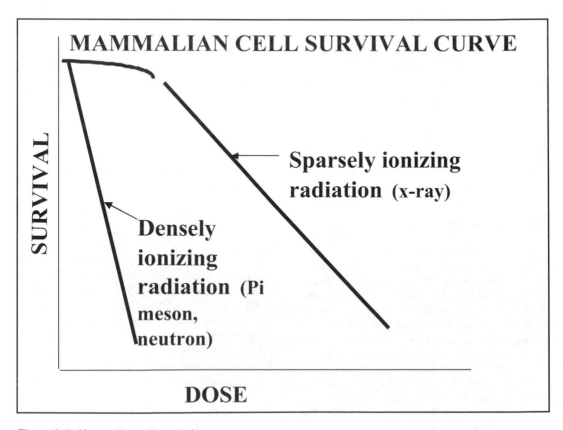

Figure 4–2. Mammalian cell survival curve.

There are other operational causes of cell death. A lymphocyte, a white blood cell of the immune system, is extremely radio-sensitive; the acinic cells of the parotid salivary gland and germinal cells also demonstrate extreme sensitivity. Apoptosis, or programmed cell death, occurs in many mammalian cells (Dewey, Ling, & Meyn, 1995). These sensitive cells (lymphocyte, germinal, acinic) demonstrate apoptosis at very low doses. The sensitivity of parotid acinic cells is clinically manifested by a dramatic acute sialoadenitis following the first dose of fractionated radiotherapy in head and neck cancer (infrequently), following mantle irradiation in Hodgkin's disease (occasionally), and following iodine 131 administration in the treatment of thyroid cancer (frequently). The patient will present with acute swelling of the parotid gland that is associated with discomfort.

Sublethal Repair

It is important to recognize that mammalian cells' exposure to radiation is not lethal in all cases. Sublethal damage can occur in normal cells and the injury is repaired within hours. This ability to repair damage within hours is demonstrated in split course experiments in Chinese hamster cells. These show that giving a similar dose split into two equal fractions 30 min apart results in a greater surviving fraction than a single dose (i.e., 15.6 Gy single dose versus 7.6 Gy given twice, 30 min apart; Elkind et al., 1965). It is thought that sublethal damage repair is present in both normal and malignant cells. Moreover, the repair of sublethal damage is compatible with the repair of DNA breaks prior to the infliction of a lethal injury.

Reassortment and Repopulation

A number of operational factors may occur during a standard course of fractionated radiation therapy. Repair of sublethal injury has already been discussed. This has obvious implications because normal cells exposed to radiation are able to overcome the radiation injury and survive. Cells may also reassort during the various cell cycle phases (mitosis, synthesis, G_1 [gap 1], and G_2 [gap 2]) and may enter into more sensitive phases (mitosis, G_2; Figure 4–3). This factor of synchronization may be of importance in tumor cells. Moreover, repopulation of rapidly growing cells may occur within 12 hr. Repopulation of these normal self-renewal cells leads to ultimate healing. This is clinically apparent in the radiation therapy clinic following a course of radiation therapy. The acute dermatitis will heal by the formation of islands of new cells that ultimately coalesce into a new layer of skin. It is this delicate balance between cell killing and repopulation that accounts for the above findings. However, tumor cells may also repopulate within 12 hr and lead to local failure to control the cancer. The inability to control tumors locally with standard, once-a-day radiation has led to the development of altered fractionation regimens. These fractionation regimens try to address tumor repopulation and to take advantage of reassortment of tumor cells. By decreasing the interval between fractions and decreasing overall treatment time, researchers have shown improvement on local control on tumors of the head and neck and lung. The clinical strategy of using hyperfractionation (splitting a daily dose of radiation into two doses spaced 6 hr apart) to spare long-term tissue injury also helps to obviate the problem of tumor cell repopulation. It is nonetheless appreciated clinically that an acute mucosal reaction is enhanced with hyperfractionation and by the use of concurrent radiosensitizing drugs (i.e., chemotherapy; Ang & Peters, 1994; Fu, 1993; Peters et al., 1988; Vokes & Weichselbaum, 1990).

Reoxygenation

A radiobiological discussion is not complete without a discussion of the oxygen effect. Of all the modifying agents that affect radiation response, oxygen has, by far, been the most studied and intriguing (Gray et al., 1953; Sartorelli, 1988). Oxygen enhances the effect of sparsely ionizing

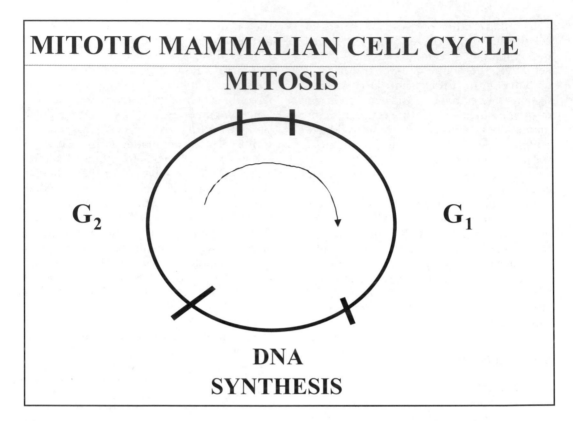

Figure 4–3. Mammalian cell cycle.

radiation by a factor of three. To work, oxygen must be present during the irradiation. Oxygen reacts with the free radicals produced during the indirect action of radiation on absorbing atoms. It is postulated that the resultant RO_2 organic peroxide fixes the lethal injury because of its nonrecuperable target.

The presence of hypoxic cells in tumors is demonstrated histologically by the presence of necrotic centers. During the course of fractionated therapy, it is postulated that hypoxic cells become oxygenated as more sensitive euoxic cells are killed first, leaving the hypoxic cells to become better oxygenated. This biological hypothesis has led to numerous clinical trials of hyperbaric oxygen and hypoxic cell radiosensitizers such as misonidazole, which to this date have not reached sufficient conclusions to warrant their routine clinical use.

Time, Dose, and Fractionation

Having briefly touched on the four Rs of radiobiology (repair, reassortment, repopulation, and reoxygenation), focus will now be given to time, dose, and fractionation factors. It is routine clinical practice to fractionate treatment over several weeks to allow sparing of normal tissues from long-term chronic late effects. This allows repair of sublethal injury and repopulation while, at the same time, greater tumor cell killing is achieved by reoxygenation and reassortment. In effect, the resultant cell survival curve becomes a composite or effective curve made up of multiple single dose curves (Figure 4–4).

The clinician chooses a fractionation scheme that takes into account normal early responding (renewal), late-responding tissues, and, increasingly, tumor kinetics. The

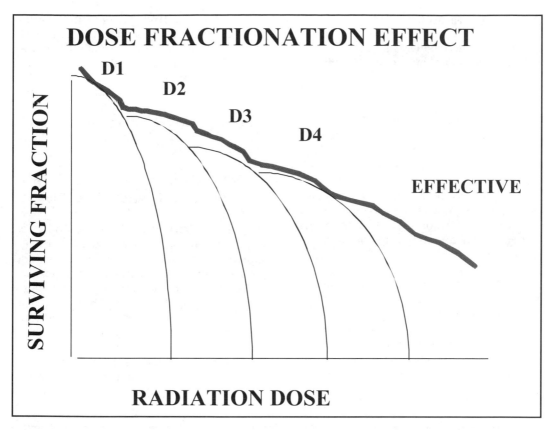

Figure 4–4. Mammalian cell effective survival curve: effect of fractionation.

focus in the past clinical radiation therapy literature has been on late-responding tissue effects. Treating to tolerance was an operational description of the strategy used by radiation oncologists to define the appropriate tumor dose. Acute reaction was felt to be self-limited and inconsequential and disassociated from late effects. Prolonged duration of treatment by interruption of treatment was frequently used to limit acute side effects. A greater appreciation of the potential adverse effect of protracted treatment on the local control of cancer in head and neck patients has emerged that refutes this attitude. The decrement in control of head and neck carcinomas is now estimated at 3% per day of interruption of treatment (Withers, Taylor, & Maciejewski, 1988). Hence, a 2-week interruption, not unusual in the past, leads to a loss of 30% of control and, ultimately,

inability to achieve cure. The analysis of the treatment parameters in a radiation therapy treatment course should include the total dose delivered, the duration of treatment, and the dose per fraction. The dose response curve for late-responding tissues (i.e., spinal cord, brain) has a broad shoulder indicating increased repair of sublethal damage. However, due to slow proliferation the biological effects of radiation are evident months to years after treatment. Therefore, damage to late-responding tissues is dependent on fraction size and total dose (higher fraction, higher incidence of late effects) rather than treatment time. However, due to early responding tissues or tumor, this indicates that fraction size is the predominant factor determining late effects, whereas both fraction size and overall time affect acute cell renewal tissue response.

Accelerated Repopulation

It has been increasingly apparent that accelerated repopulation occurs in tumors as a response to fractionated radiation therapy and that this phenomenon becomes significant during the 4th week of treatment (Withers et al., 1988). Tumors may appear to be responding in midcourse of treatment and, yet, the number of clonogenic cells will be increasing. Ultimately, failure to control the cancer is dependent on the inability to eradicate all of the clonogenic cells. Strategies to overcome accelerated repopulation have focused on the use of hyperfractionation and accelerated regimens. The intensification of regimens of radiation therapy sometimes in combination with radiosensitizing chemotherapeutic drugs has resulted in prolonged acute mucositis (Figure 4–5). It is postulated that prolonged denudation of mucosal cells of the pharynx during head and neck irradiation may be operational as the result of consequential death (Garden, Morrison,

Ang, & Peters, 1995). A putative association between prolonged acute mucositis and chronic swallowing dysfunction was found in the University of Miami A-1 study combining hyperfractionation radiation therapy, 5-fluorouracil, cisplatin, and mitomycin C in patients with locally advanced head and neck carcinoma (Abitbol et al., 1992; 1997; Schwade et al., 1992).

RADIATION THERAPY OF THE HEAD AND NECK REGION

Radiation therapy of the head and neck region is an interesting model for the application of radiobiological concepts and modern multidisciplinary management. The region contains both acute-responding (self-renewal) tissues, such as mucosa, skin, hair follicles, and parotid, and late-responding tissues, including brain, spinal cord, bone (particularly mandible), and cartilage. Additionally, salivary glands have rapidly responsive acinic cells and the

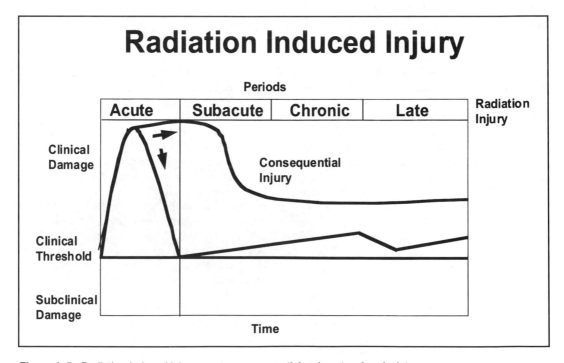

Figure 4–5. Radiation-induced injury: acute, consequential, subacute, chronic, late.

potential for late dysfunction (chronic xerostomia). Moreover, connective tissue in the subcutaneous tissues react subacutely (subcutaneous edema) and chronically, with resultant soft tissue fibrosis (ankylosing of the temporomandibular joint, with resultant trismus). Occasionally, mucosal lesions may not heal completely and may lead to soft tissue necrosis of the tongue (or other soft tissue parts). The radiation oncologist has to exercise particular caution in protecting life-sustaining or critical organs from overexposure (i.e., brain, spinal cord, eye, mandible, and lung). At the same time, the radiation oncologist manages the acute reactions associated with mucosal, skin, and salivary exposure.

The tumor kinetics of head and neck carcinoma suggest that rapid doubling of tumor cells occurs in these tumors. The analyses of potential doubling time in such tumors have been studied and correlated with a better response with the use of accelerated radiation regimens. There is a need for validation of these preliminary data.

Initial Evaluation

The initial consultation with the radiation oncologist will focus on a complete physical examination, detailed assessment of the head and neck region using palpation and fiberoptic laryngoscopy and pharyngoscopy with appropriate site-specific diagram of the tumor, staging according to the American Joint Commission for Staging Manual (Beahrs & Henson, 1989), and, lastly, prognosis and treatment. The presence of significant ethanol and cigarette abuse as etiologic agents in the causation of head and neck carcinoma in this patient population requires discussion related to cessation. The discussion will focus on the adverse effects of continued ethanol/cigarette abuse on the tolerance of the mucosa during radiation therapy and during the subacute posttherapy period. These agents exacerbate the severity of the mucositis and lead in certain laryngeal cancers to a higher likelihood of laryngeal edema. Moreover, one report suggests a worsening control rate of patients with laryngeal cancer

who continue to smoke during treatment. Perhaps even more disheartening is the significant incidence of secondary aerodigestive cancers (greater than 25%) in patients who survived their first head and neck cancer, reported by the Radiation Therapy Oncology Group Study. There is a suggestion that patients who continue to smoke will experience even higher rates of secondary aerodigestive cancers.

Patients with head and neck cancer will frequently have poor dental hygiene. A dental consultation is routinely obtained because the radiation oncologist must be concerned about preservation of dentition. Dental decay will frequently occur following head and neck radiation unless close dental surveillance and fluoride prophylactic treatment are used. The radiation-induced xerostomia and poor quality of saliva postradiation predispose these patients to dental decay. All salvageable teeth that need restorative work are attended to immediately. All nonsalvageable teeth are extracted with appropriate antibiotic prophylaxis, suturing of the dental extraction site, and smoothing of the extraction site edges. The extraction sites are allowed to heal prior to initiation of treatment. The importance of this consultation becomes apparent in the next 2 years. Dental extractions during this period may lead to osteoradionecrosis. The extraction sites serve as a portal of entry of bacteria in an already devitalized bone. The mandible is much more likely to develop osteoradionecrosis than the maxilla.

Simulation

A typical course of radiation therapy given with curative intent is illustrated below, and simulation films indicating the treatment volumes are depicted in Figures 4–6A, 6B, and 6C. The initial field uses a parallel opposed technique to treat the oropharynx in this 65-year-old female patient with a squamous cell carcinoma of the base of tongue, stage T4 N0 M0. The field is designed to encompass the primary tumor (base of tongue), direct subclinical microscopic contiguous spread to adjacent

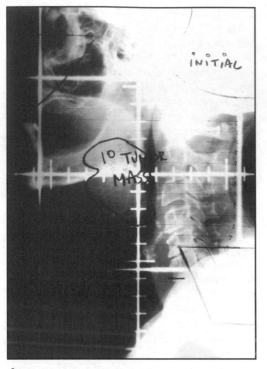

A

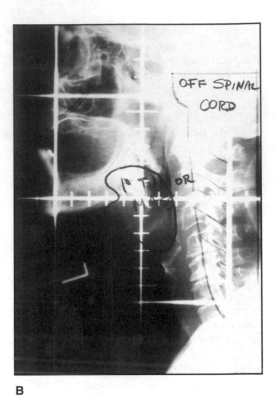

B

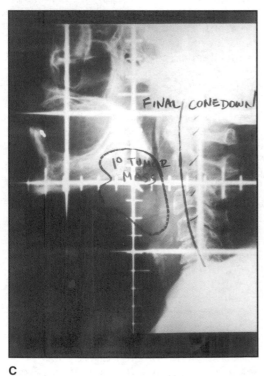

C

Figure 4–6. Base of tongue carcinoma T4 N0 M0:
(**A**) Initial shrinking field technique. (**B**) Off spinal
cord. (**C**) Final cone down.

tissues (including the root of the tongue, tonsillar fossa, middle third of the tongue, vallecula), plus the primary echelon of neck nodes depicted. The oropharyngeal field has a safety margin of 1–2 cm to allow for daily variation of setup and movement. The patient's head and neck are immobilized by means of a head holder and face-neck mask individually designed at the time of simulation. The setting up of radiation therapy, simulation, is accomplished with the patient's comfort and daily reproducibility in mind. The lower supraclavular regions are also simulated, with the intent to treat to a baseline dose of 45 Gy in 25 treatments as a safeguard against occult spread in lymphatic channels and lymph nodes. Parallel opposed treatment fields serve to homogenize the dose distribution in the oropharyngeal region as well as gain treatment of the opposite neck, where frequently occult disease is present. Hence, the radiation therapy field is much more encompassing than a surgical field (composite resection of the base of tongue and unilateral neck dissection).

Treatment

A basic concept of clinical radiation therapy is the phenomenon of dose response based on the volume of cancer (Figure 4–7). Subclinical or occult nodal disease (which is not palpable or demonstrated radiographically and is presumed to be microscopic) requires a dose of 45–50 Gy in 5 weeks (1.8–2 Gy/fraction) to ensure greater than 90% freedom from relapse. For gross tumor, a total dose of 70–74 Gy in 7–8 weeks (1.8–2 Gy/fraction) is frequently used. A shrinking field technique is used to gradually reduce normal tissue

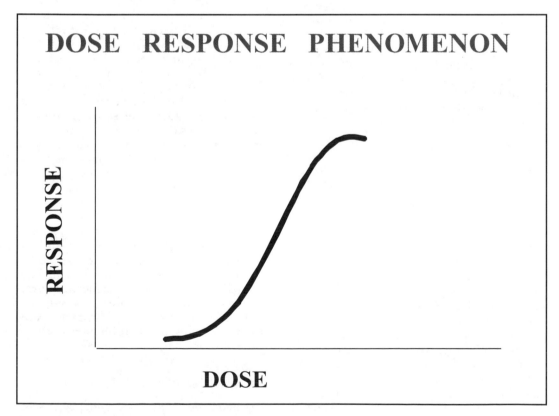

Figure 4–7. Dose response phenomenon.

exposure (to reduce acute and long-term complications) while reducing the margin around the tumor. The initial field is carried to a baseline dose of 44 Gy, at which time the spinal cord is excluded from the field and the posterior cervical lymph nodes treated with electrons of 6–12 meV energy. The electrons spare the spinal cord because of the steep falloff on dose of the electron beam. The appropriate electron energy is chosen based on the neck thickness and the distance from the skin to the spinal cord as determined from a radiograph. Precision is necessary to avoid overlapping of the upper oropharyngeal–upper neck field and the anterior bilateral supraclavicular field. This is accomplished by using appropriate shielding of the divergence of the beam from the upper fields, using a halfbeam block or independent jaw blocking, technical refinements designed to block the divergence of the radiation beam. Alternatively, a change in the location of the junction of the upper oropharyngeal–upper cervical fields and supraclavicular fields is done at set interval doses to prevent creation of a cold or hot spot. A great deal of quality assurance is required to ensure reliability of the physical dose parameters, with monitoring of critical organ dose frequently done (spinal cord, optic chiasm).

Acute Reaction

The normal acute tissue reaction will follow a dose response phenomenon. Taste alteration frequently will occur early, and rarely, acute short-lived sialoadenitis may occur. Acute-reacting tissues, including skin and mucosa, will demonstrate erythema at 20 Gy, patchy dry dermatitis and mucositis at 30–40 Gy, and frequently confluent mucositis beyond 50 Gy.

Dietary management is important. Patients are counseled to avoid acid foods, sharp-edged foods, and hot or cold liquids. Maintenance of a daily caloric count and fluid intake with daily weight recording is essential. The use of multiple small feedings is encouraged. Pain frequently accompanies mucositis and requires active pain

management with oxycodone slow release, 10–20 mg every 12 hr, supplemented by short-acting oxycodone with acetaminophen liquid (Roxicet), 1 teaspoon every 4 hr, for breakthrough pain. Analgesic dose escalation or stronger analgesic fentanyl (Duragesic), 25–75 μg/hr transdermally, is sometimes required. Adequate attention to the anticipated side effects of analgesic medication is given by ensuring adequate fluid intake and increase in fiber and encouraging exercise (to prevent constipation). A stool softener is frequently prescribed. Hoarseness will frequently be present. Dermatitis may also occur with doses of 40 Gy or greater.

Coincident with the onset of mucositis and dermatitis, there is a decrease in salivary flow, particularly the serous component, resulting in a ropy feeling and difficulty swallowing. Patients will frequently complain of waking up in the morning and experiencing difficulty expectorating their phlegm. The tenaciousness and scantiness of the saliva cause pooling in the recesses of the head and neck region (i.e., piriform sinus, vallecula). Encouragement is given to these patients to frequently gargle and rinse their mouth and throat with a baking saline solution (1 quart water with 1 teaspoon salt and 1 teaspoon baking soda). Close monitoring of the nutritional status of the patient is necessary to forestall acute dehydration and nutritional depletion. A weight loss of greater than 10% of baseline is the usual indication for insertion of a percutaneous endoscoic gastrostomy (PEG) tube for nutritional repletion. The management of these complex patients requires the active participation of a multidisciplinary team including radiation oncologist, radiation therapist, radiation oncology nurse, dietitian, social worker, and speech-language pathologist in addition to the medical physicist and dosimetrist. Emotional support and close communication with major caregivers at home are established early in order to facilitate the management.

Subacute Reaction

The acute dermatitis will typically resolve in 2–3 weeks and the oropharyngeal mucositis in 4 weeks. Return of taste function may be delayed for up to 12 weeks. Perhaps most annoying to patients is the persistence of xerostomia, which will frequently interfere with swallowing function. A therapeutic trial of pilocarpine (Salagen) to reduce xerostomia is initiated within a month of completion of radiation therapy. Dose escalation is done to achieve maximum response (initial 5 mg three or four times a day to 10 mg three or four times a day). Swallowing dysfunction during this period (1–3 months follow-up) should be vigorously evaluated by cookie swallow to exclude a rare case of cervical esophageal stricture (Figure 4–8). These strictures respond well to dilatation. The strictures may be due in part to the agglutination of mucosal surfaces in the upper cervical esophageal region related to prolonged mucositis. Mucosal adhesions are found frequently in gynecologic patients receiving high-dose external radiation therapy and uterovaginal brachytherapy (typically for

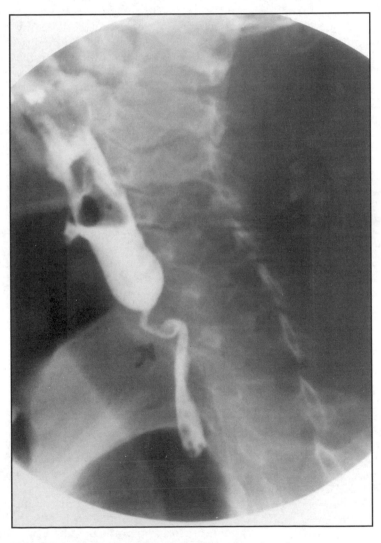

Figure 4–8. Cervical esophageal stricture.

cervical carcinoma) leading to vaginal synechia requiring vaginal dilatation (two to three times weekly for 1 or 2 years for prevention). In addition to monitoring tumor response, the radiation oncologist closely examines mucosal surfaces to look for areas of breakdown indicative of soft tissue necrosis (STN). STNs found in the tongue frequently cause pain and interfere with mastication and swallowing. The STNs are located frequently in areas of high dose and are commonly seen following interstitial implantation using iridium 192. Conservative management—including analgesic, dietary modification, oral hygiene, cessation of smoking/ethanol use, and a great deal of patience—leads to healing. Great judgment must be exercised to exclude the possibility of tumor persistence/recurrence, which can mimic this clinical situation and can only be excluded by means of a biopsy. If there is a lack of response to conservative management, hyperbaric oxygen therapy is used with great success.

An occasional patient will develop a Lhermitte's sign within the first few months posttherapy. This interesting but annoying clinical phenomenon manifests itself with shooting electriclike pains down the back, precipitated by flexion of the neck. This transient myelopathy of the cervical spinal cord is a self-limited neurological entity not unique to radiation therapy and has also been caused by trauma and, in the past, by syphilitic involvement of the spinal cord. This symptom abates within a few weeks or months and is not a harbinger of the serious radiation induced myelopathy with delayed onset (6–24 months) that leads to severe neurological deficits including quadriparesis, sensory loss, and sphincter loss of the bladder/rectum.

Chronic Reaction

The patient is followed jointly with the referring ear, nose, and throat specialist or surgical oncologist. The persistence of xerostomia requires careful management by the radiation oncologist and supportive care. The patient will report to the physician dietary restrictions (e.g., solids, peanut butter, and sandwich). The patient will almost always carry a small water bottle to moisten the mouth and throat and will liberally wash down food with water. A good strategy is to recommend using a chicken broth prior to each meal to "lubricate" the mucosa to facilitate swallowing. Continued collaboration with the dentist is essential in order to maintain dental hygiene. The radiation oncologist will confirm the persistent use of fluoride under the tutelage of the dentist and will confirm the continuity of dental surveillance. A good line of communication, preferably documented in written communications, helps the management of the patient. Likewise, any restorative dental work during the first 2 to 3 years postradiation therapy requires cross-consultation with the radiation oncologist. Any planned dental extraction must be avoided during this period because this potentially introduces bacteria into a partially devitalized mandible or maxilla, leading to nonhealing and osteoradionecrosis. Restorative work can be done during this period using root canal. Dental extractions done beyond this period should be done with caution if the site is the area of high-dose radiation (greater than 45 Gy). The use of hyperbaric oxygen therapy before and after dental extraction has been extremely useful in preventing episodes of osteoradionecrosis during the first year posttherapy and is considered useful beyond this period as well. Additionally, hyperbaric oxygen therapy is used in the treatment of osteoradionecrosis refractory to intraoral sequestrectomy. For cases refractory to hyperbaric oxygen therapy, surgical resection of the diseased portion of the bone is done. The most troublesome period of xerostomia is the first 2 years. Ultimately, patients adjust remarkably well and compensate well.

The apices of the lung are frequently included in the supraclavicular fields (designed to treat occult disease). Rarely will functional abnormalities or clinical pneumonitis ensue. Radiographs of the chest will frequently reveal fibrotic streaks a few months posttherapy, which are of little clinical importance.

Radiation-induced cervical myelopathy and cerebral injuries are late events of radiation injury. Luckily, these complications are rare because of the attention given to their prevention by the radiation oncologist. However, certain clinical situations mandate "pushing" the dose to the spinal cord beyond the conventional commonly accepted threshold dose (45 Gy/25 fractions or 50 Gy using twice-a-day regimen of 1.1 to 1.2 Gy/fraction). In the case where the tumor hugs the spinal column and achieving a satisfactory total dose of 70–76 Gy is required, the radiation oncologist will push the dose to the spinal cord to 55 Gy with careful planning. Because most myelopathies occur at greater than 60 Gy (1.8–2.0 Gy/fraction for 6 weeks), this calculated strategy is used only in an unusual case. Cerebral injuries are frequently avoided by careful attention to planning the delivery of the treatment. However, certain sites such as paranasal sinuses that abut the brain require substantial doses of radiation (greater than 55 Gy/33 fractions) to be delivered to a small portion of the brain and to the orbit. Radiation-induced injury to the brain is rare but retinopathy and optic nerve injury are not infrequent when the orbital contents are treated due to tumor extension. The optic lens is extremely sensitive to low doses (less than 2–5 Gy), leading to lens opacification (cataract), which is surgically correctable.

Combined Surgery and Radiation Therapy

A number of therapeutic strategies are used in the management of patients with locally advanced head and neck carcinoma. The current use of initial surgery followed by postoperative radiation therapy is well established. Debulking gross tumor surgically typically is accomplished by the use of a composite resection of the oral cavity/pharynx tumor or laryngopharyngectomy combined with ipsilateral neck dissection. Radiation therapy (typically delivered to total doses of 60 Gy at 2.0 Gy/fraction for 6 weeks) is used to treat occult microscopic residual disease in the primary tumor bed and necks. Significant reductions in locoregional recurrence and improvements in survival result from this combined approach (Lundahl et al., 1998).

Combined Radiation Therapy and Chemotherapy

The use of concurrent chemotherapy and altered fractionation in the radiotherapeutic management of head and neck carcinoma is currently undergoing investigation. This intensification of treatment has led to an increased and prolonged acute mucositis and increased dermatitis. Added vigilance is required in the management of pain and the resultant nutritional depletion in these patients. Potential myelosuppression with the risk of leukopenic fever and sepsis leading to death must be diagnosed early and treated aggressively with antibiotic and granulocyte colony-stimulating factor to increase circulating blood leukocytes. The University of Miami has conducted a number of combined concurrent radiation therapy-chemotherapy trials since 1988 (Abitbol et al., 1992, 1997). The patient noted above was treated in a combined twice-a-day regimen of radiation therapy (total dose 74.4 Gy; 1.2 Gy/fraction; 43-day duration) and concurrent chemotherapy (three cycles of constant-infusion 5-fluorouracil 750 mg/m^2 per day for 3 days; cisplatin 50 mg/m^2 per day; paclitaxel 70 mg/m^2 per day; A-2 protocol), which achieved control of the tumor (see computed tomography [CT] scans in Figures 9A and 9B). As expected, the patient developed severe and prolonged mucositis of 3.6 months duration. Her current swallowing function is excellent and aside from slight xerostomia is fully functional, and she is free of cancer at 1-year follow-up. The University of Miami is currently initiating the A-3 trial that uses hyperfractionated radiation therapy with constant-infusion 5-fluorouracil, cisplatin, and paclitaxel in combination with amifostine, a radiochemoprotector (Yuhas, Spellman, & Culo, 1980). This interesting compound has the potential for sparing the

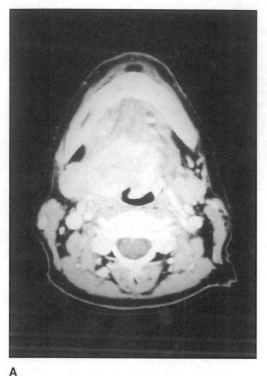

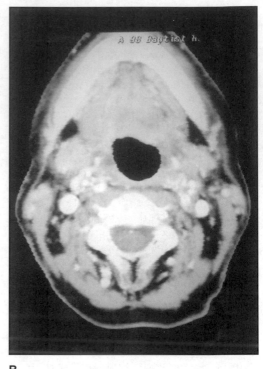

A

B

Figure 4–9. CT scan of patient with base of tongue carcinoma T4 N0 M0. **(A)** Pretreatment. **(B)** 4 months posttreatment.

mucosa, skin, salivary gland, and myelo-suppresive effects of radiation therapy and chemotherapy.

CONCLUSION

It is beyond the scope of this chapter to discuss in detail each anatomic region of the body. Suffice it to say that radiation oncology has evolved from a nascent empirical clinical field to a more scientifically based specialty. Although radiation therapy is a highly technical field, it is an intensely clinical field of medicine and an integral part of the multidisciplinary management of malignant tumors.

REFERENCES

Abitbol, A. A., Schwade, J. G., Lewin, A. A., Sridhar, K., Brandon, A. H., Markoe, A. M., et al. (1992). Hyperfractionated radiation therapy and concurrent 5-fluorouracil, cisplatin and mitomycin C in head and neck carcinoma. *American Journal of Clinical Oncology, 15,* 250–255.

Abitbol, A. A., Sridhar, K. S., Lewin, A. A., et al. (1997). Hyperfractionated radiation therapy and 5-fluorouracil, cisplatin, mitomycin-C (+/- granulocyte-colony stimulating factor) in the treatment of patients with locally advanced head and neck carcinoma. *Cancer, 80,* 266–276.

Ang, K. K., & Peters, L. J. (1994). Altered fractionation in radiation oncology. In V. T. DeVita, Jr., S. Hellman, & S. A. Rosenberg (Eds.), *Principles & practice of oncology PPO updates.* Vol. 8, No. 4 (p. 1) Philadelphia: J. B. Lippincott.

Beahrs, O. H., & Henson, D. E. (1989). *American Joint Committee on Cancer manual for staging of cancer* (3rd ed.). Philadelphia: J.B. Lippincott.

Dewey, W. C., Ling, C. C., & Meyn, R.E. (1995). Radiation-induced apoptosis: Relevance to radiotherapy. *International Journal of Radiation Oncology, Biology, Physics, 33*, 781.

Elkind, M. M., & Sutton, H. (1960). Radiation response of mammalian cells grown in culture: I. Repair of x-ray damage in surviving Chinese hamster cells. *Radiation Research, 13*, 556–593.

Elkind, M. M., Sutton-Gilbert, H., Moses, W. B. et al. (1965). Radiation response of mammalian cells in culture: V. Temperature dependence of the repair of xray damage in surviving cells (aerobic and hypoxic). *Radiation Research, 25*, 359–376.

Flam, M. S., John, M., Pajak, T., et al. (1995). Radiation (RT) and 5-fluorouracil (5FU) vs. radiation, 5FU, mitomycin-C (MMC) in the treatment of anal carcinoma: Results of a phase III randomized RTOG/ECOG intergroup trial [Abstract]. *Proceedings of the American Society of Clinical Oncology, 14*, 191.

Fowler, J. F. (1992). Brief summary of radiobiological principles in fractionated radiotherapy. *Seminars in Radiation Oncology, 2*, 16.

Fu, K. K. (1993). Integration of chemotherapy and radiotherapy for organ preservation in head and neck cancer. In J. T. Johnson & M. S. Dikolkar (Eds.), *Head and neck cancer* (Vol. 3, p. 17). New York: Elsevier Science.

Garden, A. S., Morrison, W. H., Ang, K. K., & Peters, L. J. (1995). Hyperfractionated radiation in the treatment of squamous cell carcinomas of the head and neck: A comparison of two fractionation schedules. *International Journal of Radiation Oncology, Biology, Physics, 31*, 493.

Gray, L. H., Conger, A. D., Ebert, M., et al. (1953). The concentration of oxygen dissolved in tissues at the time of irradiation as a factor in radiotherapy. *British Journal of Radiology, 26*, 638–654.

Hall, E. J. (1994). *Radiobiology for the radiologist* (pp. 2–13). Philadelphia: J. B. Lippincott.

Johns, H. E., & Cunningham, J. R. (1969). *The physics of radiology*. Springfield, IL: Charles C. Thomas.

Lundahl, R. E., Foote, R. L., Bonner, J.A., et al. (1998). Combined neck dissection and postoperative radiation therapy in the management of high-risk neck: A matched pair analysis. *International Journal of Radiation Oncology, Biology, Physics, 40*, 529–534.

Peters, L. J., Ang, K. K., Thames, H. D., Jr. (1988). Accelerated fractionation in the radiation treatment of head and neck cancer: A critical comparison of different strategies. *Acta Oncologica, 27*, 185.

Rubin, R., & Casaret, G. W. (1968). *Clinical radiation pathology*. Vol. 1. Philadelphia: W. B. Saunders.

Sartorelli, A. C. (1988). Therapeutic attack of hypoxic cells of solid tumors. *Cancer Research, 48*, 775.

Schwade, J. G., Markoe, A. M., Abitbol, A. A., et al. (1992). Accelerating hyperfractionation for carcinoma of the head and neck. *Seminars in Radiation Oncology, 2*, 51.

Van den Bogaert, W., Horiot, J.-C., & van der Schueren, E. (1989). Radiotherapy with multiple fractions per day. In G. G. Steel, G. E. Adams, & A. Horwich (Eds.), *The biologic basis of radiotherapy* (2nd ed., p. 209). New York: Elsevier Science.

Vokes, E. E., & Weichselbaum, R. R. (1990). Concomitant chemoradiotherapy: Rationale and clinical experience in patients with solid tumors. *Journal of Clinical Oncology, 8*, 911.

Withers, H. R. (1985). Biologic basis for altered fractionation schemes. *Cancer, 55*(Suppl. 9), 2086–2095.

Withers, H. R., Taylor, J. M. G., & Maciejewski, B. (1988). The hazard of accelerated tumor clonogen repopulation during radiotherapy. *Acta Oncologica, 27*, 131–146.

Yuhas, J. M., Spellman, J. M., & Culo, F. (1980). The role of WR-2721 in radiotherapy and/or chemotherapy. *Cancer Clinical Trials, 3*, 211–216.

5

Primary Brain Tumors

Joy E. Gaziano, M.A., CCC-SLP, and Rakesh Kumar, M.D.

Diagnosis and management of brain tumors present unique challenges for the medical team. Although primary brain tumors represent only 2% of all malignancies, they are a major cause of death and disability. They significantly affect physical performance and quality of life. Services must be provided that address not only the medical but also the physical, psychological, social, spiritual, and educational needs of patients. Interventions span all phases of the disease. Therefore, multidisciplinary management is critical to promote optimal outcomes at each phase.

Patient survival is being extended with advances in neuroimaging, neurosurgery, radiation therapy, and chemotherapy. Consequently, rehabilitative strategies that enhance the quality of that survival are desirable.

CLINICAL PRESENTATIONS

Brain tumors have a wide range of clinical presentations. However, there are some common clinical symptoms that may be indicative of a brain tumor. A headache is a common initial presenting symptom. Headaches associated with brain tumors usually present in the morning and resolve as the day progresses. The location of headaches in the adult population does not correlate with the specific site in the brain. They are often bilateral and are due to stretching of the pain-sensitive fibers located within the dura covering. The headaches are moderate in severity, intermittent, and exacerbated by Valsalva-like maneuvers such as bending, stooping, or coughing. Vomiting usually accompanies headaches and is related to increased intracranial pressure.

Seizures are another frequent symptom of brain tumors. The onset of a seizure in a patient over the age of 25 without a previous history of seizures immediately raises the possibility of the diagnosis of a brain tumor. An estimated 50% of patients experience seizures during the course of their illness. They are second in frequency to headaches as a presenting symptom of patients with brain tumors. Seizures are more likely to occur when the tumor arises in the frontoparietal region or temporal lobe (Harsh & Wilson, 1990). Anticonvulsant drugs used to control seizures include phenytoin (Dilantin), phenobarbital, and carbamazepine (Tegretol).

Changes in mental status may be another hallmark of a brain tumor. Deficits in memory, concentration and attention, alertness, reasoning and judgment, behavior, and personality may be evident. The patient also can show somnolence, dullness, loss of attentiveness and mental agility (abulia), emotional lability, or irritability

(Harsh & Wilson, 1990). Decreased level of consciousness is noted in up to 40% of all elderly patients with brain tumor. Speech and language deficits may also appear. Nausea and vomiting are frequent clinical manifestations as well. Often, changes in vision, including blurred or double vision or a field cut, may be a patient complaint.

Although dysphagia is rarely a presenting feature of a brain tumor, swallowing problems may exist, either directly related to brainstem or lower cranial nerve tumors or distortion, or indirectly due to vomiting and aspiration or depressed level of consciousness. Tumors infiltrating or compressing the brainstem could affect the corticobulbar tracts or medullary center and produce dysphagia. Patients with large, unilateral diffuse supratentorial tumors frequently present with swallowing problems. In these patients, the decreased level of consciousness and contralateral weakness of the face and tongue contribute to the swallowing deficit. Patients with primary brain tumors with dysphagia are likely to have impairment of swallowing out of proportion to their complaints and are therefore at risk for aspiration and nutritional compromise (Newton, Junck, Bromberg, Page, & Greenberg, 1994).

These general symptoms associated with brain tumors are usually a result of increased intracranial pressure. As a tumor grows within the skull, it causes a mass effect that may damage brain tissue by compressing and displacing it. Intracranial pressure can damage tissue in several ways. The tumor itself may press on the brain. Or it may compress the ventricles that provide fluid flow through the brain, called hydrocephalus. Finally, the brain may swell around the tumor as a result of fluid accumulation around the tumor.

These symptoms are general and nonspecific and may occur in patients with brain tumors at any site. Other site-specific clinical manifestations of brain tumors may also occur. The clinical presentation is dependent on the site of lesion and the tumor's effect on that and surrounding brain structures.

SITE-SPECIFIC DEFICITS

Tumors in the prefrontal area affect intellect, attention, problem solving, and judgment. Apathy, abulia, emotional lability, as well as impulsiveness and loss of social inhibition can be present. Motor aphasia is a result of neoplasia involving Broca's area, located in the opercular and triangular portions of the inferior frontal gyrus of the dominant hemisphere. Lesions damaging the precentral gyrus result in a contralateral hemiparesis.

Tumors in the temporal lobes can induce impairment of hearing, speech, equilibrium, vision, behavior, and movement. Tumors in the posterior part of the superior temporal gyrus lead to receptive aphasia (Wernicke's aphasia).

The parietal lobe receives and interprets sensations such as pain, temperature, pressure, and shapes. Lesions in the parietal lobe impair spatial awareness such as body orientation in space or body part recognition. Stereognosis and graphesthesia will be altered on the contralateral side. Lesions in the superior parietal lobule cause asomatognosia. The parietal lobe also controls hearing, reasoning, and memory functions. Speech and graphic disturbances may occur if the tumor is in the dominant hemisphere. Tumors in the dominant supramarginal gyrus produce conduction aphasia and ideomotor apraxia. Tumors located in the angular gyrus result in alexia and Gerstmann's syndrome of agraphia, acalculia, finger agnosia in both hands, and confusion of right and left. Tumors involving the occipital lobes characteristically impair vision. Table 5–1 lists deficits that occur as a result of brain tumors at specific locations.

TUMOR CLASSIFICATION

Gliomas are the most common type of brain tumor, accounting for approximately one half of all brain neoplasms. *Glioma* is a general term for tumors that arise from glial or neuroepithelial (supportive) tissue in the brain. They are classified into several groups according to the type of glial cell involved.

Table 5–1. Chart of Deficits

Tumor Location	Symptoms
Acoustic	Tinnitus Dizziness Hearing loss Loss of facial sensation Ipsilateral facial weakness Symptoms similar to brainstem tumor
Brainstem	Change in blood pressure, heartbeat, respiration Altered consciousness, sleeping patterns Vomiting Contralateral facial weakness Contralateral limb weakness, ataxia Dysphagia Dysarthria Vision impairment Headache
Cerebellum–posterior fossa	Headache Nausea and vomiting Ataxic gait Dizziness Ataxic dysarthria
Corpus callosum	Impaired judgment/memory in anterior corpus callosum Behavioral changes in posterior corpus callosum Tumor may invade other lobes with symptoms consistent with lesion in those locations
Frontal lobe	Contralateral weakness Seizures Communication deficit in dominant hemisphere Cognitive deficit in nondominant hemisphere
Hypothalamus	Thirst, urination, sleep, homeostasis, appetite, emotions
Occipital lobe	Blindness Visual neglect Alexia Seizures
Parietal lobe	Altered pain, temperature, pressure Decreased body awareness, spatial disorders, sensation Hearing changes Memory and reasoning Communication deficit in dominant hemisphere Object recognition
Temporal lobe	Memory loss Emotional disturbances Seizures Communication deficits Vision changes
Thalamus	Contralateral sensory loss, weakness Decreased cognition, speech, headache, nausea/vomiting Decreased urinary control Gait disturbances

Astrocytoma, the most common glioma, arises from star-shaped glial cells called astrocytes. They are graded I to IV according to degree of malignancy. Grades I and II astrocytomas, also called low-grade or well-differentiated astrocytomas, are the least malignant and may be slow growing. Grade III astrocytoma, also called midgrade or anaplastic astrocytoma, grows more rapidly and contains some malignant traits. Grade IV astrocytoma, also called high-grade or glioblastoma multiforme, grows rapidly, invades nearby tissue, and contains highly malignant cells.

DIAGNOSIS OF BRAIN TUMORS

Computed tomography (CT) and magnetic resonance imaging (MRI) should be obtained in all patients suspected of having a brain tumor. These studies allow detection of the precise location of the tumor and establish the relationship with the normal anatomy. Functional MRI is a newer technology that shows promise in tumor detection. Angiography and magnetic resonance angiography are used to identify the presence of blood vessels in the brain. They are used primarily in patients with brain tumors for planning surgery for tumors suspected of having a large blood supply. Positron emission tomography (PET) is used to evaluate cerebral blood flow, glucose metabolism, and the blood-brain barrier using a radioactive material bound to glucose and injected into the patient. As the brain converts glucose into energy, malignant tumors are identified because they consume glucose at a higher rate than normal brain tissue. Single photon emission computed tomography (SPECT) is similar to PET and may be used to distinguish between recurrent brain tumors and radiation necrosis, and it differentiates high- and low-grade tumors.

MANAGEMENT

Optimum therapy for a patient with a malignant brain tumor is trimodal: a combination of surgery, radiation therapy, and chemotherapy. Symptomatic treatment with steroids is begun at diagnosis to reduce edema in the brain surrounding the tumor. Dexamethasone (Decadron) and prednisone are commonly prescribed. Common side effects include weight gain due to water retention, increased appetite, mood changes, irritability, depression, and sleeplessness. Because steroids reduce brain swelling, they frequently improve brain functioning. Steroid use should not be stopped suddenly; rather it should be tapered slowly to reduce reemergence of symptoms. Histamine H2 receptor antagonists such as ranitidine (Zantac) or famotidine (Pepsid) are given concurrently to prevent peptic ulceration that may be induced by high doses of steroids.

Surgery

In most patients with malignant astrocytomas, a craniotomy should be performed with the goal of removing as much tumor as possible with minimal neurological deficit. There is consistent evidence in the literature that indicates the direct association between the extent of tumor resection and the length of survival (Salcman, 1985). Gross total tumor resection along with age, histology, and neurology status (Karnofsky performance score) have been identified as important prognostic factors (Medical Research Council Brain Tumor Working Party, 1990). The surgical resection of a tumor offers several advantages: (a) surgical decompression decreases the intracranial pressure and may improve the neurological function; (b) tumor removal reduces the number of cells potentially resistant to radiation or chemotherapy; and (c) surgical removal provides a wide tissue sampling for histological diagnosis in order to select the optimal adjuvant therapy and accurately estimate the prognosis.

During tumor dissection it is necessary to define the tumor location and boundaries. For cortical lesions, tumor identification is straightforward, but the localization of subcortical tumors can require the use of ultrasound or other image-guidance devices. The cortical incision should avoid damage to "eloquent areas" (e.g, the precentral gyrus, postcentral gyrus, and calcarine gyri bilaterally; the dominant posterior inferior frontal gyrus, posterior superior temporal gyrus, and inferior parietal lobule; and the nondominant superior parietal lobule and the vessels that supply these areas).

Intraoperative cortical mapping for motor and speech areas provides guidance to minimize postoperative deficits in tumors involving or adjacent to eloquent areas. The mapping is performed during craniotomy under local anesthesia and has made possible the safe resection of tumors previously considered inoperable (Black, Levine, Paling, & Cantrell, 1987). Another technique, electrocorticography, identifies any epileptogenic area in brain adjacent to the tumor. Resecting this area along with the tumor provides maximal tumor control (Berger & Ojemann, 1992). The incorporation of the surgical microscope that guarantees adequate magnification and illumination and the development of microsurgical instrumentation have greatly facilitated the removal of malignant brain tumors.

Emerging technologies to navigate the brain are available for the resection of brain tumors. These techniques not only allow precise localization but also become an interactive guidance system that tracks the position of the instruments during surgery and displays this position in the preoperatively obtained images in real time. Real time MRI permits MRI guidance during surgery to verify the amount of tumor removal. Stereotactic navigational systems use a hand-held wand that, when touched to the brain, transmits three-dimensional coordinates showing the precise location of the tumor. The application of these techniques results in a greater consistency in achieving adequate visualization and in accurately defining the extent of tumor resections (Maciunas, Berger, & Copeland, 1996). Selectively resecting "hot spots," areas of tumor suspected of being a higher grade, separately from the large tumor bulk aids in diagnosing a high-grade tumor within an otherwise low-grade tumor. This is important, as the patient's prognosis is dependent on detection of the highest grade of the tumor present.

Radiation

Conventional external beam radiation is a nonsurgical means of shrinking or controlling tumor growth. Radiation to the brain may be used to provide a cure, to prevent tumor metastasis to the brain, or to control symptoms. Many patients experience few or no side effects. Others experience temporary effects, including hair loss and skin discoloration in the radiation field, inflammation of the ear, edema, nausea, fatigue, or reduced appetite.

Some delayed reactions may also occur that may affect communication or swallowing functions. Several weeks after completion of radiation, an increase in preexisting conditions may present due to a temporary disruption in the myelin formation or a buildup of necrotic debris with associated edema. Radiation necrosis, death of brain tissue due to late effects of radiation on blood vessels, may be a late effect of treatment months or years posttreatment. Deficits may include decreased cognitive functioning or alteration in normal functioning in the radiated area.

Following surgery, radiation remains the single most effective treatment for malignant astrocytoma (Hochberg & Pruit, 1980). The value of postoperative radiation was conclusively established by the multicenter randomized trial of the Brain Tumor Study Group. The median survival of patients receiving surgery alone was 17 weeks in comparison to 37.5 weeks for those undergoing surgery plus radiation (Chang et al., 1983). The recommendation for standard postoperative treatment of a patient with a malignant glioma is focal radiation to a dose of 6,000 rads given in divided doses, called fractions, over a 5- to 6-week period, five times per week (Levin et al., 1979).

Brachytherapy represents a method by which high doses of radiation can be delivered to the target with relative sparing of the surrounding brain. It is accomplished by implanting sources of radiation into the tumor, thus attacking from inside the body. Radioactive isotopes iridium 192 and iodine 125 pellets are placed in the tumor site using CT- and MRI-directed stereotactic surgical techniques. Brachytherapy is considered particularly useful in recurrent gliomas. Leibel, Gutin, and Sneed (1987) reported a median survival of 54 weeks for grade IV tumors and 81 weeks for grade III tumors from the time of recurrence. This technique also has been used as a focal boost after external beam radiation in newly diagnosed tumors.

Lately, radiosurgery has been explored in the treatment of primary brain tumors. This is a method of stereotactic treatment that delivers a high dose of radiation in single or multiple fractions to a small, well-defined target, thus reducing the amount of radiation received by normal tissue. The gamma knife, stereotactic linear accelerator, and cyclotron are machines that are used to administer the focused dose of radiation. Small malignant gliomas can be boosted using stereotactic radiosurgery after conventional external radiation, and patients with small recurrent tumors after biopsy are also candidates for this therapy (Coffey, Lunsford, & Taylor, 1988; Coffey, Lunsford, & Flinkinger, 1991; Mehta, Masciopinto, & Rozental, 1994).

Photodynamic therapy (PDT) is another treatment modality, whereby a light-sensitive drug that concentrates in tumor cells is administered during a surgical procedure. When light penetrates the tumor, the drug is activated and kills the tumor cells.

Conformal radiation, also called intensity modulated radiation therapy (IMRT), shapes the pattern of the radiation beam to the shape of the tumor. Radiation may also be delivered via monoclonal antibodies, which insert radioactive molecules into a tumor. Various drugs serve as radioprotectors that protect brain cells during radiation therapy. Radiosensitizers may make tumor cells more sensitive to radiation, and radioenhancers are designed to increase the beneficial effects of radiation without increasing the dose.

Chemotherapy

Chemotherapy is the use of chemicals to treat tumors. It acts to cause tumor cell death either immediately or as it attempts to reduplicate. Chemotherapeutic agents affect normal cells as well as tumor cells. The normal cells that may be affected include bone marrow cells that manufacture blood products, hair cells, skin cells, and cells of the oral, esophageal, gastric, and intestinal mucosa. Common side effects include hair loss, nausea, vomiting, reduced appetite, anemia, mouth sores, skin reactions, and decreased resistance to infection. Some chemotherapy agents such as cisplatin can be ototoxic. Side effects are drug specific and are generally reversible after treatment is completed.

The use of cytotoxic drugs is now an established modality in the treatment of brain tumors. Chemotherapy has proved to prolong survival in anaplastic astrocytomas, but glioblastoma multiforme tends to be more chemoresistant. Carmustine (BCNU) and lomustine (CCNU) have been the standard drugs used for brain tumors.

A new route of drug delivery, using surgical implantation of BCNU-impregnated wafers, is promising. These wafers are biodegradable BCNU that can be directly implanted into the brain, producing high local brain concentration of BCNU for approximately 2 or 3 weeks. The wafers are currently approved by the Food and Drug Administration for human use in recurrent malignant gliomas and are implanted in the tumor cavity at the time of surgery. The wafers have been shown to prolong survival of patients with recurrent malignant gliomas and reduce the systemic toxicity that traditional routes of chemotherapy may cause (Levin et al., 1990).

Ongoing clinical trials are evaluating new agents for the treatment of brain tumors. They include procarbazine, carboplatin, and vincristine, and are used alone or in combination. PVC (a combination of procarbazine, lomustine, and vincristine) is used in clinical trials for oligodendroglioma and malignant astrocytoma. Temozolomide is a lower toxicity oral chemotherapy also being tested for malignant astrocytoma, and CPT-11 is being tested in gliomas.

In other drug delivery research, new developments are occurring in transmission of chemotherapy drugs to tumor sites through the bloodstream. Receptor-mediated permeabilizers (RMP-7) are being investigated as a way of opening the blood-brain barrier to allow more chemotherapy to permeate the brain. Phenylburerate and phenylacetate are promising as compounds that may return tumor cells to more normal behavior. All of these chemotherapies are available in clinical trials.

A great deal of research is being conducted on biological response modifiers, which alter the growth patterns of tumor cells. Drugs that impede angiogenesis (the development of new blood vessels) are being tested to control the growth of new blood vessels around tumors. Angiogenesis inhibitors currently being tested include Angiostatin, Endostatin, Suramin, and Squalamine.

Gene therapy is another promising area of brain tumor investigation; genes that are known to be sensitive to certain drugs are transferred into a tumor, after which the drug is administered in attempt to destroy the sensitized tumor. Other research focuses on the use of viruses to deliver treatment, thus protecting new blood cells from the effects of chemotherapy. Researchers also investigate the genetic manipulation of growth factors that supply nutrients to and control reproduction of tumor cells. Brain tumor research and treatment is rapidly expanding and new management options are under investigation. However, further data is required before the long-term effectiveness of many of these treatment options is understood.

MULTIDISCIPLINARY MANAGEMENT

Successful management of patients with brain tumors requires a multidisciplinary approach. From diagnosis to recovery or death, coordinated interaction from all team members encourages efficacious treatment. Through coordinated efforts by the neurologist, neurosurgeon, radiologist, radiation oncologist, medical oncologist, and pathologist, tumor detection and staging are accomplished. Consultation by other medical specialists, including otolaryngologists, pulmonologists, gastroenterologists, and psychiatrists, may be indicated for accompanying diagnoses. Medical support is provided by oncology nurses, dietitians, and respiratory services during hospitalization and subsequent outpatient treatment. Psychosocial interventions are provided by social work, psychology, and chaplaincy and may include creative programs such as art or pet therapies. Rehabilitative services including physical, occupational, and recreational therapies; speech-language pathology; and neuropsychology provide comprehensive rehabilitation during or after medical intervention. Community services including support groups, home health services, hospice, and vocational rehabilitation play an important role in the total habilitation of the patient.

Traditionally, cancer treatment has focused on prolonging a patient's life. With the development of new surgical, radiation, and chemotherapeutic modalities, cancer patients are living longer, but the adverse effects can drastically affect patients' physical, emotional, social, and financial lives. Therefore, there has been a shift in orientation from merely survival to the quality of that survival. Comprehensive cancer rehabilitation should address all aspects of a patient's cancer experience.

Deitz (1995) has developed a goal classification system that is frequently used in cancer centers. Preventative interventions are performed when disability can be predicted and education is provided to lessen its impact. Restorative techniques are introduced that may return the patient to precancer levels of function. Supportive rehabilitation assists with compensatory strategies and adaptations to cope with functional changes resulting from cancer or its treatment. Palliative measures are designed to provide physical and emotional comfort in the presence of declining ability while maintaining independence.

Dysphagia

Dysphagia is a frequent sequela of a brain tumor and may be present in one of four patients with gliomas (McKeran & Thomas, 1980). Swallowing deficits are evident in the oral preparatory, oral, pharyngeal, or esophageal phases of swallowing (Logemann, 1986). The nature, location, and severity of the brain lesion may affect the clinical manifestation. In the oral preparatory and oral phases of swallowing, deficits may include poor lip closure, which may result in loss of material from the oral cavity and drooling. Reduced buccal tone may cause loss of material into the space between the molars and the cheek. Poor lingual control may result in inability to efficiently prepare and propel the bolus into the posterior oral cavity. A delay in the trigger of the pharyngeal response or an absent swallow reflex may result in the bolus entering the pharynx and/or larynx prior to initiation of the pharyngeal phase.

One or more components of the pharyngeal phase of swallowing may also be impaired. Reduced swallowing efficiency or aspiration may occur as a result of reduced tongue base retraction and pressures on the bolus, resulting in residue in the pharynx, unilateral or bilateral pharyngeal paresis or paralysis, reduced laryngeal elevation that interferes with pharyngeal clearance, reduced anterior movement of the larynx that may limit cricopharyngeal sphincter relaxation and increase stasis in the pyriform sinuses, and reduced laryngeal closure that may encourage tracheal aspiration.

Esophageal phase dysphagia, although less common in patients with brain tumors than oropharyngeal dysphagia, has been reported in a case of central nervous system lymphoma (Benjamin, Eisold, Gerhardt, & Castell, 1982). Neuromotor disorders of the esophagus resulting from brain neoplasm are usually affected by neural disruption to the skeletal muscles of the cervical or proximal one third of the esophagus, which is under central nervous sytem control. Symptoms of esophageal dysphagia may include food sticking in the chest, heartburn, or regurgitation (Di Palma & Myers, 1987).

Evaluation of Dysphagia

Primary brain tumors cause oropharyngeal dysphagia more commonly than has been previously recognized (Newton, 1994). Additionally, patients are likely to have deficits out of proportion to their complaints, so they are at risk for aspiration and nutritional compromise. Therefore, a comprehensive evaluation is critical for dysphagia management.

Initial clinical assessment includes a complete review of medical history including tumor grade and type, location, treatment received to date, medications, results of neurological and other specialty evaluations, and patient complaints. Diet history, use of supplemental and nonoral feeding options, laboratory results, physical status, and cognitive status should be reviewed. Consultation with nursing and other support staff as well as family members can identify other factors that may affect potential for oral intake.

A thorough oromotor and cranial nerve assessment is conducted to determine rate, range of motion, and speed of voluntary and involuntary movements of the lips, tongue, palate, and pharynx and of respiration. An orosensory assessment is useful in determining presence of abnormal reflexes, awareness of stimuli such as varied temperature, taste, and texture, and elicitation of normal oral movements with the application of specific therapeutic stimuli. Clinical evaluation of laryngeal function may be accomplished by perceptually assessing voice quality. A wet, gurgly voice may indicate aspiration of secretions, liquids, or solids that penetrate the vocal folds (Linden & Siebens, 1983). Presence and strength of a reflexive and volitional cough should also be assessed. Otolaryngological evaluation, including videostroboscopy, should also be considered if laryngeal involvement is suspected.

Clinical assessment of the swallow is warranted before a physiological evaluation is administered. Using graduated amounts of varying food textures, useful clinical information is gained that assists in determining readiness for an instrumental swallow assessment and in treatment planning.

Because of the high incidence of silent aspiration in patients with neurogenic dysphagia and brain tumor patients' poor self-awareness of severity of swallowing deficits (Newton, 1994), instrumental assessment is important for accurate diagnosis and management. Instrumental assessments such as the modified barium swallow, fiberoptic endoscopic evaluation of swallowing, and ultrasound swallowing evaluation may be completed. The evaluation not only documents swallowing anatomy and physiology, but also serves as a baseline measure of swallow functions and an efficacy trial in developing appropriate treatment strategies.

Management Issues

Unique challenges exist in the management of dysphagia in patients with brain tumors. The progressive nature of many tumors, combined with the effects of multiple medical regimens, requires the clinician to reevaluate the traditional model of dysphagia rehabilitation. For many patients the goal is not long-term improvement in functional abilities. Rather, the maintenance of safe and adequate function in the presence of declining health is a reasonable outcome.

Clinicians work as part of a multidisciplinary team to evaluate function, make treatment recommendations, and implement a treatment plan. However, faced with limited potential for functional gains, clinicians are frequently asked to justify to the physicians and payers the need for costly services. Evaluation identifies the physiological deficits that cause dysphagia and determines strategies that maximize swallowing efficiency and minimize aspiration risk. Intervention by the speech-language pathologist allows for patient and family education regarding swallowing prognosis, safety of oral intake, nonoral feeding options, and emotional support.

Indirect therapy techniques may be introduced and include exercises to improve movements required for swallowing such as range of motion or strengthening exercises. Direct therapy involves incorporation of eating and drinking activities to elicit active movements of specific muscles as in thermal tactile stimulation. Often, compensatory strategies, physical maneuvers that improve swallowing efficiency or reduce aspiration risk, are introduced successfully. Facilitating techniques that change external variables such as type of utensil, bolus size, or food temperature are used with patients with brain tumors to maintain safe oral intake.

Timing of intervention with patients with brain tumors is critical. The inability to eat is a distressing concern of many patients as they begin to lose functions that were once automatic. Patients and their families need information early in the disease in order to make appropriate decisions about their care. It is critical to time management strategies so that problems are addressed as they present, but with an eye to the future to anticipate problems that may develop.

As health and swallowing functions deteriorate, the speech-language pathologist's role is to monitor swallowing function and provide modified strategies and compensations to prolong safe and pleasurable oral intake if that is a patient preference; to assist in optimizing nutrition and hydration; to keep team members apprised of swallowing status; to participate in discussions of benefits and burdens of tube feeding; and to provide education and support to the patient and family members. Patients should be encouraged to determine their health care preferences including means of nutritional intake, through an advanced directive.

Support Groups

Many patients with brain tumors benefit from attending support groups. Support groups can provide information and education, as well as psychological support and necessary community resources to help patients and their families cope with the stresses of cancer. Support groups may help reduce a patient's anxiety while offering encouragement from other survivors. They educate patients about new treatment methods, research, and resources. They also provide patients with an extended support system outside of their family that helps to alleviate a feeling of isolation and encourages hope.

Numerous national resources exist that offer a wide range of services including referral to brain tumor support groups throughout the country, phone and computer networking, patient education materials, public awareness, professional education, research, and fund-raising. Following is a noninclusive list of organizations that advocate for issues affecting individuals with brain tumors.

The Brain Tumor Society

84 Seattle Street
Boston, MA 02134-1245
(800) 770-TBTS (8287)
(617) 783-0340
Fax: (617) 783-9712
E-mail: info@tbts.org
http://www.tbts.org

American Brain Tumor Association

2720 River Road
Des Plaines, IL 60018
(847) 827-9910
Fax: (847) 827-9918
Patient Line: (800) 886-2282
E-mail: info@abta.org
http://www.abta.org

National Brain Tumor Foundation

785 Market Street, Suite 1600
San Francisco, CA 94103
(800) 934-CURE (2873)
E-mail: nbtf@braintumor.org

Brain Tumor Foundation of Canada
formerly: Brain Research Fund
Foundation of London

111 Waterloo Street, Suite 600
London, Ontario N6B 2M4
Canada
(519) 624-7755

Brain Tumor Foundation for Children, Inc.

2231 Perimeter Park Drive, Suite 9
Atlanta, GA 30341
(404) 458-5564

Brain Tumor Society

258 Harvard Street, Suite 308
Brookline, MA 02146
(617) 433-7033

Children's Brain Tumor Foundation

35 Alpine Lane
Chappaqua, NY 10514
(914) 238-4917

Acoustic Neuroma Association

P.O. Box 12402
Atlanta, GA 30355
(404) 237-8023
Fax: (404) 237-2704
E-mail: ANAusa@aol.com
http://anausa.org

National Institute of Neurological Disorders and Stroke

P.O. Box 5801
Bethesda, MD 20824
(800) 352-9424
(301) 496-5751

National Institutes of Health/ National Cancer Institute

Building 31, Room 8A52
31 Center Drive, MSC 2540
Bethesda, MD 20892-2540
http://www.nih.gov/
http://www.ninds.nih.gov/

Cancer Information Service

(800) 4-CANCER
(800-422-6237)
TTY: (800) 332-8615
E-mail: cis@icic.nci.nih.gov
http://cancernet.nci.nih.gov

Candlelighters Childhood Cancer Foundation

7910 Woodmont Avenue, Suite 460
Bethesda, MD 20814-3015
(800) 366-2223
(301) 657-8401
Fax: (301) 718-2686
E-mail: info@candlelighters.org
http://www.candlelighters.org

National Coalition for Cancer Survivorship

1010 Wayne Avenue, Suite 505
Silver Spring, MD 20910
(301) 650-8868
Fax: (301) 565-9670
E-mail: info@cansearch.org
http://www.cansearch.org

National Epilepsy Foundation of America

4351 Garden City Drive
Landover, MD 20785
(301) 459-3700
(800) EFA-1000
Fax: (301) 577-2684
http://www.efa.org/organization/where/affil.htm

REFERENCES

Benjamin, S. B., Eisold, J., Gerhardt, D. C., & Castell, D. O. (1982). Central nervous system lymphoma presenting as dysphagia. *Digestive Diseases and Sciences, 27,* 155–160.

Berger, M. S., & Ojemann, G. A. (1992). Intraoperative brain mapping techniques in neuro-oncology. *Stereotactic and Functional Neurosurgery, 58,* 153–161.

Black, W. C., Levine, P. A., Paling, M. R., & Cantrell, R. W. (1987). MRI vs high resolution CT scanning: Evaluation of the anterior skull base. *Otolaryngology—Head and Neck Surgery, 3,* 260–267.

Chang, C. H., Horton, J., Schoenfeld, D., et al. (1983). Comparison of postoperative radiotherapy and combined postoperative radiotherapy and chemotherapy in the multidisciplinary management of malignant gliomas: A joint Radiation Therapy Oncology Group and Eastern Cooperative Oncology Group study. *Cancer, 52,* 997–1007.

Coffey, R. J., Lunsford, L. D., & Taylor, F. H. (1988). Survival after stereotactic biopsy of malignant gliomas. *Neurosurgery, 21,* 21–26.

Coffey, R. J., Lunsford, L. D., & Flinkinger, J. C. (1991). The role of radiosurgery in the treatment of malignant brain tumors. *Neurosurgery Clinics of North America, 3,* 231–244.

Deitz, S. (1995). Diagnosis and treatment of pneumonia in the nursing home. *Nurse Practioner, 20,* 35–39.

Di Palma, J., & Myers, G. (1987). A rational clinical approach to esophageal motor disorders. *Dysphagia, 2,* 97–108.

Harsh, R., & Wilson, C. B. (1990). Neuroepithelial tumors of the adult brain. In J. R. Yuoumans (Ed.), *Neurological surgery: A comprehensive reference guide to the diagnosis and management of neurosurgical problems* (3rd ed., p. 3040). Philadelphia: W. B. Saunders.

Hochberg, F. H., & Pruit, A. (1980). Assumptions in the radiotherapy of glioblastoma. *Neurology, 30,* 907–911.

Leibel, S., Gutin, P. H., & Sneed, D. (1987). Interstitial irradiation for the treatment of primary and metastatic brain tumors. *PPO Update, 13,* 1–11.

Levin, V. A., Silver, P., Hannigan, J., et al. (1990). Superiority of postradiotherapy adjuvant chemotherapy with CCNU, procarbazine, and vincristine (PCV) over BCNU for anaplastic gliomas: NCOG 6G61 final report. *International Journal of Radiation Oncology, Biology, Physics, 18,* 321–324.

Levin, V. A., Wilson, C. B., Davus, R., et al. (1979). A phase III comparison of BCNU, hydroxyurea, and radiation therapy to BCNU and radiation therapy for treatment of primary malignant gliomas. *Journal of Neurosurgery, 51,* 526–532.

Linden, P., & Seibens, A. (1983). Dysphagia: Predicting laryngeal penetration. *Archives of Physical Medicine and Rehabilitation, 64,* 281–283.

Logemann, J. (1986). *Manual for the videofluoroscopic study of swallowing* (2nd ed.). Austin, TX: PRO-ED.

Maciunas, R. J., Berger, M. S., & Copeland, B. (1996). Techniques for interactive image-guided neurosurgical intervention in primary brain tumors. *Neurosurgery Clinics of North America, 7,* 245–266.

McKeran, R. O., & Thomas, D. G. T. (1980). The clinical study of gliomas. In D. G. T. Thomas & D. I. Graham (Eds.), *Brain tumors, scientific basis, clinical investigation, and current therapy* (pp. 194–230). London: Butterworth.

Medical Research Council Brain Tumor Working Party. (1990). Prognostic factors for high-grade malignant glioma: Development of a prognostic index. *Journal of Neuro-oncology, 9,* 47–55.

Mehta, M. P., Masciopinto, J., & Rozental, J. (1994). Stereotactic radiosurgery for glioblastoma multiforme: Report of a prospective study evaluating prognostic factors and analyzing long-term survival advantage. *International Journal of Radiation Oncology, Biology, Physics, 30,* 541–549.

Newton, H. B., Junck, L., Bromberg, J., Page, M. A., & Greenberg, H. S. (1990). Procarbazine chemotherapy in the treatment of recurrent malignant astrocytoma after radiation and nitrosourea failure. *Journal of Neuro-oncology, 13,* 111–117.

Salcman, M. (1985). The morbidity and mortality of brain tumors: A perspective on recent advances in therapy. *Neurologic Clinics, 3,* 1–29.

6

Effects of Surgery for Head and Neck Cancer

Marion B. Ridley, M.D.

Treatment for malignancies of the head and neck involves one or more of the three primary modalities of cancer therapy: surgery, radiation therapy, and chemotherapy. Any one of these forms of treatment can affect a patient's ability to speak and swallow. The combination of two or all three modalities increases the likelihood that function will be impaired. For many years the standard therapy for advanced malignancies of the head and neck has been surgery and postoperative radiation therapy. Most of the recently developed organ preservation protocols for head and neck cancer use a combination of radiation therapy and chemotherapy. These organ-sparing approaches reserve surgery for those who do not achieve a complete response to radiation and chemotherapy; however, anatomic preservation of structures does not necessarily ensure functional integrity.

Depending on the structures involved, speech and swallowing function are frequently already affected at time of diagnosis of a malignancy of the head and neck. Any therapy to eradicate the disease will leave scarring and fibrosis in the area that was involved by the tumor, except in cases of very small tumors where healing may occur without significant

fibrosis. The effects of radiation are related to the structures irradiated and the dose delivered to those tissues. Structures not involved by the cancer can be shielded from the radiation beam during treatment in order to prevent unnecessary side effects; however, it is frequently not possible to shield the salivary glands when treating the oral cavity or oropharynx. Xerostomia, or dry mouth, is a common sequela of radiation for head and neck tumors. The side effects of chemotherapy are mostly acute in nature (e.g., mucositis); however, fibrosis at the site of the primary tumor frequently results from tumor cell death in response to the treatment and subsequent healing.

Surgery for cancer of the head and neck affects function in two ways: the extent of the resection and the method of reconstruction. Resection of malignant tumors of the head and neck is generally based on surgical oncologic principles of complete resection of the primary tumor with a 1- to 2-cm margin of normal mucosa and en bloc resection of involved or at-risk lymphatics (e.g., an ipsilateral neck dissection). The resulting mucosal defect can be left to heal by granulation (secondary intent), closed primarily, or reconstructed using a skin graft or a local, pedicled, or free flap. A *graft* is tissue transferred from one part of the body to another that does not have a new blood supply immediately reestablished, but must develop it over a period of days from its recipient site. A *flap* is defined as tissue transferred from one body site to another that either maintains its original blood supply (local flap or pedicled flap) or has a new blood supply established in the recipient field by microvascular anastomoses (free flap). The type of reconstruction chosen depends on the location and extent of the defect. Each of these factors may affect the functional outcome of the patient's speech and swallowing following surgery.

THE SPECTRUM OF HEAD AND NECK CANCER

The term *head and neck cancer* generally refers to carcinoma of the upper aerodigestive tract arising from a mucosal site; however, it also includes other primary sites such as the skin, the thyroid and salivary glands, and sarcomas (non-epithelial malignancies; Table 6–1). The majority of upper aerodigestive mucosal malignancies are squamous cell carcinomas and are associated with tobacco and alcohol abuse. The carcinogenic effects of tobacco on squamous mucosa and the potentiating effects of alcohol are well established. Malignancies of most mucosal sites including the oral cavity, oropharynx, larynx, and hypopharynx are associated with these risk factors. Only the relatively rare mucosal tumors of the nasal cavity, sinuses, and nasopharynx are not associated with smoking. Tobacco and alcohol are also the primary risk factors for development of esophageal and lung cancer. Nonmucosal malignancies of the head and neck (thyroid, salivary gland, sarcomas) are not related to these risk factors.

Incidence

Mucosal malignancies of the upper aerodigestive tract account for approximately 7% of all cancers (Boring, Squires, & Tong,

1991). If cancers of the thyroid, the salivary glands, and the nasopharynx are excluded, over 80% of cancers of the head and neck are squamous cell carcinoma (Berg, 1982). It is this cell type that is related to tobacco and alcohol abuse. Presently these tumors are more than twice as common in men than in women; however, this gap has been narrowing in recent years as smoking rates in women have approached those of men. Squamous cell carcinoma of the head and neck typically occurs in the 6th or 7th decade of life. This is most likely related to cumulative effects of smoking over many years. Reports in recent years have suggested an association between smoking marijuana and the occurrence of squamous cell carcinoma of the upper aerodigestive tract at a much earlier age (Endicott, Skipper, & Hernandez, 1993).

Symptoms

The symptoms of head and neck cancer are extremely variable and are referable to the structure(s) involved. Cancer of the true vocal fold causes hoarseness in the early stages of disease, whereas supraglottic or tonsillar cancers may be relatively far progressed when they become symptomatic. Head and neck cancers may not present with any symptoms related to the primary tumor at all, but may present as a neck mass denoting a metastasis to a cervical lymph node. Any persistent change in voice, difficulty swallowing, lump in the neck, pain in the mouth or throat, or mucosal bleeding may be an indication of a head and neck cancer, especially in a patient in the 50- to 70-year-old age range who smokes. These symptoms must be investigated to confirm or exclude the diagnosis of malignancy.

Diagnosis

The diagnosis of head and neck cancer is made on the basis of a microscopic examination of a biopsy specimen. Squamous cell carcinoma typically appears as a mu-

TABLE 6–1. Types of Head and Neck Malignancies and Frequent Sites of Origin

Histological Type	Site of Origin
Squamous cell carcinoma (most common)	Mucosa, skin
Mucoepidermoid carcinoma	Salivary glands
Adenoid cystic carcinoma	Salivary glands
Adenocarcinoma	Salivary glands
Acinic cell carcinoma	Salivary glands
Carcinoma ex pleomorphic adenoma	Salivary glands
Papillary carcinoma	Thyroid
Follicular carcinoma	Thyroid
Medullary carcinoma	Thyroid
Anaplastic carcinoma	Thyroid
Lymphoepithelioma	Nasopharynx, tonsils
Lymphoma	Lymph nodes, adenoids, tonsils
Extramedullary plasmacytoma	Nose, nasopharynx, sinuses
Liposarcoma	Neck, cheek, orbit
Rhabdomyosarcoma	Orbit, nasopharynx, middle ear
Fibrosarcoma	Nose, sinuses, larynx
Malignant fibrous histiocytoma	Nose, sinuses, neck
Osteosarcoma	Mandible, skull, maxilla
Leimyosarcoma	Nose, sinuses, skin
Angiosarcoma	Scalp, cheek, nose
Synovial carcinoma	Neck, hypopharynx
Mesenchymal chondrosarcoma	Maxilla, mandible, orbit
Basal cell carcinoma	Skin
Malignant melanoma	Skin, mucosa, eye
Merkel cell carcinoma	Skin
Dermatofibrosarcoma protuberans	Skin
Malignant Schwannoma	Neck
Neuroblastoma	Neck
Esthesioneuroblastoma	Nose, anterior skull base

cosal irregularity with ulceration on gross inspection. A mass is frequently palpable around and beneath the ulceration. Any suspicious area of mucosal abnormality can be biopsied either in the office using local anesthesia (oral cavity and oropharynx) or in the operating room using general anesthesia (larynx and hypopharynx). The diagnostic evaluation of a suspected head and neck cancer usually includes a *panendoscopy*, or endoscopic evaluation of the larynx, bronchi, and esophagus. The biopsy may be obtained at the time of the panendoscopy. The diagnosis of malignancy is made by the head and neck pathologist based on the microscopic characteristics of biopsy and clinical characteristics documented by the otolaryngologist–head and neck surgeon. Definitive treatment is usually not performed until the final results of the biopsy are known and treatment options are discussed by the surgeon with the patient and other members of the interdisciplinary head and neck treatment group.

Staging

Head and neck cancer is staged according to the *Manual for Staging of Cancer* of the American Joint Committee on Cancer (1992). Tumors are staged according to the size and extent of the primary tumor (T), the involvement of cervical lymphatics (N), and the presence of any distant metastases (M). Based on the site of the primary and the TNM classification, the tumor can then be assigned a *stage* of I, II, III, or IV, generally corresponding to prognosis.

Each head and neck site has a different set of criteria for establishing the T classification. In the oral cavity and oropharynx the T classification is based primarily on the size of the tumor. Tumors in these locations are generally accessible and, therefore, measurable. Tumors of the larynx, hypopharynx, and nasopharynx are less accessible and are classified according to the number of subsites involved or other factors such as fixation of the vocal fold. A small tumor of larynx that involves only one vocal fold is classified as T1 unless it is causing fixation, in which case it is automatically classified as T3. Any tumor that involves bone or cartilage or extends into the deep soft tissues of the neck is automatically assigned a T4 classification.

Involvement of the cervical lymph nodes is designated by the N classification. N0 denotes no evidence of cervical metastases. Involvement of one ipsilateral lymph node less than 3 cm in diameter is designated as N1. Generally, multiple involved nodes are classified as N2, and massive lymphatic involvement is N3 (Table 6–2). The status of distant metastases is designated either M0 (none present) or M1 (present). The T, N, and M classifications are then grouped into stages I–IV (Table 6–3). The stage of disease correlates with the probability of 5-year survival following treatment, based on the site of the primary tumor and the tumor cell type.

TREATMENT PLANNING

Other procedures in addition to biopsy of the primary tumor may be performed at the time of the panendoscopy. Of primary importance is accurate, detailed documentation of the extent of tumor involvement with diagrams (tumor mapping). A fine-needle aspiration of a neck mass may be performed for cytological confirmation of the involvement of a lymph node by metastases. Central venous access procedures may be performed for administration of chemotherapy, if planned, by means of an indwelling catheter or an implantable port device. Dental extractions may need to be performed if the patient is likely to undergo radiation therapy and has poor dentition that will not tolerate the resulting xerostomia. Any questionably healthy teeth are usually extracted prior to radiation therapy because patients requiring extractions following radiation are at high risk of developing progressive necrosis and destruction of the mandible, or o*steoradionecrosis.*

After all the necessary data have been gathered, including the final biopsy results, tumor mapping, radiological studies, etc., each patient's management should be individualized by obtaining recommendations from the members of a multidisciplinary head and neck cancer team. Members of the team may include the otolaryngologist–head and neck surgeon, radiation oncologist, medical oncologist, head and neck pathologist, head and neck radiologist, speech-language pathologist, dental oncologist and/or maxillofacial prosthodontist, and representatives from nursing and psychosocial oncology (psychiatry, psychology, and social work; Ridley, 1996).

It is preferable that the necessary members of the team evaluate the patient prior to the multidisciplinary team meeting in order to accurately assess the patient's medical status, needs, capabilities, limitations, and desires regarding treatment options. The speech-language pathologist experienced in working with patients with head and neck cancer can greatly assist the treating physician by (a) counseling the patient regarding speech and swal-

TABLE 6–2. Staging Classification of Regional Lymph Nodes (N)

Classification	Definition
N1	Metastasis in a single ipsilateral lymph node, ≤3 cm
N2a	Metastasis in a single ipsilateral lymph node, >3 cm but <6 cm
N2b	Metastasis in multiple ipsilateral lymph nodes, none >6 cm
N2c	Metastasis in bilateral or contralateral lymph nodes, none >6 cm
N3	Metastasis in a lymph node, >6 cm

Source: Adapted from *Manual for Staging of Cancer*, by American Joint Committee on Cancer, 1992, Chicago: J. B. Lippincott.

TABLE 6–3. Stage Grouping

Stage	Classification		
I	T1	N0	M0
II	T2	N0	M0
III	T3	N0	M0
	T1	N1	M0
	T2	N1	M0
	T3	N1	M0
IV	T4	Any N	M0
	Any T	N2	M0
	Any T	N3	M0
	Any T	Any N	M1

Source: Adapted from *Manual for Staging of Cancer*, by American Joint Committee on Cancer, 1992, Chicago: J. B. Lippincott.

lowing issues pertinent to the patient's disease and anticipated treatment and (b) educating the patient about methods of rehabilitation following treatment, especially laryngectomy. The recommendations for the individualized treatment plan are formulated with input from the entire multidisciplinary team and presented to the patient by the responsible physician. The final decision to proceed with treatment rests with the patient.

Tracheotomy and Tracheostomy

Any patient who presents initially with a compromised airway because of a head and neck tumor may require an alternative route for ventilation. Advanced malignancies of the upper aerodigestive tract may obstruct the airway or impair the ability to intubate the patient following administration of general anesthesia because of their size. In either case the surgeon may elect to perform a tracheotomy using local anesthesia prior to the administration of general anesthesia. In this way the patient can maintain control of his or her own airway while the tracheotomy is performed and prior to the administration of any muscle-paralyzing agents. The patient is usually given an intravenous benzodiazepine to induce amnesia for the procedure. With proper local anesthetic technique the procedure is painless. Once the airway is established via the tracheotomy, general anesthesia can be given safely and the procedure can proceed.

A *tracheotomy* is an operation to make an opening (*-tome*: to cut) into the trachea. An incision is made in the skin of the midline of the neck (either vertically or horizontally) below the level of the cricoid cartilage. The incision is carried through the subcutaneous tissue down to the strap muscles overlying the cricoid cartilage and upper trachea. These are divided in the midline to reveal the isthmus of the thyroid gland, which is also divided. A horizontal incision is made in the trachea at the level of the third tracheal ring. An inferiorly based, U-shaped flap is incised in the anterior trachea and sutured to the skin of the anterior neck. At this point the patient can breathe spontaneously via the tracheotomy. A *tracheostomy tube* (*-stoma*: mouth) is then inserted into the trachea to maintain the airway, and through this the patient can be ventilated during general anesthesia. A tracheotomy may be performed at the time of panendoscopy and biopsy if necessary; however, it is preferable that it be performed at the time of the definitive resection of the malignancy because of the possibility of seeding the tracheotomy site with tumor cells. A tracheotomy is usually needed for all but the smallest of head and neck tumors requiring surgery because of the risk for postoperative airway compromise from soft tissue swelling.

A tracheotomy that is performed for airway management for the period during and after head and neck surgery is usually temporary. Once the soft tissue swelling has resolved and the incisions are healed, the tracheostomy tube can be removed and the tracheotomy site allowed to heal. This is in contrast to the *tracheostoma* (also called a *tracheostomy*) formed following a total laryngectomy, where the transected trachea is sutured directly to the skin of the anterior neck. These tracheostomas usually do not require a tube to maintain their patency; however, they are the patient's only airway. There is no longer any connection whatsoever between the respiratory and digestive tracts. The patient cannot be intubated orally or nasally, nor can he or she aspirate liquids taken orally (or smell). Likewise, the patient does not have the nose and mouth to protect the airway from the environment. Particulate matter or even flying insects may enter the trachea directly through the neck if the tracheostomy is not covered. These patients must take special precautions when showering, swimming, or boating to prevent drowning by water directly entering the trachea.

Oral Cavity

Each major site in the head and neck is divided into smaller subsites for identification of where the tumor is centered and which structures are involved. A tumor arising in the oral cavity is further classified as involving one or more of the following structures: lip, buccal mucosa, alveolar ridge (upper and lower), retromolar trigone, floor of the mouth, hard palate, and oral tongue. Staging of tumors of the oral cavity is based primarily on size (Table 6–4).

TABLE 6–4. Classification of Primary Tumor (T) for Lip and Oral Cavity

Classification	Definition
T1	Tumor ≤2 cm
T2	Tumor >2 cm, but <4 cm
T3	Tumor >4 cm
T4	Tumor invades adjacent structures (e.g., bone, skin, deep muscle of tongue)

Source: Adapted from *Manual for Staging of Cancer*, by American Joint Committee on Cancer, 1992, Chicago: J. B. Lippincott.

Lip

The lips represent a transitional zone between the skin and the oral mucosa. Carcinoma of the lip is associated with both sun exposure and tobacco use. The most common histological type is squamous cell carcinoma, and the lower lip is most frequently involved. Squamous cell carcinoma of the lip is more likely than squamous cell carcinoma of the skin to metastasize, but less likely than oral mucosal squamous cell carcinoma. The lips perform as a sensate, dynamic sphincter for the mouth and assist in the prehension of oral intake, but are elastic enough to allow wide opening of the jaw. Because of this natural elasticity small carcinomas of the lip may be excised in a wedge-shaped fashion and closed primarily without compromising function. Lip cancers requiring larger resections (up to half of the oral circumference) are usually reconstructed using only remaining lip tissue in order to preserve the sphincteric function, but may result in *microstomia*, or a small oral aperture. Microstomia following reconstruction is rarely severe enough to preclude oral intake; however, even small degrees may make the insertion of dentures difficult, if not impossible. More extensive resections of lip tissue require reconstruction with nonlip tissue, which is insensate and adynamic, severely compromising the oral sphincteric function.

Buccal Mucosa

The buccal mucosa is the mucosal lining of the cheeks and the inner surface of the lips. Despite this area's being easily accessible for examination, approximately half of the malignancies arising there present in late stages (stages III and IV). Tumors of the buccal mucosa frequently arise from areas of *leukoplakia*, a white keratotic plaque that cannot be rubbed off and cannot be given another diagnostic name (Vegers, Snow, & Van der Waal, 1979). Cancer of the buccal mucosa is associated with cigarette and cigar smoking and chewing tobacco.

Carcinomas of the buccal mucosa can invade the deep soft tissues of the cheek and the skin of the face. Involvement of the pterygoid muscles causes *trismus*, or difficulty opening the mouth secondary to pain, fibrosis, or both. These tumors may involve the mandible and maxilla. Surgery or radiation alone may be given for early lesions (stages I and II); however, surgery and postoperative radiation therapy are usually recommended for advanced disease (stages III and IV).

Recurrence is a major problem in carcinoma of the buccal mucosa. The local recurrence rate ranges from 37% to 45%, and local recurrence is frequently accompanied by regional nodal recurrence (Pop et al., 1989).

Alveolar Ridge

The alveolar ridges are the tooth-bearing processes of the mandible and maxilla. The lower alveolar ridge includes the alveolar process of the mandible and the associated attached gingiva from the gingivobuccal sulcus to the junction of the nonattached mucosa of the floor of the mouth. The upper alveolar ridge includes the alveolar process of the maxilla and the attached mucosa extending from the gingivobuccal sulcus to the junction of the hard palate.

Primary tumors of the alveolar ridges tend to involve bone early in the course of the disease and as a result are frequently stage IV on presentation. Numbness of the mandibular teeth or lower lip indicates involvement of the inferior alveolar nerve coursing through the mandible. Tumors of the maxillary alveolar ridge may invade the maxillary sinus.

Retromolar Trigone

The retromolar trigone is the area of attached mucosa overlying the ascending ramus of the mandible. It extends from the posterior surface of the last mandibular molar superiorly to the area adjacent to the maxillary tuberosity. Cancer of the retromolar trigone often behaves aggressively and frequently has invaded adjacent structures such as the tonsil, pterygoid muscles, and mandible at the time of diagnosis. Tumors in this area often require resection of the angle and ascending ramus of the mandible for adequate surgical margin.

Floor of the Mouth

The floor of the mouth is the semilunar area beneath the oral tongue within the arch of the mandible. Its boundaries are the attachment of the gingiva on the lingual surface of the mandible, the undersurface of the tongue, and the palatoglossal fold posteriorly. It is bisected in the midline anteriorly by the lingual frenulum. Its deep margin is the mylohyoid and hyoglossus muscles. The submandibular and sublingual salivary gland ducts empty into the floor of the mouth anteriorly.

Approximately half of the cancers of the floor of the mouth present with stage I or II disease, and half with stage III or IV disease (Shaha, Spiro, Shah, & Strong, 1984). Adjacent structures including the tongue and mandible are often involved in advanced disease. In the posterior floor of the mouth the mandibular division of the trigeminal nerve (cranial nerve V_3) divides into the inferior alveolar nerve and the lingual nerve. The inferior alveolar nerve enters its canal within the mandible at the lingula on the posterior medial surface of the mandible. The lingual nerve lies submucosally in the floor of the mouth and provides taste and general somatic sensation to the anterior two thirds of the tongue. Any loss of sensation in the distribution of these nerves indicates nerve involvement by the tumor. Cancer of the floor of the mouth frequently involves the mandible because of its proximity. Advanced tumors may invade over or through the mandible to involve the skin of the lip, chin, or neck.

Hard Palate

The area of the hard palate extends from the inner surface of the upper alveolar ridge to the posterior margin of the palatine bones. Whereas more than 90% of cancers of the oral cavity are squamous cell carcinoma, only about two thirds of cancers of the hard palate are (Petruzelli & Myers, 1994). Most of the rest are malignant neoplasms of the minor salivary glands, which are numerous in the hard palate. The hard palate is not only the roof of the mouth, but also the floor of the nose and the maxillary sinuses. Resections of the bone of the hard palate result in oronasal or oroantral fistulae, which are usually closed at the time of surgery with a prosthetic obturator.

Oral Tongue

The oral tongue or anterior two thirds of the tongue, is the freely mobile portion of the tongue anterior to the line of the circumvallate papillae and the attachment of the palatoglossal folds. It includes the undersurface, which extends to the junction of the tongue with the floor of the mouth. The areas of the tongue are described as the tip, the lateral aspects, the dorsum (superior or villous surface), and the undersurface (ventral or nonvillous surface). The oral tongue is the most frequent site of occurrence of cancer of the oral cavity after the lip, representing almost half of these cancers (Krupala & Gianoli, 1993). Most cancers of the oral tongue occur on its posterior lateral aspect.

Treatment for early stage (I and II) cancer of the oral tongue may be surgery, radiation, or a combination thereof, depending on the adjacent structures involved and the status of the cervical lymph nodes. Primary radiation for an oral tongue carcinoma requires treatment of a large portion of the oral cavity, and thus the adjacent major and minor salivary glands, causing xerostomia. For this reason surgery is usually recommended for stage I and II oral tongue cancer. Surgery and postoperative radiation therapy are standard therapy for stage III and IV disease.

Surgery for Cancer of the Oral Cavity

The primary goal of surgery for cancer of the oral cavity is the complete resection of the disease. The secondary goal is to provide a reconstruction that will accomplish the maximum degree of function. Surgery will affect function depending on the extent of the resection and the method of reconstruction. The decision as to which type of reconstruction to perform is based on the extent of the defect and the medical condition and desires of the patient. Simpler and less time-consuming reconstructive options (e.g., skin graft) may be chosen for a patient in whom concurrent medical conditions make an extensive and time-consuming reconstruction (e.g., free flap) too high-risk. Younger, healthier patients who are highly motivated to regain maximum function are better candidates for sophisticated, although frequently lengthier, methods of reconstruction such as free microvascular bone flaps following mandibulectomy and microneural anastomoses to restore sensation to intraoral flaps.

The pliable tissues of the oral cavity are not precisely reproducible by skin grafting or flap reconstruction. Following resection of a cancer of the buccal mucosa, the loss of native tissues and fibrosis will produce some degree of limitation in oral opening. The function of the buccinator muscle is usually impaired, causing food to accumulate in the gingivobuccal sulcus during mastication.

Bone invasion by squamous cell carcinoma of the oral cavity tends to proceed via the occlusal surface of the alveolar ridges rather than through the lingual or buccal cortices of the mandible (McGregor & McDonald, 1987). Tumors that have invaded bone are generally considered incurable by radiation alone. Recommended treatment is usually surgery and postoperative radiation therapy. Tumors that are abutting bone or have minimal radiographic evidence of bone involvement may be adequately excised by performing a marginal mandibulectomy, leaving mandibular continuity intact. Loss of alveolar height from tumor resection results in obliteration of the gingivoalveolar sulcus, making the retention of dentures difficult. A sulcoplasty using a split-thickness skin graft or a mucosal graft may be required to restore the sulcus.

More extensive bony disease or nerve involvement necessitates segmental resec-tion of the mandible, resulting in loss of mandibular continuity. Lateral mandibular defects can be left unreconstructed; however, this leaves a substantial cosmetic deformity of the face and neck and causes a shift of the remaining mandible to the opposite side, resulting in malocclusion of the teeth. The patient may be able to eat a soft diet; however, mastication is severely affected, precluding eating a normal diet. These mandibular defects can be reconstructed using a metal plate and a pedicled musculocutaneous flap or with a bone-containing free flap.

Anterior mandibular defects leave a more severe deformity if not reconstructed. Besides the severe cosmetic deformity due to the loss of mandibular projection, the anterior attachment of the tongue is lost. This allows the tongue to fall back into the oropharynx, producing airway obstruction. These patients are usually tracheotomy dependent and limited to a liquid or pureed diet. Reconstruction of the anterior mandible using alloplastic materials is unreliable due to the high incidence of plate extrusion. These defects are best reconstructed using a bone-containing free flap such as the iliac crest, scapula, or fibula flap. This restores mandibular continuity, provides anterior attachment for the tongue, allows decannulation of the tracheotomy, and greatly enhances the patient's ability to resume oral intake and speech, depending on the amount of tongue resected.

Resection of a portion of the oral tongue affects speech more severely than it does swallowing. Loss of the tip of the tongue causes articulation problems when the tip can no longer touch the palate or the teeth. A defect resulting from a resection of the anterior tongue and a portion of the anterior floor of the mouth that is then closed primarily may tether the tongue to the floor of the mouth, preventing normal elevation for articulation. These patients may benefit from an anterior tongue release and grafting of the floor of the mouth and the ventral surface of the tongue.

A hemiglossectomy is the resection of one half of the oral tongue along its midsagittal plane. This procedure usually preserves the patient's ability to swallow, and sparing the tip on the contralateral side preserves the most of the articulatory ability. Larger resections of the oral tongue may require soft tissue reconstruction. The radial forearm free flap has proved to be an excellent method for oral tongue reconstruction due to its being thin and pliable. Cutaneous nerves may be harvested with the flap and anastomosed to the lingual nerve to restore sensation to the flap (Urken & Biller, 1994). Theoretically, sensate flaps should enhance a patient's ability to speak and swallow because of the sensory feedback such flaps should provide; however, studies have not yet shown a significant benefit in the speech or swallowing of patients reconstructed in this manner as compared to those reconstructed with nonsensate flaps.

Oropharynx

The boundary between the oral cavity and the oropharynx is the posterior border of the hard palate superiorly, the palatoglossal folds laterally, and the line of the circumvallate papillae inferiorly. The dividing line between the nasopharynx and the oropharynx is an imaginary line extending posteriorly from the plane of the hard palate. The inferior limit of the oropharynx is the plane of the pharyngoepiglottic folds, which separates it from the hypopharynx. The oropharynx comprises the soft palate, the base of the tongue, the anterior and posterior tonsillar pillars (palatoglossal and palatopharyngeal folds), the tonsillar fossae and palatine tonsils, the lateral walls of the oropharynx (posterior to the posterior tonsillar pillars), and the posterior oropharyngeal wall. Staging of oropharyngeal tumors is based primarily on size (Table 6–5).

Soft Palate

In contrast to carcinomas of the hard palate, the vast majority of cancers of the soft palate are squamous cell carcinoma, which is strongly associated with tobacco and alcohol abuse. The function of the soft palate is to seal the nasopharynx by contacting the posterior pharyngeal wall to prevent nasal regurgitation during swallowing and nasal escape of air during speech. Surgery for cancer of the soft palate compromises its function depending on the amount resected. There are currently no adequate surgical techniques for reconstruction of a functional soft palate following complete excision due to its highly complex requirements for normal function. For this reason radiation is usually the preferred treatment for cancer of the soft palate except for very small lesions that can be excised without creating a full-thickness palatal defect. The cure rates for surgery are comparable to those of radiation therapy; however, the morbidity is greater because of the resulting velopharyngeal incompetence.

In the event of an incomplete response to radiation therapy or a recurrence, surgery is the only option for treatment. Swallowing and speech rehabilitation is possible using a palatal prosthesis, although the results are quite variable among patients (Fee et al., 1979).

Base of Tongue

The base of the tongue is the posterior one third of the tongue, posterior to the line of the circumvallate papillae. The sensory innervation of the base of the tongue is via the glossopharyngeal nerve (cranial nerve IX), whereas that of the oral tongue is via the trigeminal nerve (cranial nerve V). Cancer of tongue base frequently presents with *otalgia*, or pain in the ear, due to referred pain via the glossopharyngeal nerve. Tongue base carcinoma is more aggressive than that of the oral tongue and is among the most difficult head and neck malignancies to manage. These tumors are frequently advanced, with cervical metastases at the time of diagnosis due to their being relatively asymptomatic in the early stages.

Resection of more than one half of the tongue base severely impairs the pharyngeal phase of swallowing. Reconstruction of this area with an adynamic flap does not restore the complex function of tongue base. Because of the morbidity associated

TABLE 6–5. Classification of Primary Tumor (T) for Oropharynx

Classification	Definition
T1	Tumor ≤2 cm
T2	Tumor >2 cm but <4 cm
T3	Tumor >4 cm
T4	Tumor invades adjacent structures (e.g., bone, deep muscle of tongue)

Source: Adapted from *Manual for Staging of Cancer*, by American Joint Committee on Cancer, 1992, Chicago: J. B. Lippincott.

with resection of the tongue base, most patients choose to undergo primary radiation therapy. If the tumor fails to respond to radiation therapy alone or recurs, surgical excision is the only option available. Patients undergoing extensive resections of the tongue base frequently require a total laryngectomy even though the larynx itself is not involved by the tumor. Older patients with limited pulmonary reserve may not be able to tolerate the aspiration that invariably results from extensive tongue base resection and reconstruction. Patients who do not have a laryngectomy initially may require one later due to repeated episodes of aspiration pneumonia.

The hypoglossal nerves (cranial nerve XII) enter the tongue base from the upper neck and provide motor innervation to the intrinsic muscles of the tongue. Preservation of one hypoglossal nerve will preserve some function of the oral tongue and tongue base; however, swallowing may be so severely impaired that long-term tube feedings are required. If one hypoglossal nerve is spared, speech is usually intelligible.

Tonsil

Cancers arising from the tonsillar pillars, the tonsillar fossae, and the palatine tonsils are all considered cancer of the tonsil. It is the most frequent primary cancer of the oropharynx. Tonsil cancer is frequently found in patients presenting with metastatic squamous cell carcinoma of the neck who do not have an obvious primary mucosal lesion. Other sites that can be responsible for *squamous cell carcinoma of unknown primary* are the base of the tongue, the nasopharynx, and the pyriform sinuses. Patients presenting with metastatic carcinoma in a jugulodigastric lymph node are recommended to undergo a panendoscopy with biopsies of these areas if no mucosal lesion is visible. Complete excision of the tonsil on the side of the metastasis is often performed in order to rule out a small primary cancer within a tonsillar crypt.

Both surgery and radiation therapy are effective treatments for early (stage I and II) carcinoma of the tonsil (Spiro & Spiro, 1989; Wong et al., 1989). Radiation produces xerostomia due to its effects on the oropharyngeal mucosa and the salivary glands, and surgery can result in varying degrees of dysphagia and dysarthria depending on the extent of the resection. Patients with neck disease greater than N1 usually undergo a planned neck dissection 6 to 8 weeks following completion of radiation therapy. Patients with advanced (stage III and IV) disease usually undergo surgical resection followed by postoperative radiation. Treatment results for cancer of the tonsil are generally better than those for cancer of the base of the tongue, unless the tonsil cancer has invaded the tongue base, in which case it behaves more like a tongue base cancer.

Structures deep to the tonsillar fossa that may be involved by tonsillar carcinoma include the ascending ramus of the mandible, the pterygoid muscles, the internal carotid artery, and cranial nerves IX through XII. Segmental resection of the mandible may be necessary for complete excision of the tumor. Invasion by the tumor or resection of the pterygoid muscles usually results in some degree of trismus. Involvement of any of the lower cranial nerves by the tumor, requiring resection, will result in varying degrees of dysphagia, dysphonia, and dysarthria. If tumor has spread deeply to completely encase the internal carotid artery, it is generally considered to be unresectable.

Soft tissue reconstruction of the oropharynx following resection of a carcinoma of the tonsil is usually accomplished using a pedicled pectoralis major musculocutaneous flap. This flap provides excellent reconstruction of the defect, as the functional requirements are minimal. This is in contrast to poorer results obtained when reconstructing the base of the tongue, whose functional requirements are great.

Oropharyngeal Wall

Cancer of the oropharynx originating posterior to posterior tonsillar folds is referred to as cancer of the oropharyngeal wall. Because its boundaries with the nasopharynx and the hypopharynx are not distinct anatomic structures but imaginary lines, these tumors frequently extend to involve these sites as well. They are often advanced at the time of diagnosis and generally have a worse prognosis than cancer of the tonsil.

Early (stage I and II) lesions can be treated with surgery or radiation therapy. Advanced (stage III and IV) lesions are usually treated with surgery and postoperative radiation therapy. Extensive resections of the oropharyngeal walls can result in severe dysphagia secondary to the loss of function of the pharyngeal constrictor muscles, which impairs the pharyngeal phase of swallowing. As in tongue base carcinoma, the risk of aspiration may necessitate a simultaneous laryngectomy.

Larynx

The larynx is the second most frequent site of involvement by cancer in the head and neck after the oral cavity. The vast majority of malignancies of the larynx are squamous cell carcinoma. Compared to all other sites in the head and neck, laryngeal cancer has one of the highest cure rates. The risk factors for cancer of the larynx are, as for most upper aerodigestive malignancies, tobacco and alcohol; however, gastroesophageal reflux disease has also been recently implicated (Koufman, 1991). Cancers of the larynx present and behave differently depending on the site of origin within the larynx. The larynx is divided into three primary sites: supraglottis, glottis, and subglottis. Classification of the primary for staging of laryngeal tumors is slightly different for each of the three subsites (Table 6–6).

Supraglottis

The supraglottic larynx is that portion above a horizontal plane passing through the apex of the laryngeal ventricle. Supraglottic subsites include the suprahyoid epiglottis (lingual and laryngeal aspects), the infrahyoid epiglottis, the false vocal (ventricular) folds, the arytenoids, and the aryepiglottic folds.

Symptoms from cancer of the supraglottic larynx are typically sore throat and dysphagia, which may be minimal and, therefore, ignored by the patient for a long period. These tumors can grow to a very large size with a surprising paucity of symptoms. Hoarseness does not usually appear until later in the course of the disease as compared to cancer of the glottic larynx. This is one reason for supraglottic malignancies' tending to present at a more advanced stage than glottic primaries. The other is the rich lymphatic drainage supplying the supraglottic larynx.

Supraglottic cancers have a high incidence of cervical lymphatic metastases. The rate of metastases (both clinically apparent and occult) for T1 (early) supraglottic tumors is as high as 25% (Sinard, Netterville, Garrett, & Ossoff, 1996). Higher T classifications have correspondingly higher rates of cervical metastases. Bilateral neck metastases from these tumors are com-

TABLE 6–6. Classification of Primary Tumor (T) for Larynx

Classification	Definition
	Supraglottis
T1	Tumor limited to one subsite of the supraglottis, with nomal vocal fold mobility
T2	Tumor invades more than one subsite of the supraglottis or glottis, with normal vocal fold mobility
T3	Limited to the larynx, with vocal fold fixation and/or invasion of the post-cricoid area, medial wall of the pyriform sinus, or preepiglottic tissues
T4	Tumor invades through the thyroid cartilage and/or extends to other tissues beyond the larynx (e.g., to the oropharynx or soft tissues of the neck)
	Glottis
T1	Tumor limited to the vocal fold(s) (may involve anterior or posterior commissures), with normal mobility
T1a	Tumor limited to one vocal fold
T1b	Tumor involves both vocal folds
T2	Tumor extends to the supraglottis and/or subglottis, with or without impaired vocal cord mobility
T3	Tumor limited to the larynx, with vocal fold fixation
T4	Tumor invades through the thyroid cartilage and/or extends to the other tissues beyond the larynx (e.g., to the oropharynx or soft tissues of the neck)
	Subglottis
T1	Tumor limited to the subglottis
T2	Tumor extends to the vocal fold(s), with normal or impaired mobility
T3	Tumor limited to the larynx, with vocal fold fixation
T4	Tumor invades through the cricoid or thyroid cartilage and/or extends to other tissues beyond the larynx (e.g., to the oropharynx or soft tissues of the neck)

Source: Adapted from *Manual for Staging of Cancer*, by American Joint Committee on Cancer, 1992, Chicago: J. B. Lippincott.

mon because of the lack of a midline fascial plane to impede contralateral lymphatic flow. For this reason any plan for treatment of supraglottic tumors must address the cervical lymphatics.

A T1 cancer of supraglottis is defined as involvement of only one subsite. T2 tumors involve more than one subsite, with normal vocal fold mobility. Tumors that are limited to the larynx and are causing vocal fold fixation or invading the postcricoid area, the medial wall of the pyriform sinus, or the preepiglottic space are classified as T3. T4 tumors are those that have invaded the thyroid cartilage or extended outside the larynx.

Treatment of early (stage I and II) cancer of the supraglottis may be either surgery or radiation. Very small tumors can be excised endoscopically, especially those of the suprahyoid epiglottis. A supraglottic (horizontal partial) laryngectomy may be performed for T1 and T2 tumors, excising the laryngeal structures above the ventricles while preserving one superior laryngeal nerve for supraglottic sensation. Elective dissection of the internal jugular chain of lymph nodes is usually performed bilaterally because of the high incidence of ipsilateral and contralateral cervical lymphatic metastases.

Patients undergoing a supraglottic laryngectomy have a tracheostomy tube in place following surgery that is removed as soon as the postoperative swelling resolves sufficiently to allow an adequate oronasal airway. This allows the patient to begin swallowing therapy as soon as healing is adequate without the laryngeal remnant's being tethered in the neck by the tracheostomy tube. Working with a speech-language pathologist experienced in treating head and neck cancer patients is integral for maximal recovery of swallowing function in these patients. Because the patient no longer has the supraglottic structures (epiglottis, aryepiglottic folds, and false vocal folds) to assist in protecting the airway, laryngeal excursion superiorly and anteriorly beneath the base of the tongue during swallowing is critically important.

Early supraglottic tumors may also be treated with radiation therapy alone. Control rates of greater than 80% for T1 and greater than 70% for T2 supraglottic tumors using radiation therapy alone are possible (Mendenhall, Parsons, Stringer, Cassisi, & Million, 1990). These rates are even higher if surgical salvage is added for incomplete responses to radiation therapy and for recurrences. Partial laryngectomy following radiation, however, is fraught with a higher incidence of complications. These may include inability to decannulate the patient secondary to persistent edema of the airway or fibrosis in the neck, which impedes movement of the larynx and prevents achievement of an effective swallow postoperatively. For this reason most cases of persistent or recurrent disease following radiation therapy for supraglottic cancers require a total laryngectomy.

A number of factors may affect the decision of which treatment modality to use (surgery or radiation), including the subsite(s) involved, the status of cervical lymph nodes, the general medical condition of the patient, and the preferences of the patient and the treating physician. Patients with chronic lung disease and inadequate pulmonary reserve are generally considered to be poor candidates for partial laryngectomy procedures. They usually cannot tolerate the expected pulmonary aspiration that results from the surgery, especially during the early postoperative period. The ability to cough and effectively clear the trachea and bronchi is required to compensate for the aspiration that follows a supraglottic laryngectomy. If the cough mechanism is inadequate or ineffective, aspiration pneumonia will result. Repeated episodes of aspiration pneumonia following a supraglottic laryngectomy may require a completion laryngectomy.

Patients with advanced (T3 and T4) malignancies of the supraglottic larynx are frequently not candidates for supraglottic laryngectomy because of fixation of one of the true vocal folds or involvement of the postcricoid area. Combined therapy is usually indicated. Recommended primary surgical therapy is usually a total laryngectomy. Because of the high incidence of cervical lymphatic metastases, ipsilateral or bilateral neck dissection is usually indicated. Postoperative radiation therapy is generally recommended. This treatment (surgery followed by radiation) has been considered standard therapy in most centers for advanced supraglottic cancers. More recently organ preservation treatment protocols have offered an alternative to primary total laryngectomy for advanced laryngeal cancers. Recent studies have found similar survival rates for laryngeal cancers (supraglottic and glottic) treated with surgery followed by radiation and those treated with induction chemotherapy followed by radiation therapy (Department of Veterans Affairs Laryngeal Cancer Study Group, 1991). Nearly two thirds of the patients treated with chemotherapy and radiation were able to retain their larynges during the first 3 years of follow-up. This approach is now a treatment option for patients presenting with advanced lesions of the supraglottic larynx.

Glottis

The glottic larynx is composed of the true vocal folds including the anterior and posterior commissures. The glottis extends from a horizontal plane passing through the apex of the ventricles superiorly to a horizontal plane 1 cm inferiorly. The true vocal folds are covered with stratified squamous epithelium. Mucous glands within the mucosa of the true vocal folds are extremely sparse. The mucus for lubrication of the true vocal fold mucosa is produced in the mucous gland–rich mucosa of the ventricle, the laryngeal saccule, and the false vocal folds. Mucus from these areas flows downward onto the true vocal folds.

Cancers of the glottic larynx tend to present earlier than cancers of the supraglottis. These tumors cause hoarseness early in the course of the disease, prompting the patient to seek medical attention. Any patient with hoarseness of more than 1 month's duration must have laryngoscopy performed to determine the cause, especially those who smoke and are over 50 years old.

There are barriers to spread of cancer within the glottic larynx that are absent in the supraglottis. Glottic cancers have a lower incidence of lymphatic metastases than comparable supraglottic cancers because of the sparse lymphatics in that area. The chance of metastatic disease with a T1 glottic cancer is less than 5% and less than 10% for a T2 (Johnson & Myers, 1991). Spread to contralateral lymphatics is unusual except in very large tumors.

Early (T1 and T2) cancers of the glottis can be treated with either surgery or radiation therapy. Small glottic cancers can be effectively managed with endoscopic excision (e.g., cordectomy) or open vertical hemilaryngectomy. Vertical hemilaryngectomy is a form of partial laryngectomy in which one half of the larynx is excised including the anterior two thirds of one true vocal fold, one false vocal fold, the ipsilateral paraglottic space, and one ala of the thyroid cartilage. The hemilarynx is reconstructed using the outer perichondrium of the thyroid cartilage and the strap muscles. Laryngeal function is preserved by the mobile contralateral vocal fold approximating the reconstructed hemilarynx. As with supraglottic laryngectomy, early decannulation and swallowing therapy by an experienced speech-language pathologist are essential for optimal rehabilitation and prevention of aspiration pneumonia.

Radiation therapy alone results in very good cure rates for early glottic cancers. Control rates are 85% to 95% for T1 tumors and 65% to 75% for T2 tumors (Fein, Mendenhall, Parsons, & Million, 1993). Tumors that fail to respond completely to radiation or recur may be salvaged by conservation laryngeal surgery (e.g., hemilaryngectomy) or may require total laryngectomy. Radiation therapy is frequently chosen for treatment of early glottic cancers because of the high cure rates and the better resulting voice quality as compared to surgery for similar tumors. Radiation therapy, however, requires daily treatments over a period of 6 weeks or more, as compared to surgery, which may require no more than 5–7 days of hospitalization. Postoperative radiation therapy following surgery is frequently avoided in early glottic cancers.

Standard therapy for advanced glottic cancers (T3 and T4) has been laryngectomy followed by radiation therapy. As noted with supraglottic tumors, induction chemotherapy followed by radiation therapy achieves comparable survival rates in these patients, with preservation of the larynx in about two thirds.

Subglottis

The subglottic larynx extends from the inferior border of the glottic larynx (a horizontal plane 1 cm below a horizontal plane passing through the apex of the ventricle) to the inferior border of the cricoid cartilage. Tumors originating in this area are rare; however, advanced glottic tumors frequently extend to involve this region of the larynx. From the subglottis tumors may extend to involve the cervical trachea, the postcricoid region of the hypopharynx, or the soft tissue of the neck via the cricothyroid membrane. The subglottic region has a richer lymphatic drainage than the glottic larynx, and lymphatic metastases are much more common when this area is involved either by a primary tumor or by extension from a glottic primary.

Tracheoesophageal Puncture

Restoration of speech is possible in the great majority of patients undergoing total laryngectomy. Previously, options were limited to learning esophageal speech or using an electrolarynx. Fewer than one third of patients with laryngectomies are able to develop fluent esophageal speech, and many patients consider the monotone speech produced by the electrolarynx to be objectionable. Singer and Blom (1980) introduced a method of voice restoration following laryngectomy that allows most patients to regain speech that is comparable to esophageal speech.

This technique involves creation of a tracheoesophageal puncture in the back wall of the tracheostomy through which a catheter is placed until healing of the fistula tract has occurred. The catheter is then replaced with a one-way valve that allows exhaled air to be diverted from the trachea through the fistula and into the pharynx. The stream of air causes vibration of the mucosa of the pharynx, which serves as a sound generator for speech. The structures necessary for resonance and articulation are unaffected by laryngectomy, and speech is produced using the sound produced by pharyngeal mucosal vibration just as it is using the sound produced by vibration of the vocal folds. The one-way valve prevents leakage of saliva from the pharynx into the trachea.

Patients undergoing laryngectomy who will require postoperative radiation therapy do not usually have a tracheoesophageal puncture performed until at least 6 weeks following radiation. Patients who have already been treated with radiation may have the tracheoesophageal puncture performed at the time of the laryngectomy (primary tracheoesophageal puncture).

Preoperative assessment for tracheoesophageal puncture includes assessment of stomal adequacy. A stoma less than 2 cm in diameter may require a stomaplasty to increase the size of the stoma in order to adequately accommodate the prosthesis. A stomaplasty can be performed at the same time as the tracheoesophageal puncture.

A Taub test determines if sufficient pressure can be generated in the thorax to inject air into the pharynx and cause mucosal vibration. It is performed by placing a catheter through the nose and into the pharynx to the level of the tracheal stoma. The free end of the catheter is attached to an airtight housing placed over the stoma. Occlusion of the housing over the stoma will divert exhaled air through the catheter and into the pharynx. The ability to produce sound predicts successful development of speech using the tracheoesophageal prosthesis.

Patients who are unable to generate sound using this technique may be experiencing spasm of the pharyngeal constrictor muscles in response to air being injected into the pharynx. Blocking the pharyngeal constrictors with lidocaine injected percutaneously into the muscle may allow the production of sound. This confirms the presence of muscle spasm and predicts successful development of speech if a pharyngeal myotomy is performed at the time of the tracheoesophageal puncture.

Hypopharynx

The hypopharynx, also called the laryngopharynx, is that portion of the pharynx from the level of pharyngoepiglottic folds to the cricopharyngeus muscle. This muscle, which is the upper esophageal sphincter, attaches to cricoid cartilage anteriorly and surrounds the pharynx posteriorly at its junction with cervical esophagus. The subsites of the hypopharynx are the pyriform sinuses, the postcricoid area (the mucosa covering the posterior aspect of the cricoid lamina and forming the anterior wall of the hypopharynx), and the posterior wall of the hypopharynx. Classification of the primary tumor in hypopharyngeal sites is primarily based on the number of subsites involved (Table 6–7). Endoscopic evaluation under general anesthesia is usually required to determine the extent of involvement.

The pyriform (pear-shaped) sinuses lie on either side of the larynx and are shaped somewhat like an inverted, three-sided

TABLE 6–7. Classification of Primary Tumor (T) for Hypopharynx

Classification	Definition
T1	Tumor limited to one subsite of the hypopharynx
T2	Tumor invades more than one subsite of hypopharynx or an adjacent site, without fixation of hemilarynx
T3	Tumor invades more than one subsite of hypopharynx or an adjacent site, with fixation of hemilarynx
T4	Tumor invades adjacent structures (e.g., cartilage or soft tissues of neck)

Source: Adapted from *Manual for Staging of Cancer,* by American Joint Committee on Cancer, 1992, Chicago: J. B. Lippincott.

pyramid, with the apex at the level of the inferior border of the cricopharyngeus muscle. The three sides are referred to as the anterior, medial, and lateral walls. The pyriform sinuses are collapsed at rest and are opened during swallowing by anterior and superior movement of the larynx.

T1 tumors of the hypopharynx are those limited to one subsite. T2 tumors involve more than one subsite, without vocal fold fixation. A hypopharyngeal lesion causing fixation of a vocal fold denotes a T3 tumor. A tumor that has invaded adjacent structures such as cartilage or the soft tissue of the neck is designated T4.

Diagnosis of early (T1 or T2) hypopharyngeal cancers is unusual. These tumors are relatively asymptomatic when small. Even as a tumor in this area increases in size enough to cause obstruction of one pyriform sinus, symptoms may remain minimal because of shunting of the swallowed bolus to the contralateral side. Patients may not present for treatment until the tumor is causing obstruction of the entire hypopharyngeal lumen or hoarseness develops as a result of invasion into the larynx. Direct extension of hypopharyngeal cancers into the soft tissues of the neck is common.

Early cancers (T1 and T2) of the hypopharynx are usually treated with radiation therapy in order to preserve the larynx, although tumors in this area may not be as radiosensitive as those in other sites of the head and neck. Tumors that persist or recur following radiation therapy and advanced cancers (T3 and T4) of the

hypopharynx generally require total laryngectomy. An ipsilateral neck dissection is usually performed simultaneously. Postoperative radiation therapy is recommended for advanced cancer of the hypopharynx.

The hypopharynx is reconstructed using the remaining hypopharyngeal mucosa if there is sufficient mucosa present to produce an adequate hypopharyngeal lumen. The circumference of the reconstructed hypopharynx can be augmented using a pedicled musculocutaneous flap such as the pectoralis major musculocutaneous flap. Tumors that extend to the apex of the pyriform sinus or into the cervical esophagus require circumferential pharyngectomy in order to obtain adequate surgical margins around the tumor. Reconstructive options include a jejunal free flap (interposition of a segment of small bowel between the pharynx and esophagus with anastomosis of its vascular supply to vessels in the neck) or a radial forearm free flap (soft tissue and skin harvested from the volar aspect of the forearm supplied by the radial artery).

UNILATERAL VOCAL FOLD PARALYSIS

The motor innervation of the laryngeal muscles is primarily via the recurrent laryngeal nerves, which are branches of the vagus nerves (cranial nerve X). The vagus nerve arises from rootlets on the brainstem, which coalesce and pass superiorly through the foramen magnum into the cranium. It then exits via the jugular foramen with the internal jugular vein and cranial nerves IX, XI, and XII. The vagus then descends in the neck in the carotid sheath adjacent to the carotid artery. The origin of the recurrent laryngeal nerves is different for the right and left sides.

On the right side the recurrent laryngeal nerve arises from the vagus at the level of the thoracic inlet and passes around the subclavian artery before ascending in the neck to reach the larynx. On the left side it arises at the level of the arch of the aorta in the chest and loops around the aorta before returning superiorly. The left recurrent laryngeal nerve typically lies deep in the tracheoesophageal groove in the neck and has a more vertical ascent, whereas the right recurrent laryngeal nerve may lie outside the tracheoesophageal groove and has a more oblique ascent from lateral to medial toward the larynx. Vocal fold paralysis may result from injury or tumors anywhere along the course of the vagus and recurrent laryngeal nerves.

Neoplasms that may present as a vocal fold paralysis include skull base tumors, paragangliomas (carotid body tumors and glomus tumors), thyroid tumors, and laryngeal, pharyngeal, and esophageal tumors. Paralysis of the left vocal fold may result from cancer of the lung, mediastinum, or thoracic esophagus, or from enlargement of the left atrium of the heart. Trauma, either accidental or iatrogenic, to the vagus or recurrent laryngeal nerves in the head, neck, or chest may cause paralysis of a vocal fold (Table 6–8).

Unilateral paralysis of a vocal fold typically produces a weak, breathy voice secondary to incomplete apposition of the functional vocal fold to the paralyzed fold. This results from excess air escape during phonation. Vocal efficiency is decreased, with fewer words produced per breath. Unilateral vocal fold paralysis does not compromise the airway if the contralateral vocal fold is able to fully abduct.

Rehabilitation of a symptomatic unilateral vocal fold paralysis involves medialization of the paralyzed vocal fold so that the contralateral functional vocal fold can appose it. The paralyzed vocal fold should be medialized to the midline in order to achieve maximal vocal efficiency. In the past, medialization of a paralyzed vocal fold was performed by injecting Teflon paste laterally into the thyroarytenoid muscle of the vocal fold.

Isshiki described techniques of thyroplasty, including medialization, using an implant placed through a window in the thyroid ala (Isshiki, Okamura, & Ishikawa, 1975). This technique was popularized by Koufman in the United States using a Silastic block implant to medialize a paralyzed vocal fold (Koufman, 1986). Over the past 10 years many authors have confirmed the benefits of vocal fold medialization using Silastic implants including its low rate of complications. The advantages of this procedure include the preservation of the mucosal wave on the medialized fold, the ability to perform the procedure under local anesthesia, and its reversibility. These are in contrast to injection of Teflon, which usually results in loss of the mucosal wave, generally requires general anesthesia, and is irreversible. The Silastic implant can be sized at the time of surgery to produce maximum vocal quality.

A temporary method of vocal fold medialization is Gelfoam injection. A thick paste is made from Gelfoam powder (absorbable gelatin), which is used as a surgical hemostatic agent. The Gelfoam paste is then injected laterally into the paralyzed vocal fold, medializing it to the midline. The medialization lasts from 1 to 3 months, after which the gelatin is absorbed. This procedure is indicated for patients with vocal fold paralysis who are not candidates for medialization thyroplasty because of medical status or limited life expectancy. Gelfoam injection of the vocal fold can be performed under general or local anesthesia in the operating room using direct laryngoscopy, or in the office using local anesthesia and indirect (mir-

TABLE 6–8. Causes of Vocal Fold Paralysis

Accidental trauma (blunt and sharp)
        Neck injury
        Chest injury
        Head injury

Iatrogenic
        Intubation injury (arytenoid subluxation, recurrent nerve injury)
        Neck surgery (thyroid, parathyroid, carotid, cervical disc, larynx, cricopharyngeal myotomy)
        Chest surgery (heart, lung, trachea)
        Skull base surgery (jugular foramen, temporal bone)
        Neurosurgery (posterior fossa, brainstem)

Idiopathic
        Viral neuritis?
        Autoimmune disease?

Neoplasm
        Brain tumor
        Skull base tumor (glomus tumor, nasopharyngeal carcinoma)
        Vascular tumor (carotid body tumor)
        Nerve tumor (Schwannoma, neurofibroma)
        Larynx malignancy (squamous cell carcinoma)
        Thyroid malignancy (papillary, follicular, medullary, anaplastic)
        Pharyngeal malignancy (squamous cell carcinoma)
        Neck malignancy (metastatic squamous cell carcinoma)
        Esophageal malignancy (squamous cell carcinoma)
        Tracheal tumor (squamous cell carcinoma)
        Lung malignancy (squamous cell carcinoma, adenocarcinoma, small cell carcinoma)

Congenital
        Central nervous system lesions
        Arnold-Chiari malformation
        Meningomyelocele
        Birth trauma

Other
        Cricorytenoid joint arthritis
        Left atrial enlargement
        Mediastinal adenopathy
        Cerebrovascular accident
        Multiple sclerosis
        Lyme disease
        Poliomyelitis
        Postpolio syndrome

ror) laryngoscopy. Patients with inoperable lung or esophageal cancer who have vocal fold paralysis are greatly helped by this simple procedure, which improves the voice and enhances the efficiency of the cough. The procedure is safe and reversible because, unlike with Teflon, any overcorrection of the vocal fold that occurs will resolve because of the eventual resorption of the gelatin.

BILATERAL VOCAL FOLD PARALYSIS

Patients with bilateral vocal fold paralysis present with airway obstruction. The voice is generally fair or good; however, there is marked inspiratory stridor, especially on exertion. This is due to the inability to abduct to vocal folds during inspiration. The diagnosis may be made when a patient is unable to tolerate extubation following endotracheal intubation or is unable to be decannulated following tracheotomy.

Voice quality is a secondary consideration to maintaining an adequate airway in these patients. Any procedure to increase the size of the glottic aperture may result in a deterioration of voice quality; however, maintaining a safe airway is of primary importance. Procedures for enlarging the laryngeal airway in the presence of bilateral vocal fold paralysis include arytenoidectomy with vocal fold lateralization and transverse laser cordotomy (Kashima, 1991).

CONCLUSION

Any surgical procedure performed in the head and neck may affect the patient's ability to speak and/or swallow. Knowledge of the normal anatomy, the physiology of speech and swallowing, the behavior of neoplasms in the head and neck, and the effects of treatments and reconstructive procedures will provide the ability to assess a patient's degree of dysfunction, develop a plan of treatment, and determine the prognosis for recovery.

REFERENCES

American Joint Committee on Cancer. (1992). *Manual for staging of cancer* (4th ed.). Chicago: J. B. Lippincott.

Berg, J. W. (1982). Morphologic classification of human cancer. In D. Schottenfeld & J. G. Fraumeni (Eds.), *Cancer epidemiology and prevention* (pp. 74-89). Philadelphia: W. B. Saunders.

Boring, C. C., Squires, T. S., & Tong, T. (1991). Cancer statistics. *CA: A Cancer Journal for Clinicians, 41,* 19–36.

Department of Veterans Affairs Laryngeal Cancer Study Group. (1991). Induction chemotherapy plus radiation compared with surgery plus radiation in patients with advanced laryngeal cancer. *New England Journal of Medicine, 324,* 1685–1690.

Endicott, J. N., Skipper, P. M., & Hernandez, L. (1993). Marijuana and head and neck cancer. In H. Friedman, T. W. Klein, & S. Specter (Eds.), *Advances in experimental medicine and biology: Vol.* 335. *Drugs of abuse, immunity, and AIDS.* (pp. 107–113). New York: Plenum Press.

Fee, W. F., Schoeppel, S. L., Rubenstein, R., Goffinet, D., Goode, R., & Boles, R. (1979). Squamous cell carcinoma of the soft palate. *Archives of Otolaryngology, 105,* 710–718.

Fein, D. A., Mendenhall, W. M., Parsons, J. T., & Million, R. R. (1993). T1-T2 squamous cell carcinoma of the glottic larynx treated with radiotherapy: A multivariate analysis of variables potentially influencing local control. *International Journal of Radiation Oncology, Biology, Physics, 25,* 605–611.

Isshiki, N., Okamura, H., & Ishikawa, T. (1975). Thyroplasty type I (lateral compression) for dysphonia due to vocal cord paralysis or atrophy. *Acta Otolaryngologica, 80,* 465–473.

Johnson, J. T., & Myers, E. N. (1991). Cervical lymph node disease in laryngeal cancer. In C. E. Silver (Ed.), *Laryngeal cancer.* New York: Thieme.

Kashima, H. K. (1991). Bilateral vocal fold motion impairment: Pathophysiology and management by transverse cordotomy. *Annals of Otology, Rhinology, and Laryngology, 100,* 717–721.

Koufman, J. A. (1986). Laryngoplasty for vocal cord medialization: An alternative to Teflon. *Laryngoscope, 96,* 726–731.

Koufman, J. A. (1991). The otolaryngologic manifestations of gastroesophageal reflux disease (GERD): A clinical investigation of 225 patients using ambulatory 24-hour pH monitoring and an experimental investigation of the role of acid and pepsin in the development of laryngeal injury. *Laryngoscope, 101* (Suppl. 53), 1–78.

Krupala, J. L., & Gianoli, R. (1993). Carcinoma of the oral tongue. *Journal of the Louisiana State Medical Society, 145,* 421–426.

McGregor, I. A., & MacDonald, D. G. (1987). Spread of squamous carcinoma to the nonirradiated edentulous mandible: A preliminary study. *Head and Neck Surgery, 9,* 157–161.

Mendenhall, W. M., Parsons, J. T., Stringer, S. P., Cassisi, N. J., & Million, R. R. (1990). Carcinoma of the supraglottic larynx: A basis for comparing the results of radiotherapy and surgery. *Head and Neck, 12,* 204–209.

Petruzelli, G. J., & Myers, E. N. (1994). Malignant neoplasms of the hard palate and upper alveolar ridge. *Oncology, 8,* 43–48.

Pop, L. A. M., Eijkenboom, W. M. H., deBoer, M. F., de Jong, P. C., Knegt, P., Levendag, P. C., Meeuwis, C. A., Reichgelt, B. A., & van Putten, W. L. J. (1989). Evaluation of treatment results of squamous cell carcinoma of the buccal mucosa. *International Journal of Radiation Oncology,16,* 483–487.

Ridley, M. B. (1996). Clinical practice guidelines for malignancies of the head and neck: Larynx, oropharynx, and oral cavity. *Cancer Control, 3,* 442–447.

Shaha, A., Spiro, R., Shah, J., & Strong, E. (1984). Squamous carcinoma of the floor of the mouth. *American Journal of Surgery, 148,* 455–459.

Sinard, R. J., Netterville, J. L., Garrett, C. G., & Ossoff, R. H. (1996). Cancer of the larynx. In E. N. Myers & J. Y. Suen (Eds.), *Cancer of the head and neck* (3rd ed., p. 385). Philadelphia: W. B. Saunders.

Singer, M. I., & Blom, E. D. (1980). An endoscopic technique for restoration of voice after laryngectomy. *Annals of Otology, Rhinology, and Laryngology, 89,* 529–533.

Spiro, J. D., & Spiro, R. H. (1989). Carcinoma of the tonsillar fossa. *Archives of Otolaryngology—Head and Neck Surgery, 115,* 1186–1189.

Urken, M. L., & Biller, H. F. (1994). A new bilobed design for the sensate radial forearm flap to preserve tongue mobility following significant glossectomy. *Archives of Otolaryngology—Head and Neck Surgery, 105,* 26–31.

Vegers, J. W. M., Snow, G. G., & Van der Waal, I. (1979). Squamous cell carcinoma of the buccal mucosa: A review of 85 cases. *Archives of Otolaryngology, 105,* 192–195.

Wong, C. S., Ang, K. K., Fletcher, G. H., Thames, H. D., Peters, L. J., Byers, R. M., & Oswald, M. J. (1989). Definitive radiotherapy for squamous cell carcinoma of the tonsillar fossa. *International Journal of Radiation Oncology, Biology, Physics, 16,* 657–662.

7

Esophageal Carcinoma

Umesh Choudhry, M.D.

Carcinoma of the esophagus is a malignancy associated with considerable debilitation, compromise of quality of life, and mortality. Due to the unique anatomic features of the esophagus, delayed onset of symptoms, and lack of an effective screening strategy in Western countries, it is often diagnosed far too late to be curable. Historically, cancer of the esophagus was almost exclusively of the squamous cell type, accounting for almost 95% of cases. Recent decades have seen an epidemic of the hitherto infrequent adenocarcinoma in the United States and other countries of the industrialized West (Blot, Devesa, & Fraumeni, 1993). Adenocarcinoma nearly always arises in columnar-lined esophagus (CLE), or Barrett's esophagus, a complication of long-standing gastroesophageal reflux disease (Haggitt, 1992). Adenocarcinoma of the esophagus now accounts for approximately 65% of all cases at our center. This dramatic change has resulted in a renewed interest in this disease. A detailed yet simplified discussion of esophageal cancer follows. Emphasis is placed on the diagnostic, therapeutic, and rehabilitation aspects and the role played by the entire dysphagia team.

EPIDEMIOLOGY

Recent studies estimate that in 1997 there were 12,500 new cases and 11,500 deaths due to esophageal cancer in the United States (Parker, Tong, Bolden, & Wingo, 1997). It is one of the top five killer malignancies between ages 55–74 years. These statistics continue to show an increase over the previous years. The incidence of adenocarcinoma of the esophagus is rising faster than any other malignancy in the White population in the United States (Blot et al., 1993).

Although historically relatively infrequent in the United States, squamous cell type is one of the commonest cancers worldwide (Day, 1984). This cell type is discussed first. Distinguishing features of squamous cell cancer (SCCA) and adenocarcinoma are discussed at various points and later under the section dealing specifically with adenocarcinoma. SCCA displays very high geographical variation in incidence. There are pockets of high incidence of SCCA in various parts of the world and within various countries. Among the most well known of these is the Asian esophageal cancer belt, which includes the Henan province in China, Caspian region of Iran, India, and Sri Lanka (Silber, 1985; Wynder, Reddy, McCoy, Weisberger, & Williams, 1976). Other regions of high prevalence include regions of South Africa inhabited by the Bantu tribe (Rose, 1973). Within the United States there are areas of high incidence in Alaska, South Carolina, and around Washington, DC (Brown et al., 1988).

ETIOLOGY

As is the case with many neoplastic conditions, more than one etiologic factor is likely. Epidemiological data are used to understand their role. Geographic variation discussed above points to a probable role of environmental and lifestyle factors. Various etiologic factors incriminated in the causation of esophageal carcinoma are given in Table 7–1. SCCA appears to have a multifactorial causation, whereas nearly all adenocarcinomas appear to arise in Barrett's esophagus, a condition resulting in metaplastic replacement of the normal squamous epithelium of the esophagus with columnar epithelium. Tobacco and alcohol in conjunction are considered to be the most important risk factors for SCCA in the United States (Weinbeck, & Berges, 1981; Wynder & Mabuchi, 1973). The type of alcohol consumed or the tar content of cigarettes may also have a role (Brown et al., 1988; La Vecchia, Liati, Decarli, Negrello, & Franceschi, 1986). In contrast, little alcohol is consumed in Iran and northern China. Interaction between genetic and environmental factors is also not uniformly understood. Australia, a country with similar ethnic population and lifestyle as the industrialized West, has a relatively low prevalence of esophageal carcinoma. Studies conducted in Linxian County in northern China provide some

intriguing insight into the causation of this disease (Li et al., 1989). This county has one of the highest rates for SCCA in the world (161 and 103 per 100,000 for men and women, respectively). The high tumor rate appears to be related to the consumption of pickled vegetables contaminated with the fungus *Geotrichum candidum* (Chang, Syrjanen, Wang, & Syrjanen, 1992). The high incidence of SCCA in humans is also closely paralleled by a high incidence of pharyngoesophageal tumors in domestic fowls, indicating a common soil factor. Human papillomavirus infection appears to be remarkably prevalent in these regions and may play a role in the etiology of these tumors.

Various conditions associated with a high risk of developing SCCA have been identified and are listed in Table 7–1. Of these, tylosis, a rare genetic disorder with autosomal dominant inheritance, has a 100% chance of developing into esophageal carcinoma, often at a young age (Schwindt, Berhardt, & Johnson, 1970). Over a period of 15–20 years, SCCA develops in 2–7% of cases of achalasia (Wychulis, Woolman, Anderson, & Ellis, 1981).

PATHOLOGY

There is a slow progression from a normal cell to various intermediate morphologies before a frank malignancy develops. This

TABLE 7–1. Risk Factors For Esophageal Cancer

Squamous Cell Cancer	Adenocarcinoma
Alcohol, tobacco	Columnar-lined esophagus
Geotrichum candidum	(or Barrett's esophagus)
(fungus)	
Human papillomavirus	
Lye ingestion	
Head and neck cancer	
Achalasia	
Celiac disease	
Tylosis	
Plummer-Vinson syndrome	

transformation occurs through a sequence of inflammation, atypia, dysplasia, and carcinoma in situ followed by an invasive carcinoma that is seen in both SCCA and adenocarcinoma. In the Western world the early forms of esophageal carcinoma are usually not seen because of the delay in diagnosis. Typically, carcinoma is diagnosed after spread to adjacent structures has already occurred (Ohta, Nakazawa, Segawa, & Yoshino, 1986).

Squamous carcinoma typically involves the mid-thoracic region of the esophagus and invades the submucosa and lymph nodes before becoming symptomatic. Histology varies from well-differentiated type with keratinization and pearl formation to poorly differentiated. There is no apparent relationship between differentiation and prognosis (Ohta et al., 1986).

Most lesions are more than 4 cm long at the time of diagnosis. Occasionally, massive tumors measuring more than 10 cm are also seen. Rapid lymphatic spread, especially in cephalad direction, occurs well beyond the macroscopic margins of the tumor. The nearest periesophageal lymph nodes belong to the common mediastinal nodal system and transport lymph bilaterally, thus facilitating multicentric spread (Akiyama, Tsurumaru, & Ono, 1981). The growth pattern is longitudinal and extramural rather than circumferential. An intramural tumor measuring more than 5 cm has a 90% chance of having metastasized to regional nodes. Absence of the serosal layer facilitates spread of esophageal carcinoma into the periesophageal tissue.

Metastasis occurs most commonly to trachea, bronchi, lungs, pleura, major vessels, and the diaphragm, with formation of esophagopulmonary or tracheoesophageal fistulae in 6–12% of cases. Figure 7–1 is a barium study showing a large tracheoesophageal fistula secondary to a squamous cell carcinoma. Figure 7–2 is an endoscopic photograph of the same lesion (the fistula is seen as a black, round opening). Distant metastasis occurs less commonly and is not clinically significant for SCCA (Boyce, 1993).

CLINICAL MANIFESTATIONS

Dysphagia, or difficulty in swallowing, is the classic symptom of esophageal cancer and indicates extensive involvement of the esophagus and surrounding structures in about 90% of patients (McKeown, 1986). Most patients have had the tumor for months to years before the onset of dysphagia. Onset of dysphagia often indicates that more than two thirds of the circumference of the esophageal wall is involved with tumor (Boyce, 1993; Edwards, 1974). Most patients delay seeking medical assistance. About 10% of patients have had warning symptoms such as retrosternal pressure, discomfort, or transient sense of fullness. Many patients unknowingly alter their eating habits and avoid tough/hard foods such as beef and unpeeled apples before even noticing or complaining of dysphagia. Others slow their speed of eating and chew their food more carefully, in effect converting solid food into pureed consistency in the mouth to overcome the esophageal obstruction. A careful history with detailed questioning of the patient regarding his or her food habits often reveals the progressive nature of dysphagia. As emphasized by Boyce, health professionals including physicians, nurses, and speech-language pathologists should be alert to the fact that dysphagia is never psychogenic (Boyce, 1993). In a normal individual a food bolus reaches the stomach within 10 s of initiation of swallow. A feeling of delay in passage of the bolus beyond a few seconds thus warrants investigation.

Odynophagia, or painful swallowing, is often not a prominent symptom. When present, pain may be in the form of chest pressure/ache due to passage or impaction of solid food. This is described as impact pain. Pain may also be burning in nature due to topical effects of irritant substances such as alcohol and citrus juice. A third type of pain experienced during swallowing is due to mediastinal involvement by the mass, occurs late in the disease process, and often requires narcotic analgesics (Boyce, 1993).

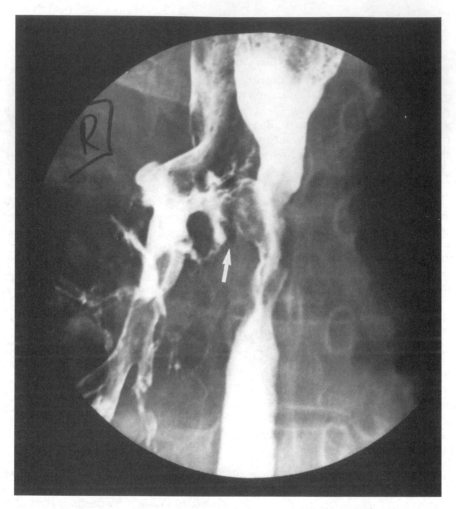

Figure 7–1. Barium radiograph showing a large tracheoesophageal fistula.

Other symptoms that often accompany or precede dysphagia include sialorrhea, or increased salivation. This results from an increased output of saliva from the salivary glands as an attempt to clear the obstruction of the esophageal lumen. During late stages, blockage of the lumen by impacted food and mass also reduces the clearance of salivary secretions, thus resulting in excess foamy mucus. Inconvenience of swallowing in association with anorexia due to the disease state results in reduced caloric intake, lassitude, weakness, and weight loss. All of these set off a vicious cycle resulting in malnutrition, anemia, and cachexia.

Pulmonary sequelae of esophageal carcinoma may be secondary to fistula formation or due to regurgitation of the retained esophageal contents into the pharynx and aspiration. These symptoms may often result in involvement of the speech-language pathologist for evaluation of the swallowing mechanism. Thus, familiarity with these symptoms is essential. Unexplained cough in a patient with SCCA may result from mediastinal/tracheal involvement. Pulmonary symptoms and pneumonia are often terminal events in debilitated patients.

Dysphonia, or vocal breathiness, in patients with esophageal cancer is likely due

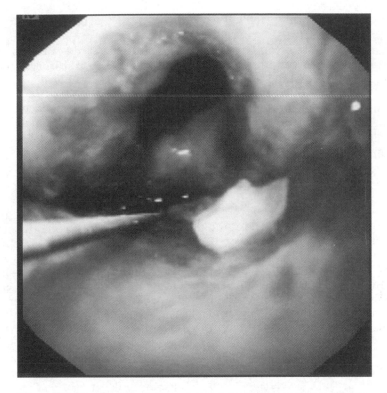

Figure 7–2. Endoscopic photograph showing a tracheoesophageal fistula.

to involvement of the recurrent laryngeal nerve, especially on the left side. During the embryonal stage, as the arch of aorta develops on the left side, it prevents the cephalad migration of this nerve on the left. Thus, in adult life, the left recurrent laryngeal nerve is more prone to be involved by mediastinal tumors. In practice, vocal hoarseness is a more prominent feature after patients have received radiation therapy to the chest cavity. Excessive pooling of tenacious secretions in the hypopharynx, inability to manage even normal or reduced quantity of secretions due to poor motor function after radiation, or a debilitated state may be other causes of dysphonia in patients with esophageal carcinoma.

DIAGNOSIS

Diagnosis of the cancer can often be made based on age group, history of alcohol and tobacco use, and clinical symp-toms. A typical scenario is a 50- to 60-year-old male with rapidly progressive dysphagia and weight loss. Radiographic techniques aid in establishing a clinical suspicion. Plain radiograph of the chest can often reveal subtle signs such as indentation of the tracheal air shadow posteriorly or deviation of trachea away from the midline. Mediastinal lymphadenopathy may be another useful sign. An air-contrast barium esophagram is an extremely sensitive technique in the diagnosis of esophageal cancer. It is also accurate in delineating the length of tumor and spatial contour of the esophagus. Endoscopy with biopsy and brush cytology is the most sensitive and specific means of diagnosing esophageal carcinoma (Graham, Schwartz, Cain, & Gyorkey, 1982; Winawer, Sherlock, Belladonna, Melamed, & Beattie, 1975). The procedure is performed under intravenous sedation and is well tolerated.

Computed tomography (CT) is a fairly sensitive and specific technique in identifying and accurately locating esophageal masses. It provides useful information regarding lymph node involvement and distant metastasis to liver and other abdominal organs. The technique is very widely available in the United States but has limitations in accurately identifying the depth of intramural invasion and lymph node metastasis (Tio, Cohen, & Coene, 1989).

STAGING

Currently, the most accepted staging classification for esophageal cancer is that given by the American Joint Committee for Cancer Staging. This classification follows the TNM method of classification based on the depth of tumor invasion, lymph node involvement, and distant metastasis (Beahrs, Hensen, Hutter, & Meyers, 1988).

All patients diagnosed with esophageal cancer should undergo staging, initially with a CT scan. If the CT scan does not show any regional/distant metastasis, endoscopic ultrasonography should be considered, if available.

Role of Endoscopic Ultrasonography in Cancer Staging

Endoscopic ultrasonography, a recent innovation in endoscopy, incorporates an ultrasonic probe into an endoscope. This technique is the most accurate means of identifying the depth of invasion and lymph node involvement in esophageal cancer. It has been shown to be superior to CT scanning in these respects (Botet et al., 1991; Tio et al., 1989). Figure 7–3 is a photograph showing a large esophageal mass extending to the muscle layer. A round, hypoechoic lymph node is shown in Figure 7–4. It is now possible to obtain aspiration cytology specimens from the lymph nodes using this technique. This has resulted in enhanced accuracy of diagnosing lymph node metastasis. The technique, however, is not universally available as yet and is not useful for identifying distant metastasis.

TREATMENT

As outlined above, most patients in the Western Hemisphere present with advanced/incurable disease. A minority of patients are fortunate to have their malignancy diagnosed early enough to receive a curative surgical resection. The remaining majority must look to palliative measures as their only recourse.

Surgery

Esophagogastrectomy with primary anastomosis (esophagogastrostomy) is the treatment of choice for this condition (Ellis, Gibb, & Watkins, 1983). Despite significant advances made in postoperative intensive care management of patients, this procedure continues to have a high operative morbidity and mortality. Although differing claims have been made, with postoperative mortality rates varying between 10–33%, the overall 5-year survival has remained around 6% (Galandiuk, Hemann, Cosgrove, & Gassman, 1986). In a review of 122 published reports Earlam found that, of 100 patients presenting with esophageal carcinoma, 58 will undergo surgery; of these, only 26 will leave the hospital and only 4 will survive for 5 years (Earlam & Cunha-Melo, 1980). Complications include anastomotic leakage, tumor recurrence, and stricture formation. Periprocedure complications and mortality depend on a host of factors such as the location of the tumor, type of surgery, colon interposition, stapling, experience of the surgeon, and nutritional status of the patient. Distal lesions usually have a better outcome. Diligent preoperative staging is important in selecting patients for surgery and improving survival. Figure 7–5 is a graphic representation of effect of preoperative stage on patient survival.

Radiation Therapy

Patients undergoing radiation therapy alone are usually not surgical candidates due to tumor stage or coexisting medical illnesses. The overall results of radiation ther-

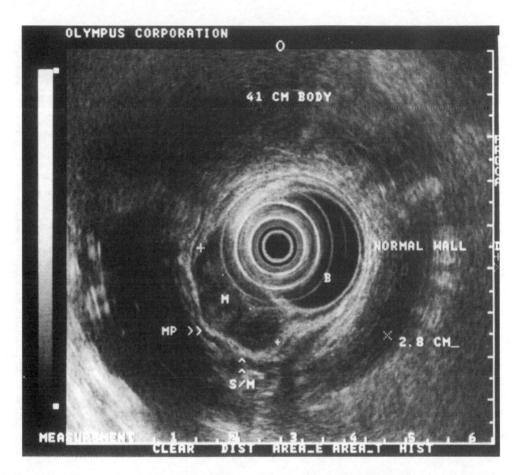

Figure 7–3. Endoscopic ultrasound photograph showing an esophageal tumor (M) confined to the muscle layer (MP).

apy alone, however, are comparable to those of surgery alone (Okawa, Kita, Tanaka, & Ikeda, 1989). This mode of therapy by itself is palliative, with duration of relief of dysphagia ranging from 2–12 months (Kelsen, 1984). A combination of chemotherapy and radiation therapy is currently the preferred modality in patients who are able to withstand the associated morbidity.

Intraluminal radiation therapy (brachytherapy) may be provided using a nasally introduced delivery system (Figure 7–6). This form of therapy is used either in patients who cannot receive external beam radiation or to provide higher doses of radiation without overexposing the adjacent

organs. A radium or cobalt 60 source is used to provide 1,200 to 2,500 cGy in two to three sessions over a period of weeks. Esophageal damage including severe esophagitis, ulceration, stricture formation, and tracheoesophageal fistula formation may occur as a result of radiation therapy. The acute esophagitis seen after radiation therapy is shown in Figure 7–7, and Figure 7–8 is a composite photograph of a patient with a malignant stricture. The patient received radiation therapy and developed a smooth contoured radiation stricture at the same site. This was followed, 2 years later, by recurrence of carcinoma at the distal end of the radiation stricture.

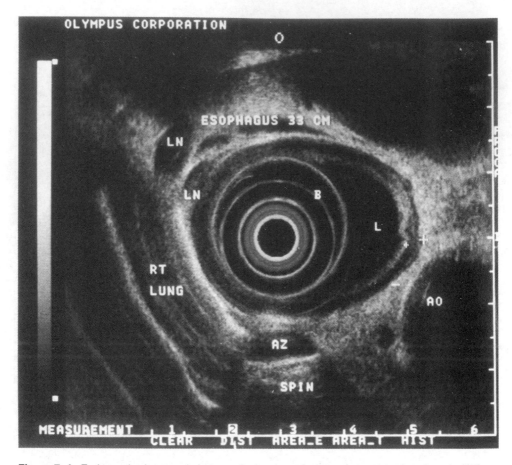

Figure 7–4. Endoscopic ultrasound photograph showing a malignant-appearing lymph node (LN).

Chemoradiation Therapy

A combination of chemotherapy and radiation therapy employed either sequentially or concomitantly has now been shown to be superior to radiation therapy alone. In these regimens, chemotherapy usually consists of two or three agents (Herskovic et al., 1992; Hukku, Fernandes, Vasishta, & Sharma, 1989; Sischy et al., 1990). Chemoradiation therapy may be provided after surgical resection of tumor (adjuvant) or prior to surgery (neoadjuvant). The median survival with chemoradiation therapy is about 12 months as compared to about 9 months with radiation alone (Herskovic et al., 1992). Chemoradiation therapy is also being employed as a primary modality, with comparable results, in patients who either cannot undergo surgery or refuse surgery. No trials have been done comparing surgery alone and chemoradiation therapy alone in tumors limited to the esophagus or to regional nodes. Using high doses of radiation therapy (5,000–6,400 cGy) in combination with chemotherapy has obvious local and systemic adverse effects. Therefore, smaller doses of radiation are being used in clinical trials, and preliminary data appear to be comparable.

ADENOCARCINOMA OF THE ESOPHAGUS

Adenocarcinoma of the esophagus differs greatly from squamous cell carcinoma. The United States, and the Western world

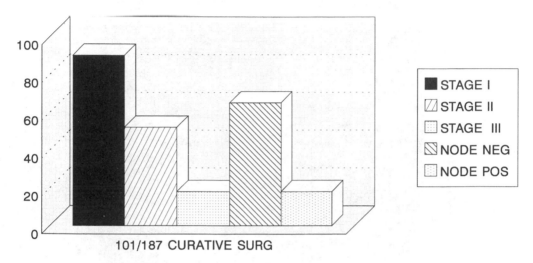

Figure 7–5. Esophageal cancer: Effect of preoperative staging on survival. (Data from "Does Esophagectomy Cure a Respectable Cancer?" by I. El Nakadi, J.-J. Jouben, F. Gay, J. Closset, M. Gelin, and J.-P. Lambilliotte, 1993, pp. 760–765, *World Journal of Surgery, 17.*)

in general, is currently seeing an unexplained epidemic of this disease (Blot et al., 1993; Haggitt, 1992). Although SCCA continues to be the predominant cell type in African American males, adenocarcinoma currently forms the majority of esophageal cancer seen in White males. The annual incidence of this tumor in White males is 1–2 per 100,000 (Blot et al., 1993). As outlined earlier, this cell type arises almost exclusively in a premalignant condition called Barrett's esophagus or CLE (Haggitt, Tryzelaar, Ellis, & Colcher, 1978). As the name suggests, in CLE the normal squamous epithelium of the esophagus is replaced by columnar epithelium containing goblet cells. This metaplastic epithelium thus resembles the intestinal epithelium, hence the name intestinal metaplasia. CLE is widely acknowledged to occur in response to long-standing gastroesophageal reflux disease. Why CLE and adenocarcinoma

occur primarily in White males is unknown. The cancer develops over a period of several years, being preceded by low- and high-grade dysplasia. Patients with CLE have nearly a 6% lifetime risk of developing esophageal cancer (Phillips & Wong, 1991).

Clinical Manifestations

In initial stages, adenocarcinoma may be completely asymptomatic. Ninety-eight percent of patients have symptoms of reflux disease but no symptoms specific to the malignancy. In later stages, symptoms are due to obstruction and are similar to those of SCCA.

Adenocarcinoma typically occurs in the distal esophagus. It has a softer consistency and has a more polypoid growth pattern (Figure 7–9). Coexisting CLE can often be seen. Its radiographic and endoscopic appearance thus differs greatly

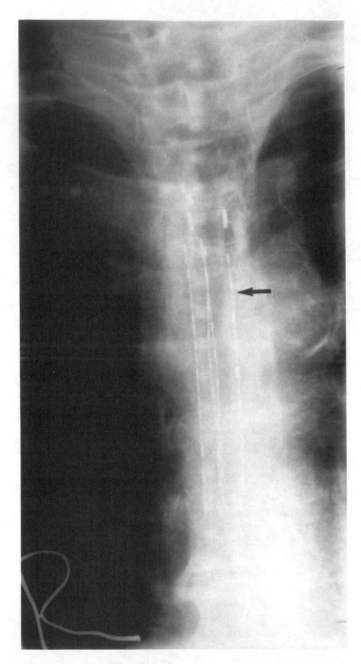

Figure 7–6. Radiograph showing a brachytherapy applicator in place.

from that of SCCA. Distant metastasis to the liver occurs more frequently and invasion of the bronchial tree and fistula formation are much less common than with SCCA.

Diagnosis

Diagnosis is typically made by endoscopic biopsy. Early stages of this cancer can be detected by periodic surveillance of patients

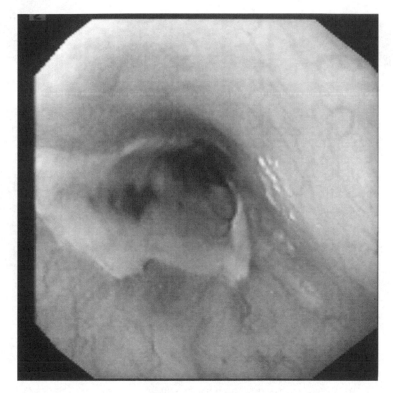

Figure 7–7. Endoscopic photograph showing radiation-induced esophagitis.

with CLE. Brush cytology and flow cytometry are special techniques, which provide higher accuracy when used in conjunction with biopsy (Reid, Sanchez, Blount, & Levine, 1987, 1991). CT is useful in assessing distant metastasis. As previously outlined for SCCA, endoscopic ultrasonography is superior to CT in assessing local and regional spread. At present, diagnosis is typically made after the cancer has spread beyond the muscular layer of the esophagus. Emphasis is thus being placed on developing effective surveillance of CLE and prevention and early detection of adenocarcinoma.

Treatment

Treatment strategies and results are similar to those seen in SCCA. These patients receive chemotherapy more often because of higher incidence of metastasis to the liver. Surgery is technically easier due to the distal location of the lesion; however, overall reported 5-year survival is comparable (Law, Fok, Cheng, & Wong, 1992). Several studies have reported that the response to chemoradiation therapy is similar to that seen with SCCA, with a 3-year survival of about 35% (Coia, Engstrom, & Paul, 1987; Naunheim et al., 1995; Orringer, 1993).

PALLIATIVE STRATEGIES IN ESOPHAGEAL CARCINOMA

Because the diagnosis of both cell types of esophageal cancer is typically made at a fairly late stage, a complete cure is often not possible. Thus, in many patients, palliation of symptoms becomes the primary goal of intervention. Several modalities including surgery, radiation therapy, chemotherapy, and chemoradiation therapy can be used for this purpose. The guiding prin-

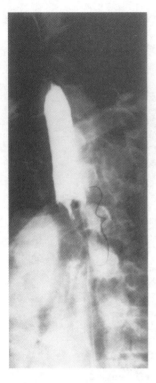
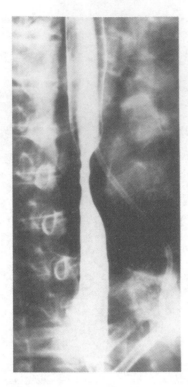
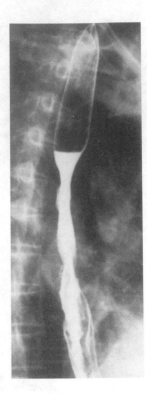

Figure 7–8. Composite photograph showing (from left to right) a malignant stricture, a radiation stricture, and the same after recurrence of cancer at distal end.

ciples of palliative therapy should be patient comfort, quality of life, availability of expertise, and maintaining nutritional adequacy. Because some of the palliative modalities achieve comparable results, individual selection and patient preference may play a role. With the recent advances in endoscopic techniques, several endoscopic palliative options have become available. These include peroral esophageal dilation, laser or thermoablation of tumor, photodynamic therapy, and esophageal endoprosthesis or stent placement.

Of all the palliative therapies, esophageal dilation is the most basic. It can temporarily provide the patient with the ability to swallow salivary secretions, liquids, or soft diet. Even if no other intervention is planned, a regimen of repeated dilations can be evolved to provide a good quality of life. Esophageal dilation can also be performed while other strategies are being planned. Performed properly, esophageal dilation is a safe

modality even in the most constricting lesions (Boyce, 1984, 1993).

The next class of endoscopic palliation techniques involves ablation of the tumor mass and consequent restoration of the luminal patency of the esophagus. This group of therapies includes laser therapy using neodymium: yttrium-aluminum-garnet (Nd:YAG) laser, where the tumor is coagulated using heat from the laser source (Lightdale, Zimbalist & Winawer, 1987). A similar approach is used when the tumor is ablated using other sources of heat such as a thermal probe or electrocautery. A more recent technique called photodynamic therapy uses photosensitizing agents and laser light from an argon laser. The sensitized tumor is thus ablated by absorbed light (Lambert, 1990). Chemoablation using 100% alcohol injection into the tumor has also been used. These ablative therapies are comparable in terms of the results achieved, but vary in cost and expertise

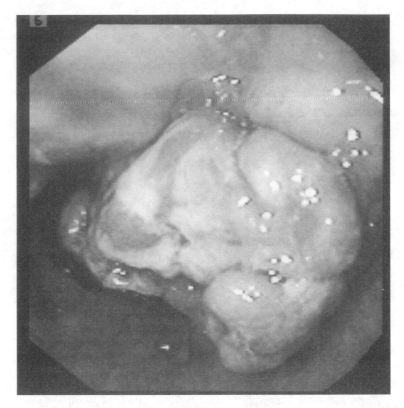

Figure 7–9. Endoscopic photograph of an adenocarcinoma in the distal esophagus.

required. These modalities also share a common shortcoming in that they require repeated sessions and may result in increased pain (Tytgat, den Hartog Jager, & Bartelsman, 1986).

Esophageal endoprosthesis or stent placement (Figure 7–10) is the palliative technique of preference at our center. This type of palliation often prevents the patient from undergoing repeated procedures, and provides quick relief of dysphagia while maintaining the nutritional status (Low & Kozarek, 1988). The availability of newer varieties of stents has considerably reduced the incidence of serious complications traditionally associated with these devices. However, the success of this modality depends on the proper training of the endoscopist, site and morphology of the lesion, and selection of the prosthesis (Kozarek, Ball, & Patterson, 1992). Stents are the only modal-ity available for patients who develop tracheoesophageal fistulas resulting from tumor invasion into the respiratory tract.

EFFECTS OF CANCER TREATMENT ON SWALLOWING

The derangement of normal swallowing function caused by cancer therapy is often poorly understood by the physicians. This may lead to the patient's trading one type of dysphagia for another. In our experience speech-language pathologists, rehabilitation services personnel, and nutritionists often have very useful insight into these problems. A true dysphagia team approach should be adopted for dealing with these problems. Consultation and assistance should be sought from these quarters whenever indicated.

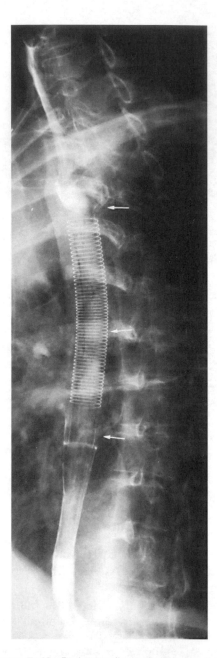

Figure 7–10. Barium radiograph showing a mid-esophageal prosthesis (plastic type).

Patients undergoing chemotherapy and/or radiation therapy may have a worsening of their dysphagia immediately after the start of the treatment. This occurs due to acute erosive esophagitis that often accompanies therapy. Odynophagia, or painful swallowing, occurs, further reducing oral intake and worsening the nutritional and hydration status of the patient. Treatment is symptomatic using lidocaine gel and/or sucralfate and acid suppressing drugs, and providing an alternative route of nutrition. Nausea and vomiting associated with therapy may further aggravate the patient's general condition. Hematemesis can result from a mucosal tear (Mallory-Weiss syndrome) occurring during forceful vomiting episodes.

External beam radiation therapy may cause a constellation of adverse effects in patients who survive longer than a few months. These include xerostomia, loss of taste buds, decreased range of movement and laxity of the oropharyngeal connective tissue, stiffening of epiglottis, fibrosis of tissue in the vallecula and pyriform sinuses, and reduced elevation of larynx during swallowing. Xerostomia, or dry mouth, inhibits the ability to form a food bolus. Reduced elasticity and fibrosis of the oropharyngeal tissue further impede the oral and pharyngeal phases of swallowing (Rhodus, Moller, Colby, & Bereuter, 1995). A stiff epiglottis and immobile larynx increase the risk of aspiration. Similarly a fibrotic cricopharyngeus may not allow the passage of the food bolus. Radiation therapy can result in pharyngeal and esophageal stricture formation requiring repeated dilations. Pooling of secretions proximal to the stricture may result in aspiration and related morbidity. A loss of taste buds reduces the patient's desire to eat, thus contributing to weight loss and malnutrition. Loss of saliva will frequently result in halitosis, further reducing the self-esteem of the patient. Lymphedema occurs due to inadequate drainage of the lymphatics from the scarred cervical tissue. This causes further stiffening of the skin and soft tissue around the neck and worsening of dysphagia.

QUALITY-OF-LIFE ISSUES

Many patients who are diagnosed at a later stage do not live long enough to suffer from the delayed effects described above. Patients undergoing palliative management for nonresectable disease have a mean survival of a few months (Coia, Engstrom & Paul, 1987). It is, therefore, of utmost importance that all attempts be made to add a life to the days and not just add days to the life. Pain must be avoided and minimized whenever possible. Inclusion of the patient in all major and minor decisions relating to his or her treatment may provide a sense of control. Education of the patient at every step of the treatment may greatly reduce the fear of the unknown. Patience and a keen understanding of the physiology of various symptoms are required of all involved. Recent emphasis on enrollment of these patients in a hospice program has greatly reduced the burden of care of both family and the physicians. Unfortunately, in the present scenario of shrinking health care funding, a significant proportion of patients may not be able to avail themselves of this crucial assistance.

DEPRESSION IN PATIENTS WITH ESOPHAGEAL CANCER

Depression may result from the knowledge of having an incurable illness, debilitating treatment, pain, economic instability, and excessive dependence on family members/health care providers. The depression may be made worse by the inability to participate in one of the most basic pleasures of living: EATING! Depression often affects the patient's desire to participate in rehabilitation, thus making the job of the dysphagia team even more difficult. Antidepressants should be prescribed when indicated.

ROLE OF THE DYSPHAGIA TEAM

An attempt has been made throughout this chapter to emphasize the debilitation caused by esophageal cancer and its treatment. It is of utmost importance to adopt a team approach to the care of these patients. This is a common practice at many tertiary care centers including ours. The team consists of a core group formed by gastroenterologists, oncologists, speech-language pathologists, and nutritionists. Additional support is obtained from physicians from other specialities such as otolaryngology, radiology, pain management/anesthesiology, and psychiatry as well as from home health care personnel and social workers. In our experience, the support of speech-language pathologists, nutritionists, and home health care personnel working in concert with physicians and family members is critical to the care of these patients. This approach results in better management of the patient's dysphagia, rapid decision making, and avoidance of unnecessary investigations. The patient and his or her family also receive a more personalized and compassionate treatment during a very difficult phase of these malignancies.

CONCLUSION

In conclusion, esophageal cancer, when diagnosed in later stages, is a very debilitating disease with significant morbidity and dismal 5-year survival rates. Strategies need to be developed to detect the disease early in its course. Recent times have seen a virtual epidemic of adenocarcinoma in White males, thus exponentially compounding the scale of the problem. Advances in molecular biology may hold the key to preventing the progression of CLE to adenocarcinoma. Palliation and enhancement of the quality of life should be the pillars of treatment strategies in patients with an advanced form of the disease.

REFERENCES

Akiyama, H., Tsurumaru, T., & Ono, T. (1981). Principles of surgical treatment of carcinoma of the esophagus. *Annals of Surgery, 194*, 438.

Beahrs, O. H., Hensen, D. E., Hutter, R. V., & Meyers, M. H. (American Joint Committee on Cancer) (1988). *Manual for staging cancer* (3rd ed). Philadelphia: J. B. Lippincott.

Blot, W. J., Devesa, S. S., Fraumeni, J. F. (1993). Continuing climb in rates of esophageal adenocarcinoma: An update. *JAMA, 270,* 1320.

Botet, J. F., Lightdale, C. J., Zauber, A. G., et al. (1991). Preoperative staging of esophageal cancer: Comparison of endoscopic US and dynamic CT. *Radiology, 181,* 419.

Boyce, H. W., Jr. (1984). Palliation of advanced esophageal cancer. *Seminars in Oncology, 11,* 186.

Boyce, H. W., Jr. (1993). Tumors of the esophagus. In M. H. Sleisenger & J. S. Fordtran (Eds.), *Gastrointestinal disease: Pathophysiology/diagnosis/management* (pp. 401-418). Philadelphia: W. B. Saunders.

Brown, L. M., Blot, W. J., Schuman, S. H., et al. (1988). Environmental factors and high risk of esophageal cancer among men in coastal South Carolina. *Journal of the National Cancer Institute, 80,* 1620.

Chang, F., Syrjanen, S., Wang, L., & Syrjanen, K. (1992). Infectious agents in the etiology of esophageal cancer. *Gastroenterology, 103,* 1336–1348.

Coia, L. R., Engstrom, P. F., & Paul, A. (1987). Nonsurgical management of esophageal cancer: Report of a study of combined radiotherapy and chemotherapy. *Journal of Clinical Oncology, 5,* 1783.

Day, N. E. (1984). The geographic pathology of cancer of the oesophagus. *British Medical Bulletin, 40,* 329.

Earlam, R., & Cunha-Melo, J. R. (1980). Oesophageal squamous cell carcinoma: I. A critical review of surgery. *British Journal of Surgery, 67,* 381.

Edwards, D. A. W. (1974). Carcinoma of the esophagus and fundus. *Postgraduate Medicine, 50,* 223.

Ellis, F. H., Jr., Gibb, S. P., & Watkins, E., Jr. (1983). Esophagogastrectomy: A safe, widely applicable, and expeditious form of palliation for patients with carcinoma of the esophagus and cardia. *Annals of Surgery, 198,* 531.

Galandiuk, S., Hemann, R. E., Cosgrove, D. M., & Gassman, J. J. (1986). Cancer of the esophagus. The Cleveland Clinic experience. *Annals of Surgery, 203,* 101.

Graham, D. Y., Schwartz, J. T., Cain, G. D., & Gyorkey, F. (1982). Prospective evaluation of biopsy number in the diagnosis of esophageal and gastric carcinoma. *Gastroenterology, 82,* 228.

Haggitt, R.C. (1992). Adenocarcinoma in Barrett's esophagus: A new epidemic. *Human Pathology, 23,* 475.

Haggitt, R. C.,Tryzelaar, J., Ellis, H., & Colcher, H. (1978). Adenocarcinoma complicating columnar epithelium-lined (Barrett's) esophagus. *American Journal of Clinical Pathology, 70,* 1.

Herskovic, A., Martz, K., Al-Sarraf, M., et al. (1992). Combined chemotherapy and radiotherapy compared with radiotherapy alone in patients with cancer of the esophagus. *New England Journal of Medicine, 326,* 1593.

Hukku, S., Fernandes, P., Vasishta, S., & Sharma,V. K. (1989). Radiation therapy alone and in combination with bleomycin and 5-fluorouracil in advanced carcinoma of the esophagus. *Indian Journal of Cancer, 26,* 131.

Kelsen, D. (1984). Current concepts in the treatment of esophageal cancer. In J. J. DeCosse & P. Sherlock (Eds.), *Clinical management of gastrointestinal cancer* (p. 123). Boston: Martinus Nijhoff.

Kozarek, R. A., Ball, T. J., & Patterson D. J. (1992). Metallic self-expanding stent application in the upper gastrointestinal tract: Caveats and concerns. *Gastrointestinal Endoscopy, 38,* 1.

Lambert, R. (1990). Photodynamic therapy for esophageal cancer. *Canadian Journal of Gastroenterology, 4,* 612.

La Vecchia, C. L., Liati, P., Decarli, A., Negrello, I., & Franceschi, S. (1986). Tar yields of cigarettes and the risk of oesophageal cancer. *International Journal of Cancer, 38,* 381.

Law, S. Y., Fok, M., Cheng, S. W., & Wong, J. (1992). A comparison of outcome after resection for squamous cell carcinomas and adenocarcinomas of the esophagus and cardia. *Surgery, Gynecology and Obstetrics, 175,* 107.

Li, J. Y., Ershow, A. G., Chen, Z. J., et al. (1989). A case-control study of cancer of the esophagus and gastric cardia in Linxian. *International Journal of Cancer, 43,* 755.

Lightdale, C. J., Zimbalist, E., & Winawer, S. J. (1987). Outpatient management of esophageal cancer with endoscopic Nd:YAG laser. *American Journal of Gastroenterology, 82,* 46.

Low, D. E., & Kozarek, R. A. (1988). Esophageal endoscopy, dilation and intraesophageal prosthetic devices. In L. E. Hill, R. W. McCallum, D. E. Mercer, & R. A. Kozarek (Eds), *The esophagus: Medical and surgical management* (pp. 47-59). New York: W. B. Saunders.

McKeown, K. C. (1986). Clinical presentation of carcinoma of the oesophagus. *Journal of the Royal College of Surgeons in Edinburgh, 31,* 199.

Naunheim, K. S., Petruska, P. J., Roy, T. S., Schlueter, J. M., Kim, H., & Baue, A. E. (1995). Multimodality therapy for adenocarcinoma of the esophagus. *Annals of Thoracic Surgery, 59,* 1085.

Ohta, H., Nakazawa, S., Segawa, K., & Yoshino, J. (1986). Distribution of epithelial dysplasia in the cancerous esophagus. *Scandinavian Journal of Gastroenterology, 21,* 392.

Okawa, T., Kita, M., Tanaka, M., & Ikeda, M. (1989). Results of radiotherapy for inoperable locally advanced esophageal cancer. *International Journal of Radiation Oncology, Biology, Physics, 17,* 49.

Orringer, M. B. (1993). Multimodality therapy for esophageal carcinoma—Update. *Chest, 103,* (Suppl. 4), 406–409.

Parker, S. L., Tong, T., Bolden, S., & Wingo, P. A. (1997). Cancer statistics, 1997. *CA: A Cancer Journal for Clinicians, 47*, 5–27.

Phillips, R. W., & Wong, R. K. H. (1991). Barrett's esophagus: Natural history, incidence, etiology and complications. *Gastroenterology Clinics of North America, 20*, 791.

Reid, B. J., Sanchez, C. A., Blount, P. L., & Levine, D. S. (1987). Barrett's esophagus: Correlation between flow cytometry and histology in detection of patients at risk for adenocarcinoma. *Gastroenterology, 93*, 1.

Reid, B. J., Sanchez, C. A., Blount, P. L., & Levine, D. S. (1991). Barrett's esophagus: Cell cycle abnormalities in advancing stages of neoplastic progression. *Gastroenterology, 105*, 119.

Rhodus, N. L., Moller, K., Colby, S., & Bereuter, J. (1995). Dysphagia in patients with three different etiologies of salivary gland dysfunction. *Ear, Nose and Throat Journal, 74*, 39.

Rose, E. (1973). Esophageal cancer in the Transkei: 1955-1969. *Journal of the National Cancer Institute, 51*, 7.

Schwindt, W. D., Berhardt, L. C., & Johnson, S. A. M. (1970). Tylosis and intrathoracic neoplasms. *Chest, 57*, 590.

Silber, W. (1985). Carcinoma of the oesophagus: Aspects of epidemiology and etiology. *Proceedings of the Nutrition Society, 52*, 24.

Sischy, B., Ryan, L., Haller, D., et al (1990). Interim report of EST 1282 phase III protocol for the evaluation of combined modalities in the treatment of patients with carcinoma of the esophagus, stage I-II. *Proceedings of the American Society of Clinical Oncology, 9*, 105.

Tio, T. L., Cohen, P., & Coene, P. P. (1989). Endosonography and computed tomography of esophageal carcinoma. *Gastroenterology, 96*, 1478.

Tytgat, G. N. J., den Hartog Jager, F. C. A., & Bartelsman, J. F. W. M. (1986). Endoscopic prosthesis for advanced esophageal cancer. *Endoscopy, 18*, 32.

Weinbeck, M., & Berges, W. (1981). Oesophageal lesions in the alcoholic. *Clinical Gastroenterology, 10*, 375.

Winawer, S. J., Sherlock, P., Belladonna, J. A., Melamed, M., & Beattie, E. G., Jr. (1975). Endoscopic brush cytology in esophageal cancer. *JAMA, 232*, 1358.

Wychulis, A. R., Woolman, G. L., Anderson, H. A., & Ellis, F. H. (1981). Achalasia and carcinoma of the esophagus. *JAMA, 266*, 1638.

Wynder, E. L., & Mabuchi, K. (1973). Cancer of the gastrointestinal tract. Etiological and environmental factors. *JAMA, 266*, 1546–1548.

Wynder, E. L., Reddy, B. S., McCoy, G. D., Weisberger, J. H., & Williams, G. M. (1976). Diet and gastrointestinal cancer. *Gastroenterology, 5*, 463.

8

Lung Cancer

*Carole S. Mackey, M.S., R.D.,
and John C. Ruckdeschel, M.D.*

Carcinoma of the lung is the commonest lethal malignancy in the United States (Boring, Squires, Tong, & Montgomery, 1994). Indeed, more patients die of lung cancer each year than of the next five most common cancers together. Lung cancer is primarily a disease of cigarette smokers, with over 90% of lung cancer patients having a significant smoking history, either primary or secondary (Shopland, Eyre, & Pechacek, 1991). Because lung cancer originates in the thorax (oftentimes adjacent to the mediastinum) and because a primary lymphatic drainage site is the mediastinal lymph nodes, lung cancer is often associated with significant compromise of swallowing and communicative processes. There are several avenues by which lung cancer can affect swallowing and speech: (a) due to direct extension or compression of local structures in the thorax, (b) due to the effects of extrathoracic metastases (e.g., brain), (c) due to several different paraneoplastic syndromes, and (d) as a direct or indirect consequence of therapy. This chapter will consider each of these in turn. In order to understand how lung cancer affects speech and swallowing we need to know how it presents, how we treat it, and how the organs involved are affected.

CLINICAL PRESENTATION AND TREATMENT OF LUNG CANCER

The earliest symptoms of lung cancer, cough and shortness of breath, are commonly ignored by patients and their physicians because they appear to represent only incremental changes in preexisting, smoking-related symptoms (e.g., smoker's cough). The commonest presenting sign of lung cancer, weight loss, is in actuality a late finding and is frequently ascribed to a new-found success in dieting. The end result of this self-deluding behavior is that only 7% of patients present with asymptomatic lesions, 27% present with signs of local advancement, and the remainder present with overt (brain, bone, liver) metastases (32%) or signs of systemic disease without overt metastases (e.g., weight loss, anorexia; 34%; Carbone, Frost, Feinstein, Higgins, & Selawry, 1970). The so-called early warning signs of lung cancer (change in cough, hemoptysis, hoarseness) are, by and large, late findings indicative of advanced disease.

Staging of Lung Cancer

The staging system was rationalized in 1985 with the description of four stages based on the usual therapeutic approaches

117

(e.g., surgery, radiation, or chemotherapy; Mountain, 1986). With the proliferation of combined modality approaches and the increasing sophistication of staging procedures, it became apparent that there was a need for a revision and this was accomplished in 1997 (Mountain, 1997). The stages of lung cancer are based on the TNM (tumor, node, metastases) nomenclature as defined in Table 8–1. Basically T status is represented first by tumor size and then by whether or not the tumor invades local intrathoracic structures. T3 lesions can be resected in toto and T4 lesions cannot be, but the definitions of *can* and *cannot* vary between surgeons and institutions despite the guidelines. Nodal status is the major aspect of intrathoracic disease that determines prognosis. N1 nodes are in the hilum of the lung or within the lung itself. N2 nodes involve the ipsilateral medi-

TABLE 8–1. International Staging System (TNM Classification)

Classification	Definition
Primary Tumor (T)	
T0	No evidence of primary tumor
TX	The tumor is identified cytologically by malignant cells in sputum samplings or bronchial washings. No specific site of origin can be recognized radiographically or bronchoscopically. Tumors that cannot be adequately assessed in retreatment staging are identified with this descriptor.
Tis	Carcinoma in situ
T1	The tumor is an invasive lesion 3.0 cm or less in greatest dimension, surrounded by lung or intact visceral pleura and without evidence of invasion proximal to or including a lobar bronchial orifice.*
T2	The tumor is more than 3.0 cm in greatest dimension, invades the visceral pleura, or has associated atelectasis or pneumonitis extending to the hilum. The proximal extent may include the lobar bronchial orifice, bronchus intermedius, or main-stem bronchus but must be at least 2 cm distal to the carina. Any associated atelectasis must involve less than an entire lung.
T3	The tumor is any size and involves the parietal pleura, chest wall, diaphragm, mediastinal pleura, mediastinal fat, parietal pericardium, phrenic nerve, or vagus nerve; or a tumor in the main bronchus within 2 cm of the carina* without involving the carina; or a tumor-associated atelectasis or obstructive pneumonitis of the entire lung.
T4	The tumor is any size and invades the structures of the deep mediastinum including heart, great vessels, trachea, esophagus, vertebral body, or carina; or a tumor associated with a pleural effusion containing malignant cells.
Nodal Involvement (N)	
N0	No demonstrable metastasis to regional lymph nodes.
N1	Metastases to lymph nodes in the peribronchial or the ipsilateral hilar region, including nodes affected by direct extension of the tumor.
N2	Metastases to lymph nodes in the ipsilateral mediastinum or subcarina, including nodes affected by direct extension.
N3	Metastases to lymph nodes in the contralateral mediastinum, contralateral hilum, ipsilateral or contralateral scalene or supraclavicular regions.
Distant Metastasis (M)	
M0	No known distant metastasis
M1	Metastases to distant organs or other lymph node sites

Note: The uncommon superficial tumor of any size with its invasive component limited to the bronchial wall, which may extend proximal to the main bronchus, is also classified T1.

Source: Adapted from "A New International Staging System for Lung Cancer," by C. F. Mountain, 1986, *Chest, 89,* pp. 225S–233S.

astinum, and N3 nodes involve either contralateral mediastinal nodes or supra-clavicular nodes. The prognosis following surgery drops sharply when any lymph nodes are involved and falls to zero when N3 nodes are involved. The M category refers to the presence or absence of distant metastatic disease, and, when present, this finding overwhelms most of the local factors in its impact on survival. The final staging classification and its various TNM subsets are listed in Table 8–2.

Histologic Characteristics of Lung Cancer

The bronchopulmonary tree is, in fact, a highly complex organ with gas exchange, secretory, immunologic, and endocrine functions (Jetten, 1991). The various cells making up the bronchial epithelium appear to arise from a common progenitor cell, with subsequent differentiation to specific functions (Gazdar et al., 1990). Virtually all lung cancers appear to arise in these differentiation-committed cells so that the histology of lung cancer mirrors these functions. The specific cell types of lung cancer (Table 8–3) are broadly characterized into small cell or non-small cell lung cancer (SCLC or NSCLC). The SCLC subset (approximately 20–25% of lung cancers) arise from neuroendocrine cells in the bronchial epithelium and tend to behave somewhat differently. They tend to spread very early in their course and are considered widespread in virtually all instances (Ihde, 1985). They were also considered to be a favorable subset due to their increased sensitivity to chemotherapy. However, stagnation in the development of new drugs for SCLC and a proliferation of new agents for NSCLC have almost eliminated any differences in outcome. By tradition, SCLC has been staged as limited (confined to the hemithorax) or extensive without regard to the TNM staging system (Table 8–2).

Adenocarcinomas and large cell carcinomas arise primarily from glandular elements of the mucosa, and squamous cell cancers from the more proximal lining

TABLE 8–2. Stage Grouping—TNM Subsets

Stage	TNM Subset
0	Carcinoma in situ
IA	T1N0M0
IB	T2N0M0
IIA	T1N1M0
IIB	T2N1M0
	T3N0M0
IIIA	T3N1M0
	T1N2M0
	T2N2M0
	T3N2M0
IIIB	T4N0M0
	T4N1M0
	T4N2M0
	T1N3M0
	T2N3M0
	T3N3M0
	T4N3M0
IV	Any T Any N M1

Note: Staging is not relevant for occult carcinoma, designated TXN0M0.

Source: Adapted from "Revisions in the International System for Staging Lung Cancer," by C. F. Mountain, 1997, *Chest, III,* pp. 1710–1717.

TABLE 8–3. Histological Subtypes of Lung Cancer

Non-small cell lung cancers
Squamous cell carcinoma
Adenocarcinoma
Large cell carcinoma
Bronchoalveolar carcinoma
Large cell neuroendocrine
Adenosquamous, clear cell, giant cell
Carcinosarcoma, adenocystic (all uncommon)
Small cell lung cancers
Small cell anaplastic
Small cell or oat cell type
Intermediate cell type
Carcinoids
Atypical carcinoids

cells. Broncheoalveolar carcinomas arise from the terminal gas-exchange cells and tend to be multicentric in origin. They are usually lumped with adenocarcinomas for analysis (Gould & Warren, 1995).

Overview of Treatment

Table 8–4 lists the generally accepted approaches to treating both NSCLC and SCLC on a stage-by-stage basis. It is often stated that surgery is the only curative treatment for NSCLC, but upwards of 25% of patients with locally advanced NSCLC may be cured by nonoperative approaches (combined chemotherapy and radiation; Wagner, 1993). Increasingly, lung cancer is treated by a combination of therapies. The need to include many of the organs involved in speech and swallowing in the field of treatment results in the significant impact of therapy on speech and swallowing.

ETIOLOGY AND MANAGEMENT OF SPEECH/SWALLOWING DYSFUNCTION IN PATIENTS WITH LUNG CANCER

Syndromes Due To Local Invasion and Compression

Dysphagia

Dysphagia is a symptom of an underlying condition that affects the swallowing pro-cess. It is defined as any difficulty with chewing or swallowing foods, beverages, or medications.

The origins of dysphagia can be neurogenic, myogenic, or obstructive, and it is categorized as either oropharyngeal or esophageal. Oropharyngeal dysphagia affects the transfer of food from the mouth or the pharynx, whereas esophageal dysphagia involves obstructive or motor disorders that interfere with the transfer of food from the mouth to the stomach.

The cause and extent of the dysphagia need to be identified and interventions planned, when possible, because malnutrition due to the inadequate intake of calories, protein, and even water can occur. Also, aspiration can occur as a result of an inadequate or painful swallow.

Usually dysphagia is diagnosed by patient complaint, and the cause is determined by a temporal relationship to the disease or a recent treatment. A patient may complain of a sore throat, or that food seems to get stuck in the throat or chest. Health care providers and patient caretakers can evaluate the dysphagia by noting how frequently the difficulty with swallowing occurs, what types of food are tolerated, where the pain is located, and if choking and coughing occur with the swallow. Also a daily food record will help to determine the adequacy of the intake,

TABLE 8–4. Current Treatment Regimens for Lung Cancer

Stage	First-line Therapy	Other
IA	Surgery	None
IB	Surgery	Preop chemo
IIA	Surgery	Adjuvant RT ± chemo
IIB	Surgery & postop RT	Adjuvant chemo
IIIA	Surgery alone Preop chemo ± RT	Adjuvant RT ± chemo
IIIB	Chemo + RT	RT only Altered fractionation
IV	Chemo	Palliative care

Small cell
  Limited
  Extensive
	
	Chemo + RT
	Chemo
		
		± PCI
		± PCI

Note: chemo = chemotherapy; PCI = prophylactic cranial irradiation; RT = radiation therapy.

identifying when further nutrition intervention is needed (Grant & Rivera, 1995).

Dysphagia can occur due to direct invasion of the esophagus, which is quite rare, or due to extrinsic compression by regional lymph nodes (more common), but only 2–3% of lung cancer patients present with dysphagia (Hyde & Hyde, 1974). In this case patients will present primarily with difficulty swallowing solids and initial management can be directed at modifying the texture and consistency of food and avoiding bulky foods (Table 8–5). Nutritionally enhanced liquids can restore a significant component of the patient's nutritional needs.

Dysphagia for liquids exclusively or for both liquids and solids (with or without subsequent aspiration) signals interference with the nerve supply to the esophagus. This can occur as a result of brain metastases or carcinomatous meningitis, as discussed later, or due to involvement of the recurrent laryngeal nerve, which partly innervates the cricoid muscles and the upper esophagus (Doyle & Aisner, 1995). It is vital to distinguish local involvement of the recurrent laryngeal nerve from the more ominous central nervous system lesions, as the treatment differs dramatically.

Hoarseness

A deepening or huskiness to the voice is quite common in lung cancer (approximately 19%), but true hoarseness is seen in only 3% of patients (Hyde & Hyde, 1974). It is invariably due to recurrent laryngeal nerve compression and is commoner in left-sided cancers due to the longer intrathoracic route for the left recurrent laryngeal nerve. On the left side it extends down to and under the aortic arch to an area of common lymph node involvement known as the aortopulmonary window. On the right side the recurrent laryngeal nerve only loops below the subclavian artery in the neck. Management of recurrent laryngeal nerve palsy is discussed elsewhere.

Syndromes Due to Extrathoracic Metastases

Central Nervous System Metastases

BRAIN METASTASES. Lung cancer is one of the commonest malignancies that metastasize to the brain. Ten percent of patients with lung cancer have brain metastases at presentation and 15–20% of patients develop brain metastases during the course of their illness (Newman & Hansen, 1974).

TABLE 8–5. Dietary Interventions for the Patient Suffering from Dysphagia

Avoid overwhelming the patient with too many choices

Provide only those food choices the patient has indicated they like and think they can manage

Serve snacks throughout the day, rather than three large meals

Modify food textures to soft or pureed foods

Avoid extremes of either hot or cold foods; serve foods at room temperature

Avoid acidic or bitter foods that may burn the throat

Avoid hard foods that may scratch

Serve mildly spiced, lightly salted, or sweet foods

Avoid foods that break up in the mouth or contain small pieces that may lodge in ulcerated tissues on swallowing

Drink beverages with foods

Provide a relaxed atmosphere for the patient to enjoy the meal and not feel pressured to eat

Source: Adapted from "Anorexia, cachexia, and dysphagia: The symptom experience," by M. M. Grant and L. M. Rivera, 1995, *Seminars in Oncology Nursing, 11,* pp. 266–271.

Brain tumor symptoms are of two basic types: nonfocal, which are symptoms related to the generalized effect of increased intracranial pressure, and site-specific/focal, which are symptoms of dysfunction of the particular area of brain that is affected.

Neurological deficits are dependent on location of the lesion, extent of brain edema, and intracranial pressure. Radiation therapy to the brain can also cause edema and brain swelling with resultant dysfunction, although this is poorly documented.

Extensive edema surrounding brain tumors or ventricular obstruction by the tumor can result in increased intracranial pressure with nausea and vomiting. Because there are no lymphatics in the brain to drain edematous fluid, it can accumulate and increase intracranial pressure, causing severe brain dysfunction.

About 20% of metastatic lesions occur in the posterior fossa where cranial nerves V, VII, IX, X, and XII make up a brainstem swallowing center which is usually triggered by either cortical influences or peripheral sensory stimuli, and, with interference, swallowing difficulties can occur (Newman & Hansen, 1974). As noted earlier, this will usually manifest itself as difficulty swallowing both liquids and solids.

LEPTOMENINGEAL METASTASES. Although uncommon, this devastating complication of lung cancer can seriously disrupt speech and swallowing. Changes in mental status, limb weakness and pain in a nonradicular pattern, neck and back pain, and loss of bowel/bladder function are common presenting signs (Rosen et al., 1982). Lesions often involve the base of the brain, however, resulting in highly specific loss of cranial nerve function, including that controlling swallowing.

GASTROINTESTINAL METASTASES. Metastases to the gastrointestinal tract occur in up to 12% of patients with lung cancer, but most are not diagnosed antemortem (Burbige, Radigan, & Belber, 1980). The commonest metastases are to the proximal large bowel and can be accompanied by apparent bowel obstruction, as the serosal metastasis leads either to paralytic ileus or intussusception of the metastatic lesion. Although metastases to the esophagus and proximal stomach are extremely rare, the obstructive symptoms from more distal lesions present with a similar inability to ingest food.

Management of speech and swallowing disorders due to extrathoracic metastases is directed at the metastatic lesions, not the esophagus. Brain metastases are treated with parenteral or oral steroids followed by cranial irradiation. Up to 70% of patients will have control of brain metastases, but the more advanced the presenting deficit, the less likely it is to improve. It is vital for therapists to remember that the steroids need to be tapered promptly after radiation, or severe candidal esophagitis can occur.

Leptomeningeal disease responds very poorly to treatment (Grossman et al., 1993). It usually incapacitates the patient and has an average life expectancy of 6 weeks. When symptoms are minimal, and life expectancy due to other metastatic lesions is reasonable, the disease is treated with an intraventricular reservoir and intrathecal chemotherapy. If cranial nerves are compromised the patient will need base of brain radiation as well as intrathecal chemotherapy, as the chemotherapy is poorly effective in this area.

Gastrointestinal metastases are an ominous sign in lung cancer. They are usually treated conservatively with suction but on occasion require extirpation of an obstructing site, or a diverting colostomy.

Paraneoplastic Syndromes

Anorexia/Cachexia Syndrome

Cancer cachexia is a syndrome of progressive wasting associated with weight loss, anorexia, early satiety, anemia, marked asthenia, and metabolic abnormalities (Table 8–6; Grant & Rivera, 1995). It has been directly associated with the presence of uncontrolled malignancy. The signs and symptoms are interrelated and are identifiable as a response to the tumor, as a response to the diagnosis of cancer,

TABLE 8–6. Characteristic Features of Cachexia

Wasting associated with malignancy, chronic disease, chronic infection

Weight loss continues despite adequate nutrient intake

Disproportionate loss of lean body mass, less effect on body fat and extracellular water

Resting energy expenditure and metabolic rates are increased or normal

Cytokine production is increased (e.g., tumor necrosis factor)

Hyperalimentation increases body weight by adding body fat and/or water, not lean body mass

Reversed by treating the cancer, treating the infection

and as side effects of antitumor treatment. Therefore it can be difficult to pinpoint cause and prescribe effective treatment (Table 8–7).

Cachexia is associated with most tumors and with all stages of disease, both localized and advanced. The exact etiology is unknown and cachexia is referred to as a paraneoplastic syndrome because the symptoms that are produced are often distant from the original tumor or its metastases (Albrecht & Canada, 1996; Grant & Rivera, 1995).

Weight loss is a frequent presenting symptom and continual problem with malignancies and is associated with poor response to treatment, reduced quality of life, and decreased survival. Weight loss is multifactorial and needs to be evaluated for possible intervention. Weight loss can be due to physiological, psychological, and/or social issues. Physiological issues include inadequate substrate intake due to an inability to eat caused by nausea, vomiting, dysphagia, esophagitis, and altered taste and smell, or altered substrate metabolism due to increased basal metabolic rate or increased cytokine release either by the tumor or in response to the tumor (Albrecht & Canada, 1996). Psychological and social issues related to the cancer diagnosis and prognosis, mental health status, and family support also contribute.

The treatment plan must continually provide for a review of patient medical, nutritional, and mental health indices for treatable causes of signs and symptoms in both patients being treated for disease and those in remission.

Research in anticachectic, or appetite-stimulating, therapies does not presume to affect survival, but reversing cachexia may increase a patient's quality of life. Two goals in using an anticachectic therapy are symptomatic care and improved nutrition intake. Eating fulfills more than just a physiological need, and by providing the ability to share meals with significant others again, nutrient intake with the resulting gain of a pound or two may result as well. For patients with anorexia-cachexia but with a functioning gastrointestinal tract, the target of therapy is the lack of desire to eat (Tchekmedyian, Halpert, Ashley, & Heber, 1992).

One of the first hypotheses for the lack of appetite in cancer patients was the role of serotonin and its precursor, tryptophan, and their close relationship to feeding behavior. Animal model experiments suggested a direct relationship between brain levels of serotonin and cachexia (Kardinal et al., 1990). The suppression of the activity of serotonin in the brain was theorized to possibly reverse cachexia. To this end, the antihistamine cyproheptadine was given as an appetite stimulant, and its use continues based more on anecdotal results than any results that could be proved with clinical trials (Kardinal et al., 1990).

Steroids are known to induce an increase in the appetite for several weeks, but for longer periods of time there are unacceptable side effects, such as muscle weakness, dysphoria, decreased potassium levels, hyperglycemia, edema, and immune dysfunction (Tchekmedyian et al., 1992).

TABLE 8–7. Factors Associated With Cachexia

Secretion of host-derived cytokines

Metabolic alterations

Decreased caloric intake

Nausea and vomiting

Gastrointestinal obstruction or dysfunction

Esophageal obstruction

Dysphagia

Depression

Source: Adapted from "Weight Loss and Human Immunodeficiency Virus Infection: Cachexia Versus Malnutrition," by S. L. Gorbach and T. A. Knox, 1992, *Infectious Diseases in Clinical Practice, 1,* pp. 224–229.

Megace, the semisynthetic derivative of progesterone, is used to stimulate appetite based on its use and resultant weight gain in patients with breast cancer (Rowland et al., 1996). An increase in appetite and weight gain have been seen in most patients who take the drug. A dose of 800 mg/day is associated with the highest level of appetite enhancement, with a median weight gain in one study of underweight patients of 9 kg. A liquid suspension is available, allowing increased tolerance to the therapy. Weight gain has been documented in patients regardless of their pretreatment weight, the extent or location of metastases, or tumor response to therapy. Studies show an increase in absolute body mass, appetite, and quality of life, with less nausea and vomiting. Patients need a normal swallowing function to benefit. Side effects include slight edema, which would be contraindicated in patients with congestive heart failure. The mechanism is not fully understood, but it appears to affect the receptors for progestins throughout the body, involving a variety of different and interrelated target sites (Gorter, 1991; Tchekmedyian et al., 1992).

The cannabinoid derivative dronabinol is also used as an appetite stimulant as well as an antiemetic (Gorter, 1991). It has been found to increase food intake, provide a sense of well-being, and promote weight gain. Side effects include a slight dizziness that is unpleasant to some and somnolence. Dronabinol given at bedtime has the effect of allowing a good night's sleep with the patient awaking with a ravenous appetite (Gorter, 1991). Dosing was at first recommended at 15 mg/day, but 2.5 mg two or three times per day seems more effective, or 5.0 mg at bedtime.

Taste and Smell Alterations

Whether from cachexia, by-products produced from the tumor, side effects of the antitumor treatments (both chemotherapy and radiation), or even inadequate body zinc or other trace elements, patients with cancer complain of alterations to taste and smell. These are a contributing factor to poor nutritional intake; patients find it difficult to enjoy their meals because foods don't smell or taste as expected. A decreased appreciation for sweets or salt and an increased sensitivity to urea are often described, with the former causing foods to taste bland and the latter producing a bitter taste with red meat (Valencius, 1978). Simple measures include increased spicing of foods and avoidance of red meats, but a significant improvement is not usually seen until the cancer is brought under control.

Learned Food Aversions

Nausea and vomiting is still a common but less severe side effect of antitumor therapies. Failure to control nausea and vomiting negatively affects the quality of life of patients, and increases the chances of patients' refusing further treatments (Beck et al., 1992). Anticipatory nausea and vomiting can occur with just the thought of the impending chemotherapy. Learned food aversions occur when patients relate an episode of nausea and vomiting (either anticipatory or posttreatment) with particular foods. In a patient who is having trouble finding any food that appeals to him or her, both of these problems need to be dealt with, both through the use of effective antiemetics and through nutritional counseling.

Therapy-Induced Swallowing and Speech Disorders

Xerostomia

ETIOLOGY. Xerostomia is defined as dryness of the mouth caused by a lack of salivary stimulation that contributes to altered taste and comfort. It is a frequently seen side effect of radiation treatment to the head and neck and upper thoracic area (Dose, 1995). It tends to occur early in treatment and to persist indefinitely.

Salivary secretion decreases when salivary glands, particularly the parotid and submandibular glands, are included in the radiation field. The radiation injures the parenchyma of the salivary glands, leading to fibrosis and secretory hypofunction (Johnson et al., 1993). The decrease in salivary flow leaves the patient with a dry mouth that affects mucosal health, affects maintenance of adequate nutrient intake, and may interfere with sleeping. With a decrease in the production of saliva, the pH of the mouth decreases and there is a loss of protective electrolytes and immunoproteins. This can cause a shift in the microflora, allowing colonization by nosocomial microbes. The patient becomes more prone to dental decay and to opportunistic infections. Saliva plays an important role also in chewing and swallowing. Saliva is needed to form a bolus of food and aids in moving the bolus around the mouth and into position to swallow (Dose, 1995).

Other factors that complicate and worsen the xerostomia include oral breathing, continuous flow with nasal oxygen, intermittent suction by mechanical means, taking nothing by mouth over a 5-hr period due to an inability to swallow complicated by esophagitis, dehydration, cigarette smoking, alcoholic beverages or mouthwashes, and any drugs that are drying to the oral mucosa.

TREATMENT OF XEROSTOMIA. Treatment includes reviewing all factors listed above for those that can be avoided, as well as the use of moistening agents, salivary substitutes, and sialogogues (agents that increase salivary flow). To enhance oral moisture and provide temporary symptom relief, patients can chew sugarless gum, suck sugarless candy, or frequently sip liquids. Sugarless rather than sugar-containing gums and candies should be used because of the possibility of promoting dental decay (Dose, 1995).

Saliva substitutes that attempt to duplicate the properties of saliva include products that contain a carboxymethyl cellulose base with added sorbitol. These agents may be costly and may change taste perception but offer temporary relief.

Sialogogues, such as pilocarpine, have been found to improve the production of saliva and relieve symptoms, even months after completing radiation therapy. Pilocarpine is a parasympathomimetic agent that functions as a muscarinic agonist with mild beta-adrenergic activity. It is an alkaloid that causes pharmacological stimulation of exocrine glands, resulting in diaphoresis, salivation, lacrimation, and gastric and pancreatic secretion (Johnson et al., 1993). Some functioning salivary glands must be present, though, for pilocarpine to be effective. Pilocarpine should not be used with patients who have a history of cardiovascular disease, gastrointestinal ulcers, or unstable hypertension. Sweating is a usual side effect.

Anecdotal reports of providing relief for xerostomia include coating the mouth two or three times a day and at bedtime with a small amount of butter, oil, or margarine. Reports say the oil at bedtime promotes longer periods of sleep. Using an air humidifier to increase the level of moisture in the air may help also.

To prevent oral caries and maintain the health of the few oral mucosa, oral hygiene measures should be performed every 2 hr. Keeping the mouth tasting fresh and relatively moist may help with appetite also.

Acute Radiation or Radiation/Chemotherapy Esophagitis

ETIOLOGY. Radiation therapy to the mediastinum causes esophageal mucosal injury leading to esophagitis. It is manifested by dysphagia and odynophagia, characterized by a retrosternal burning when swallowing liquids or solids and frequently with subsequent weight loss. The development of the irritation and ulcerations corresponds to the rapid cell turnover time of the vulnerable tissue.

The esophagus is a relatively radiation-tolerant organ, but it is the most radiosensitive in the mediastinum (Mascarenhas et al., 1989). It is affected by direct irradiation as well as by radiation scatter during treatment of other cancers in the vicinity of the esophagus (Vanagunas, Jacob, & Olinger, 1990). Appropriate shielding of vital structures in the mediastinum is attempted unless disease involvement necessitates otherwise.

The radiation dosage is a key factor along with radiation dosimetry, differences in radiation technique, and concomitant use of potentially radiosensitizing chemotherapy. However, sequential chemotherapy-radiation therapy treatment has not shown an increase in the occurrence of esophagitis (Dillman, Herndon, Seagren, Eaton, & Green, 1996).

Generally, it can be assumed that the occurrence and severity of esophagitis will increase with increasing doses of radiation and radiosensitizing chemotherapy, and reports of cases range anywhere from 3–100%. Most reported cases are mild to moderate and resolve with the termination of therapy. Esophagitis usually isn't evaluated with either endoscopy or biopsy, but rather it is diagnosed by the temporal relationship between the onset of the symptoms and treatment. Symptoms of irritation usually appear within 2 to 6 weeks of initiating therapy and begin with a decreased salivary flow (Franzen, Henriksson, Littbrand, & Zackrisson, 1995).

Because symptoms mimic peptic esophagitis, opportunistic mucositis, and drug mucositis, it is important to rule out possible causes because treatment for each differs. Substance abuse (e.g., cigarette smoking and chronic alcohol use) in a population of older adults with frequent peptic acid disease also causes difficulty in identifying incidence.

The importance of identifying and treating esophagitis is due to the pain and discomfort that it causes the patient. It may cause interruption in treatment or a patient's request to terminate treatment, and it usually interferes with ingestion of adequate nutrition and can lead to dehydration and fatigue.

TREATMENT OF ESOPHAGITIS. A common treatment agent is sucralfate, a basic aluminum salt of sulfated sucrose. It treats the pain of esophagitis, but doesn't heal the mucosal lining when seen visually with endoscopy. It is taken as either a swish and swallow or a thicker slurry that adheres to the exposed protein in the inflamed mucosal surface. It appears to provide a protective coating that chemically binds to the protein through acid contact. The limited amount of acid in the esophagus may explain its temporary advantage (Franzen et al., 1995).

In response to the conflicting reports of sulcralfate's benefits, the North Central Cancer Treatment Group chose to randomize patients to receive either a sulcralfate solution or a similar placebo to evaluate the prevention or alleviation of symptoms of radiation-induced esophagitis in patients receiving thoracic radiation therapy. They concluded that the sulcralfate not only did not alleviate esophagitis, based on doctor and patient evaluation, but it caused substantial gastrointestinal upset (McGinnis et al., 1997). Our personal experience has been more positive, however. Other agents used in the treatment of symptoms of esophagitis include either anesthetizing agents or antacids if acid-induced pain is involved.

Dietary recommendations begin with the use of an esophagitis diet, which omits foods that are obvious irritants to the throat. Semisolids, purees, and liquids are encouraged, all noncitrus and taken at room temperature. Enteral or parenteral support is indicated if the esophagitis is severe, precluding oral intake for more than 10 days in an already malnourished patient with weight loss of 10% of usual body weight. Nasogastric tubes may irritate and prolong the healing of the esophagus. Parenteral nutrition requires a dedicated venous line and has other complications, including a lack of strong evidence in support of its use in moderately malnourished patients without oral intake for 10 days. The decision to use nutrition support must be individualized for each patient. Probably the best form of nutrition intervention should begin at baseline, with frequent nutrition assessment and counseling throughout treatment. We have outlined our recommendations in a clinical pathway (Figure 8–1) that guides clinicians through this process. Many clinicians place a nasogastric feeding tube to bypass the esophagitis and permit usage of the otherwise normal gut. We feel, however, that this further irritates the esophagus and prolongs the recovery.

Chronic Esophagitis

ETIOLOGY. Chronic esophagitis is characterized by dysphagia or odynophagia occurring more than 2 months after radiation therapy. Endoscopic findings reveal esophageal strictures or, less often, ulcerations. It is a result of progressive endarteritis and slow fibrosis.

The strictures usually develop 6 to 8 months following radiation therapy and are seen in patients who are in poor general medical condition with histories of alcohol and cigarette use. The tolerance of the esophageal mucosa and submucosa to the radiation therapy is thought to be decreased due to the assault through the years of substance abuse.

Acute esophagitis is not always a predisposing factor for developing chronic esophagitis; however, it does occur more often with those who suffered with acute esophagitis, and the severity of the acute esophagitis can foretell the severity of the chronic inflammation.

Chronic esophagitis may be underestimated because neoplasia recurrence can mimic it. It must be identified and treated because it can progress to irreversible esophageal stenosis. Other long-term, but rare, complications include tracheo-esophageal fistulas, which are treated with an esophageal stent.

TREATMENT OF CHRONIC ESOPHAGITIS. Peroral dilatations are used to allow oral feedings with chronic esophagitis, with long-term gastrostomy tube feedings sometimes the only solution.

Secondary Infections

Also interfering with adequate intake due to pain with chewing or swallowing are infections caused by bacteria, viruses, or fungi. Ruling out the cause of the dysphagia may result in identifying an organism that can be treated, allowing adequate nutritional intake to resume.

For example, there may be a direct relationship between the onset and severity of oral complications from the fungus *Candida* and the severity of bone marrow suppression, with granulocyte nadirs commonly occurring 12–14 days after chemotherapy administration. Candidiasis may show up as symmetrical erosions and cracking of the labial junction, or as subacute thrush with cream-colored, flaking, loose plaque over a red inflamed mucosa. Chronic thrush can also present with a dry, red buccal mucosa and a reddened, swollen, shiny, dry cracked tongue. A decrease in the oral pH can also cause candidiasis.

Treatment choices include the topical agent chlorhexidine, which also seems helpful in the treatment of xerostomia. Nystatin, an antifungal antibiotic available as an oral suspension or a tablet, is also used to treat candidiasis and may be soothing to esophagitis as well. Clotrimazole troches, which are high in sucrose, may exacerbate oral decay with concomitant xerostomia, and may not be tolerated by patients with altered taste sensations to sweet things. A systemic antifungal agent, such as ketoconazole, may be necessary and would ensure a higher compliance rate, protect against systemic fungal spread, and treat inaccessible pharyngeal and esophageal lesions (Dose, 1995).

Herpetic esophagitis can also be a source of severe esophageal pain. We

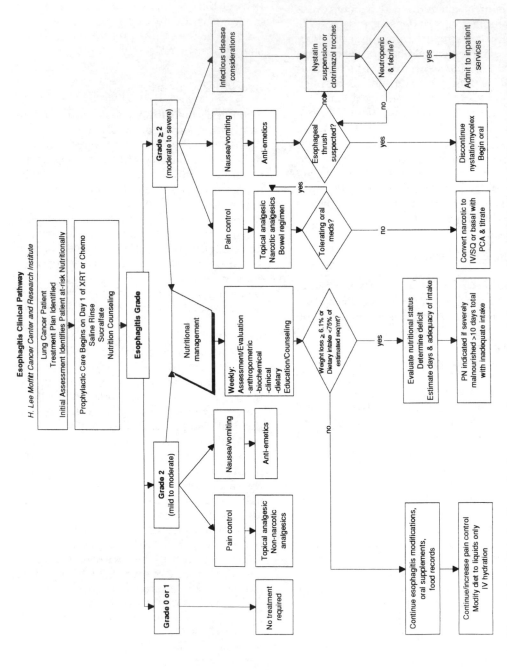

Figure 8–1. A clinical pathway for the prospective management of acute esophagitis associated with either combined modality therapy or radiation alone at the Moffitt Cancer Center. XRT = radiation therapy; chemo = chemotherapy; IV = intravenous; PN = parenteral nutrition; SQ = subcutaneous; and PCA = patient-controlled analgesia.

usually begin therapy for radiation/ chemotherapy-related esophagitis with the topical measures described earlier. Failure to respond over several days, fever, or the onset of symptoms at an exceptionally early time in treatment leads us to endoscopic evaluation. We rarely employ endoscopy when the patient first presents.

Malnutrition and the Enteral/Parenteral Debate

Incidence of Malnutrition

It was recognized as early as 1920 that malnutrition was a major cause of death in cancer patients (Heber, Byerly, & Tchekmedyiahn, 1992). Up to 40% of patients with cancer will die from complications of starvation, and about 50% of patients with lung cancer experience weight loss that shortens their survival (DeWys et al., 1980). Median survival for patients with non-small cell lung cancer who had a 6% weight loss from their usual body weight was 50% that of patients who were within 5% of their usual body weight (Heber et al., 1992).

Weight loss is frequently the presenting symptom for the patient with lung cancer. However, it is frequently disproportionate to the decrease in nutrient intake and it may occur in the presence of normal intake. It usually occurs at a rate faster than seen in starvation, suggesting an alteration in the host metabolism, a decreased efficiency in nutrient use, or competition for nutrients between the host and the tumor. It is assumed that tumor growth continues at the host's expense (Zeman, 1983). The normal adaptation to a decrease in food intake is a decrease in the basal metabolic rate, an adaptation that is not always seen in patients with cancer who eat inadequate calories and protein. The basal metabolic rate frequently remains normal, supporting the theory of altered host metabolism (Heber et al., 1992).

However, because some of the most powerful prognostic factors for survival in individuals with lung cancer relate to food intake, appetite, and quality of life, nutrition assessment is of primary importance to identify those areas of deficit where intervention can make a difference (Rowland et al., 1996; see Table 8–8).

Nutritional Assessment

Malnutrition begins when the patient fails to eat enough to meet anabolic and energy expenditure needs. The malnourished body progresses through a series of func-

TABLE 8–8. Identification of Clinical Malnutrition

Inadequate intake of nutrients caused by:

    Starvation

    Anorexia

    Intestinal malabsorption

        Metabolic rate decreased in response to decreased intake

        Lean body mass spared at expense of fat and extracellular water

        Protein synthesis decreased

        Cytokine production normal or decreased

        Cell-mediated immunity is suppressed

        Reversed by replenishing nutrients

Source: Adapted from "Weight Loss and Human Immunodeficiency Virus Infection: Cachexia Versus Malnutrition," by S. L. Gorbach and T. A. Knox, 1992, *Infectious Diseases in Clinical Practice, 1,* pp. 224–229.

tional changes that precede any changes in body composition. The extent of functional changes is related to the duration and severity of the reduced intake. The nutrition assessment at diagnosis, for those patients whose therapy will place them at risk for esophagitis, should include an evaluation of anthropometric, biochemical, clinical, and dietary factors. The goal is to identify those high–nutritional risk patients who may suffer increased morbidity and mortality or prolonged functional starvation following antitumor treatments that may interfere with maintaining adequate nutritional intake (Meguid, 1990). Nutritional assessment at diagnosis establishes a baseline that can identify pretreatment weight loss that represents an alteration in nutritional status.

The assessment begins with subjective data collected from interviews with the patient and/or significant others and it should include an evaluation of usual appetite, how it has changed over time, food intake based on food records or a complete 24-hr recall and food frequency analysis, and a weight history. Dentition, problems chewing or swallowing, and cultural, ethnic, or religious preferences should be documented. Substance use, such as cigarette smoking, alcohol intake, or illicit drug use, should be identified as well because it can interfere with adequate intake or predispose to increased nutritional risk.

Objective data collection begins with a review of the medical record and attendance at patient rounds to diagnosis, prognosis, tumor staging, and treatment modality. Weight and height should be measured as well as other anthropometrics. Fat and muscle stores are determined by tricep skin fold and midarm muscle circumference measurements. Lean body mass can be assessed by measuring creatinine and comparing it to the creatinine-height index. Indirect calorimetry using a bioelectrical impedance analyzer will measure lean body mass more accurately, even though all standards are based on a normal healthy population. Biochemi-cal lab data measuring visceral protein stores determined by serum albumin and transferrin, total iron-binding capacity, serum electrolytes, nitrogen balance, hemoglobin and hematocrit, and total lymphocyte count may need to be included.

Estimates of caloric and protein needs can be made using standard formulas (Harris and Benedict Equation; Henshaw & Schloerb, 1995) plus stress and activity factors and compared to analyses of the patient's current dietary intake.

Nutritional Intervention

The possible outcomes of nutrition intervention include nitrogen retention, weight gain, decreased susceptibility to infection by supporting the body's immune system, and continued antitumor therapy by minimizing many of the side effects of radiation and chemotherapy. Patients will also feel more active, with an increased feeling of well-being and improved quality of life (Zeman, 1983). Recommendations can be made to the patient and/or significant other on how to either maintain the current intake or increase intake to meet the estimated requirements. Weight gain can be attempted with recommendations on how to increase calories with oral intake through calorically dense foods and/or nutritional supplements. A multivitamin can be added to the daily intake to ensure all nutrients are at recommended levels.

The collected data must be evaluated and a care plan individualized for each patient. An initial counseling session should be held to review the findings and educate on the importance of maintaining a healthy diet. Patients should be told of possible side effects with radiation or chemotherapy treatments and nutrition interventions that are used. Patient education materials on the esophagitis diet, the use of nutrition supplements, and nutrition support can be introduced, with the reassurance that if the patient needs intervention, the dietitian will be available for assistance. Weekly or biweekly contact with each patient should be maintained to document usual dietary intake and monitor when intake begins to decrease.

The Enteral/Parenteral Debate

Parenteral and enteral nutrition support are much-discussed and fairly controversial therapies in oncology. Most reports of outcomes, including the Veterans Administration Cooperative Study, identify only the most severely malnourished patient as benefiting from parenteral support. Parenteral nutrition has not been shown to have therapeutic benefits to the well-nourished or modestly malnourished patient (Copeland, 1990). Of course, parenteral nutrition cannot alter the events of the terminal stages of cancer and it should not be a part of the treatment plan of patients with far-advanced disease.

Patients with cancer who would benefit from parenteral nutrition include those patients with potentially responsive tumors, but whose antitumor treatment could not continue if they were not to receive parenteral nutrition. These are patients who would not be able to tolerate the toxicity of the treatment because of the preceding malnutrition. This includes those patients who will remain without adequate nutritional intake (ranging from 60–75% of estimated requirements) due to side effects of antitumor treatment (e.g., radiation esophagitis).

The therapy must be estimated to be needed for at least 10 days, and preferably longer. Two weeks or more of parenteral nutrition therapy has been shown to stimulate anabolism, whereas less than 10 days does little good, and may be harmful secondary to marked fluid and electrolyte shifts (Grant, 1990). Also, potential parenteral nutrition candidates should be anergic to recall skin-test antigens (Copeland, 1990) and should have had a recent unintentional weight loss of more than 10% of their usual body weight. Of course, percentage of body weight lost must take into account what usual body weight had been. For example, losing 10% when a patient weighs 250

pounds may not be deleterious compared to losing 10% from 110 pounds.

It is difficult to pinpoint the role that the deficit of calories, the length of time of that deficit, and other stresses play in determining what the human body will accept until it cannot continue to function or cannot be returned to normal functioning. Caloric adequacy and length of time not meeting that adequacy must be decided on and used to determine when the patient requires nutrition support. As referred to earlier, it must be determined what length of time the nutrition support will be needed. Less than 10 days of nutrition support is not beneficial to the body, and may be detrimental.

Complications from the mechanics of providing parenteral nutrition are known and include sepsis, as well as complications from giving a wrong prescription (either too much or too little) of calories and protein. Increased calories given to a patient with lung cancer with poor pulmonary function results in fluid overload and will be more costly than allowing the patient to go without any nutrition support (Weiner, Kramer, & Clamon, 1985).

Enteral nutrition carries with it many of the same concerns as parenteral nutrition. The benefits of using enteral nutrition begin with the issue of providing nutrients in a more physiological way, through a functioning gastrointestinal tract, as compared to parenteral. Enteral nutrition stimulates the gut mucosa, preventing atrophy and bacterial and toxin translocation.

A surgical jejunostomy or gastrostomy tube may be indicated in preference to a nasoenteric tube for many reasons. Of course, a tube hidden under clothes is more appealing than a tube protruding from one's nose. Further, a nasoenteric tube may interfere and cause continued pain and discomfort while lying in an irritated esophagus. Feeding tubes placed directly into the intestine can be used with those severely malnourished patients with functioning gastrointestinal tracts who it is foreseen will suffer from long periods of poor to no oral intake.

CONCLUSION

Because both the disease itself and the treatments directed against it directly affect the organs of speech and swallowing, they have a profound impact on both functions. It is, therefore, vital to have the appropriate nutritional and rehabilitation teams involved in treatment planning rather than just in symptom management.

REFERENCES

Albrecht, J. T. & Canada, T. W. (1996). Cachexia and anorexia in malignancy. *Hematology/Oncology Clinics of North America, 10,* 791–800.

Beck, T. M., Hesketh, P. J., Madajewicz, S., Navari, R. M., Pendergrass, K., Lester, E., Kish, J. A., Murphy, W. K., Hainsworth, J. D., Gandara, D. R., Bricker, L. J., Keller, A. M., Mortimer, J., Galvin, D. V., House, K. W., & Bryson, J. C. (1992). Stratified, randomized, double-blind comparison of intravenous ondansetron administered as a multiple-dose regimen versus two single-dose regimens in the prevention of cisplatin-induced nausea and vomiting. *Journal of Clinical Oncology, 10,* 1969–1975.

Boring, C. C., Squires, T. S., Tong, T., & Montgomery, S. (1994). Cancer statistics. *CA: A Cancer Journal for Clinicians, 44,* 7–26.

Burbige, E. J., Radigan, N., & Belber, J. P. (1980). Metastatic lung carcinoma involving the gastrointestinal tract. *American Journal of Gastroenterology, 74,* 504–506.

Carbone, P. P., Frost, J. K., Feinstein, A. R., Higgins G. A., Jr., & Selawry, O. S. (1970). Lung cancer: Perspective and prospects. *Annals of Internal Medicine, 73,* 1024–1033.

Copeland, E. M. (1990). Total parenteral nutrition in the cancer patient: The present as viewed from the past. *Nutrition, 6,* 2S–3S.

DeWys, W. D., Begg, C., Lavin, P. T., Band, P. R., Bennett, J. M., Bertino, J. R., Cohen, M. H., Douglass, H. O., Engstrom, P. F., Ezdinli, E. Z., Horton, J., Johnson, G. J., Moertel, C. G., Oken, M. M., Perlia, C., Rosenbaum, C., Silverstein, M. N., Skeel, R. T., Sponzo, R. W., & Tormey, D. C. (1980). Prognostic effect of weight loss prior to chemotherapy in cancer patients. *American Journal of Medicine, 69,* 491–497.

Dillman, R. O., Herndon, J., Seagren, S. L., Eaton, W. L., & Green, M. R. (1996). Improved survival in stage III non-small cell lung cancer: Seven year follow-up of Cancer and Leukemia Group B (CALGB) 8433 trial. *Journal of the National Cancer Institute, 88,* 1210–1215.

Dose, A. M. (1995). The symptom experience of mucositis, stomatitis, and xerostomia. *Seminars in Oncology Nursing, 11,* 248–255.

Doyle, L. A., & Aisner, J. (1995). Clinical presentation of lung cancer. In J. A. Roth, J. C. Ruckdeschel, & T. H. Weisenburger (Eds.), *Thoracic oncology* (2nd ed., pp. 26–31). Philadelphia: W. B. Saunders.

Franzen, L., Henriksson, R., Littbrand, B., & Zackrisson, B. (1995). Effects of Sucralfate on mucositis during and following radiotherapy of malignancies in the head and neck region. *Acta Oncologica, 34,* 219–223.

Gazdar, A. F., Linnoila, R. I., Kurita, Y., Oie, H. K., Mulshine, J. L., Clark, J. C., & Whitsett, J. A. (1990). Peripheral airway cell differentiation in human lung cancer cell lines. *Cancer Research, 50,* 5481–5487.

Gorter, R. (1991). Management of anorexia-cachexia associated with cancer and HIV infection. *Oncology, 5,* 14–17.

Gould, V. E., & Warren, W. H. (1995). Epithelial neoplasms of the lung. In J. A. Roth, J. C. Ruckdeschel, & T. H. Weisenburger (Eds.), *Thoracic oncology* (2nd ed., pp. 49–67). Philadelphia: W. B. Saunders.

Grant, J. P. (1990). Proper use and recognized role of TPN in the cancer patient. *Nutrition, 6,* 6S–7S.

Grant, M. M., & Rivera, L. M. (1995). Anorexia, cachexia, and dysphagia: The symptom experience. *Seminars in Oncology Nursing, 11,* 266–271.

Grossman, S. A., Ruckdeschel, J. C., Moynihan, T., Finkelstein, D., Ettinger, D. S., Mahoney, E., & Trump, D. L. (1993). Randomized prospective comparison of intraventricular methotrexate and thiotepa in patients with previously untreated neoplastic meningitis. *Journal of Clinical Oncology, 11,* 561–569.

Heber, D., Byerly, L. O., & Tchekmedyiahn, N. S. (1992). Hormonal and metabolic abnormalities in the malnourished cancer patient: Effects on host-tumor interaction. *Journal of Parenteral and Enteral Nutrition, 16,* 60S–64S.

Henshaw, E. C., & Schloerb, P. R. (1995). Nutrition and the cancer patient. In *American Cancer Society textbook of clinical oncology* (1st ed., pp. 490–496). Atlanta: American Cancer Society.

Hyde, L., & Hyde, C. I. (1974). Clinical manifestations of lung cancer. *Chest, 65,* 299–306.

Ihde, D. C. (1985). Staging evaluation and prognostic factors in small-cell lung cancer. In J. Aisner (Ed.), *Contemporary issues in clinical oncology: Lung cancer* (pp. 241–268). New York: Churchill Livingstone.

Jetten, A. M. (1991). Growth and differentiation factors in tracheobronchial epithelium. *American Journal of Physiology, 260,* L361.

Johnson, J. T., Ferretti, G. A., Nethery, W. J., Valdez, I. H., Fox, P. C., Ng, D., Muscoplat, C. C., & Gallagher, S. C. (1993). Oral pilocarpine for post-irradiation xerostomia in patients with head and neck cancer. *Cancer, 329*, 390–395.

Kardinal, C. G., Loprinzi, C. L., Schaid, D. J., Hass, A. C., Dose, A. M., Athman, L. M., Mailliard, J. A., McCormack, G. W., Gerstner, J. B., & Schray, M. F. (1990). A controlled trial of Cyproheptadine in cancer patients with anorexia and/or cachexia. *Cancer, 65*, 2657–2662.

Mascarenhas, F., Silvestre, M. E., Sa da Costa, M., Grima, N., Campos, C., & Chaves, P. (1989). Acute secondary effects in the esophagus in patients undergoing radiotherapy for carcinoma of the lung. *American Journal of Clinical Oncology, 12*, 34–40.

McGinnis, W. L., Loprinzi, C. L., Buskirk, S. J., Sloan, J. A., Novotny, P. J., Drummond, R. G., Frank, A. R., & Shanahan, T. G. (1997). *Phase III evaluation of Sucralfate for radiation-induced esophagitis*. Abstract presented at ASTRO 1997 meeting.

Meguid, M. M. (1990). Identifying the at-risk cancer patient using inadequate oral nutrition intake period. *Nutrition, 6*, 10S–11S.

Mountain, C. F. (1986). A new international staging system for lung cancer. *Chest, 89*, 225S–233S.

Mountain, C. F. (1997). Revisions in the International System for Staging Lung Cancer. *Chest, 111*, 1710–1717.

Newman, S. J., & Hansen, H. H. (1974). Frequency, diagnosis and treatment of brain metastases in 247 consecutive patients with bronchogenic carcinoma. *Cancer, 33*, 492–496.

Rosen, S. T., Aisner, J., Makuch, R. W., Matthews, M. J., Ihde, D. C., Whitacre, M., Glatstein, E. J., Wiernik, P.H., Lichter, A. S., & Bunn, P. A., Jr. (1982). Carcinomatous leptomeningitis in small cell lung cancer. *Medicine, 61*, 45–53.

Rowland, K. M., Loprinzi, C. L., Shaw, E. G., Maksymiuk, A. W., Kuross, S. A., Jung, S., Kugler, J. W., Tschetter, L. K., Ghosh, C., Shaefer, P. L., Owen, D., Washburn, J. H., Webb, T. A., Mailliard, J. A., & Rett, J. R. (1996). Randomized, double blind placebo-controlled trial of cisplatin and etoposide plus megestrol acetate/placebo in extensive stage small-cell lung cancer: A North Central Cancer Treatment Group study. *Journal of Clinical Oncology, 14*, 135–141.

Shopland, D. R., Eyre, H. J., & Pechacek, T. F. (1991). Smoking-attributable cancer mortality in 1991: Is lung cancer now the leading cause of death among smokers in the United States? *Journal of the National Cancer Institute, 83*, 1142–1148.

Tchekmedyian, N. S., Halpert, C., Ashley, J., & Heber, D. (1992). Nutrition in advanced cancer: Anorexia as an outcome variable and target of therapy. *Journal of Parenteral and Enteral Nutrition, 16*, 88S–92S.

Valencius, J. C. (1978). Nutritional support of the cancer patient. In C. Kellogg & B. Sullivan (Eds.), Current perspectives in oncologic nursing (pp. 45–55). Philadelphia: C. V. Mosby.

Vanagunas, A., Jacob, P., & Olinger, E. (1990). Radiation-induced esophageal injury: A spectrum from esophagitis to cancer. *American Journal of Gastroenterology, 85*, 808–812.

Wagner, H. (1993). Rational integration of radiation and chemotherapy in patients with unresectable stage IIIA or IIIB NSCLC: Results from the Lung Cancer Study Group, Eastern Cooperative Oncology Group and Radiation Therapy Oncology Group. *Chest, 103* (Suppl. 1), 35S–42S.

Weiner, R. S., Kramer, B. S., & Clamon, G. H. (1985). Effects of intravenous hyperalimentation during treatment in patients with small-cell lung cancer. *Journal of Clinical Oncology, 3*, 949–957.

Zeman, F. J. (1983). *Clinical nutrition and dietics*. Lexington, MA: Collamore Press.

9

Leukemia and Lymphoma

Lynn C. Moscinski, M.D., and Ruben Saez, M. D.

The leukemias and lymphomas are malignant tumors of the hematopoietic system, commonly involving the bone marrow, blood, and lymph nodes. They can be separated into two broad categories: leukemias, which are tumors that predominantly involve the bone marrow and blood, and lymphomas, which are tumors that predominantly involve the lymph nodes and lymphoid tissues of the body (Hoffbrand & Pettet, 1993). They can cause swallowing and communication disorders by a variety of mechanisms. They can locally invade the soft tissues of the neck, or they can infiltrate the brain and peripheral nerves, resulting in neurological impairment. The most frequent and important mechanism by which these tumors cause dysphagia or speech problems, however, is the result of treatment. Chemotherapy and radiation therapy can produce tissue damage, and patients can develop severe infections from the complications of treatment. This chapter provides an overview of the hematopoietic neoplasms and discusses their primary sites of involvement. Additionally, it describes the common problems that result from tumor therapy, with a focus on those most common in the patient with leukemia/lymphoma. Many of the complications of treating hematopoietic neoplasms are common to other tumors, and the reader is encouraged to refer to general sections on these topics to provide additional information.

AN OVERVIEW OF HEMATOPOIETIC NEOPLASMS

Leukemia

The leukemias are a group of disorders that are characterized by the accumulation of abnormal white blood cells in the bone marrow. These abnormal cells can escape from the marrow and circulate in the peripheral blood. The leukemias have been divided into two categories, the so-called acute leukemias, which have a rapidly progressive and aggressive course, and the chronic leukemias, which have a longer and more indolent course. Additionally, within these subdivisions, the leukemias can also be grouped as to their cell of origin. Thus, acute leukemias include acute lymphoid leukemias (acute lymphoblastic leukemia, or ALL) and acute myeloid leukemia (acute myelogenous leukemia, or AML). The chronic leukemias are divided in a similar fashion, with chronic lymphocytic leukemia (CLL) and chronic myelogenous leukemia (CML) being the two most common disorders. Additionally, many other diseases are included in the acute and chronic leukemias. These are presented in Table 9–1.

The acute leukemias are identified by the presence of very immature cells in the bone marrow and blood. These immature cells are called *blasts* and constitute more than 30% of the cells present when a bone

TABLE 9–1. Types of Acute and Chronic Leukemia

Myeloid Leukemias	Lymphoid Leukemias
Acute Leukemias	
Acute myelogenous leukemia* (includes promyelocytic, monoblastic, erythroid, and megakaryoblastic subtypes)	Acute lymphoblastic leukemia* (includes B and T cell subtypes)
Chronic Leukemias	
Chronic myelogenous leukemia*	Chronic lymphocytic leukemia*
Chronic myelomonocytic leukemia	Hairy cell leukemia (and other myelodysplasias)
	Prolymphocytic leukemia
	Large granular lymphocytic leukemia
	Sezary syndrome (and other subtypes of non-Hodgkin's lymphomas with blood involvement

Note. The most common leukemias are identified by *.

marrow aspiration is performed. The distinction between AML and ALL is made on the basis of morphology, cytochemical staining properties, immunophenotyping by flow cytometry, and chromosome analysis. These tests can provide valuable diagnostic and prognostic information to help identify patients who will have an unusually good or an unusually poor prognosis. Information as to the subtype of acute leukemia may also help guide the physician's choice of treatment, or help to predict a specific complication. As an example, some subtypes of acute leukemia have a greater or lesser tendency to involve the brain or soft tissues, requiring local therapies.

ALL is the most common form of acute leukemia in children, with the highest incidence at 3–4 years of age. In this age group, the most common phenotype of ALL is that of an immature B lymphocyte (termed precursor B-ALL), with an equal sex incidence. There is a second slight increase in incidence of ALL in teenagers, with a male predominance and a predominantly T lymphoid phenotype. The incidence of ALL then decreases progressively, although it again increases after the age of 50–60 years. AML, however, occurs in all age groups, with a gradual progres-

sive increase in incidence with advancing age. It is the most common form of acute leukemia in adults, including the elderly, and is the most common secondary form of leukemia to develop after chemotherapy, myelodysplasia, or chronic leukemia.

The clinical features of acute leukemia, both AML and ALL, are predominantly a result of bone marrow failure from progressive accumulation of malignant cells. Normal white cells, red cells, and platelets decrease, causing infections, anemia, and bleeding. The leukemic cells can leave the bone marrow and circulate in the peripheral blood, thereby allowing them to infiltrate many tissues of the body. ALL, and more rarely AML, can cause enlargement of lymph nodes throughout the body, or can cause splenomegaly and hepatomegaly. Gum and mucosal hypertrophy and infiltration, skin involvement, and renal infiltration are more commonly seen in subtypes of AML that have monocytic features. Meningeal infiltration is particularly common in ALL, but is also noted in subtypes of AML with monocytic features, and can result in headache, nausea and vomiting, blurring of vision, and diplopia. Other organs can also be infiltrated; enlargement of the thymus with mediastinal compression is most commonly noted in the T lymphoid subtype of ALL.

CML comprises approximately 20% of all leukemias, and is seen most frequently in adults of middle age. This leukemia is characterized by replacement of the normal bone marrow by cells identified by the presence of the Philadelphia (or Ph) chromosome. This abnormal chromosome is the result of a translocation of part of one arm of chromosome 22 to another chromosome, usually chromosome 9. It is an acquired mutation that occurs in an early bone marrow progenitor (stem cell), and is therefore found in all dividing granulocytic, erythroid, and megakaryocytic cells of the marrow, as well as some B and T lymphocytes. The resultant leukemia is characterized by a rapid proliferation of all bone marrow lineages, with the most prominent increase noted in granulocytes (white cells). These abnormal granulocytes escape the bone marrow and cause a rapid and high increase in the patient's peripheral blood white cell count, often to values greater than 100,000 cells/µl of blood. These cells infiltrate the spleen, causing marked splenic enlargement associated with discomfort, pain, and early satiety, leading on occasion to weight loss. Infiltration of other tissues is uncommon unless the peripheral blood white cell count becomes extremely high, immature white cells predominate, or an acute leukemia secondarily develops.

CLL accounts for 25% or more of the leukemias seen, occurring primarily in older adults. There is a close clinical and morphological association between CLL and the low-grade non-Hodgkin's lymphomas. CLL results from the accumulation of large numbers of mature lymphocytes in the bone marrow, blood, spleen, lymph nodes, and liver. The vast majority of CLLs are neoplasms of B lymphocytes. They are diagnosed using a combination of cytology and immunophenotyping. The clinical features of CLL are primarily due to the tendency of these neoplastic B lymphocytes to infiltrate and enlarge normal lymphoid structures. Therefore, there is generalized and symmetrical enlargement of lymph nodes, as well as enlargement of the liver and spleen. If sufficient numbers of these neoplastic lymphocytes accumulate, they can replace normal bone marrow elements, resulting in anemia, neutropenia, and thrombocytopenia similar to the acute leukemias. Skin infiltration is present in a small number of patients. Tonsillar enlargement may be prominent, and involvement of salivary and lacrimal glands can be a rare complication.

Many other, less common subtypes of the CLLs exist. Each of these subtypes has a unique cytology and immunophenotype, and causes a unique pattern of clinical signs and symptoms. These disorders are relatively uncommon, and will not be covered in detail.

Lymphoma

The lymphomas are neoplastic disorders in which lymphocytes accumulate in the lymph nodes and other lymphoid tissues of the body. They are generally subdivided into Hodgkin's disease and the non-Hodgkin's lymphomas (Table 9–2). Although division of lymphomas into discrete subtypes may be important for prognosis and treatment planning, all of these disorders have similar clinical presentations. There is replacement of the normal lymphoid structures by collections of abnormal cells, Hodgkin's disease being characterized by the presence of Reed-Sternberg cells, and the non-Hodgkin's lymphomas by diffuse or nodular collections of neoplastic B and T lymphocytes.

Lymphomas can present at any age, but they are unusual in children. There appears to be a bimodal age incidence, with one peak in young adults (age 20–30 years) and a second that increases gradually after the age of 50 years. Hodgkin's disease tends to be more prevalent in younger adults, whereas the non-Hodgkin's lymphomas are more prevalent in older adults. There is generally a two-to-one male predominance. Most patients present with painless, nontender, and asymmetrical enlargement of the superficial lymph nodes. Enlargement of

TABLE 9–2. Types of Lymphoma

A. **Hodgkin's disease**
   Nodular sclerosis
   Lymphocyte predominant
   Mixed cellularity
   Lymphocyte depleted

B. **Non-Hodgkin's lymphomas**
   Low grade (indolent)
   Small lymphocytic lymphoma
   Lymphoplasmacytoid lymphoma (Waldenstrom's macroglobulinemia)
   Follicular lymphoma
   Marginal zone B cell lymphoma (including MALT type)

   Intermediate grade (aggressive)
   Mantle cell lymphoma
   Diffuse large B cell lymphomas
   Peripheral T cell lymphomas
   Angiocentric T cell lymphomas
   Anaplastic large cell lymphoma (Ki-1 type)

   High grade (very aggressive)
   Burkitt's lymphoma
   High-grade lymphoma, Burkitt-like (lymphomas in immunocompromised people,
      including HIV-positive and organ transplant patients)
   Lymphoblastic lymphoma

the liver and spleen, infiltration of the gastrointestinal tract or other soft tissue sites, and oropharyngeal involvement may be present. Involvement of Waldeyer's ring has been described in 5–10% of patients with non-Hodgkin's lymphomas and a lesser proportion of patients with Hodgkin's disease. Skin and brain involvement are also seen.

Hodgkin's disease is histologically subdivided by morphological features alone. Non-Hodgkin's lymphomas are also subdivided by morphological features, and these features have a direct correlate with the patient's clinical course (Harris et al., 1994). Generally speaking, lymphomas can be either low grade (indolent) or aggressive. The aggressive lymphomas occur with a higher incidence in young adults or in patients with acquired immunodeficiencies. Both T and B cell lymphomas are described. In the late stages of the disease, lymphomas, both Hodgkin's and non-Hodgkin's types, can involve the bone marrow and result in significant impairment of normal bone marrow function. In some cases, the normal bone marrow can be entirely replaced by neoplastic lymphoid cells, resulting in significant anemia, neutropenia, and thrombocytopenia. At this stage of the disease, symptoms of bone marrow failure are similar to those found with the acute leukemias.

Incidence of Dysphagia and Speech Disorders

The incidence of speech and other communication disorders with hematologic cancers is not well documented. The estimated incidence from clinical experience is low, however. When identified, speech disorders most often coexist with symptoms of dysphagia and are secondary to the inflammation and associated mucosal pain. Occasionally, they can occur independently of dysphagia. In these instances, they may be secondary to involvement of the brain or peripheral nerves (e.g., the laryngeal or recurrent laryngeal nerves).

Patients with hematologic malignancies (leukemia and lymphoma) develop dysphagia (including mucositis and infectious complications) at a rate two to three times that of patients with solid tumors (Sonis, Sonis, & Lieberman, 1978). This is most likely a consequence of the fact that these patients are immunosuppressed and myelosuppressed with very low white blood cell and platelet counts—a consequence of the malignancy and its therapy (Lockhart & Sonis, 1979). The rate of dysphagia has been estimated at between 30% and 100% (Ramirez-Amador et al., 1996; Sonis et al., 1978), depending on the patient age and type of malignancy. Young patients tend to develop mucositis more frequently than older patients. Several studies have estimated that almost 90% of pediatric patients between the ages of 1 and 20 years develop mucositis with chemotherapy, whereas many fewer geriatric patients over the age of 60 develop similar problems (Sonis et al., 1978). This difference in incidence between age groups holds when patients with the same malignancy and same chemotherapeutic regimen are studied. One explanation has been that cell proliferation and epithelial growth are slower in older patients, so the toxic effects of chemotherapy may be less in this population (Baraket, Toto, & Choukas, 1969).

However, this is not to say that all groups of patients with hematologic malignancies have a high incidence of oral complications. Each hematologic malignancy is treated with a unique combination of chemotherapeutic agents, which may or may not be supplemented with external radiation. The reported rates of dysphagia are lowest with chronic and acute leukemias, although several intensive regimens for acute leukemia (especially those containing high-dose ara-C) also have high rates of mucositis. However, the highest reported rates are with Hodgkin's disease. Patients with non-Hodgkin's lymphomas of various subtypes have an intermediate risk. This most likely is a result of the fact that patients with leukemia tend to be treated with chemotherapy alone, whereas many patients with Hodgkin's disease have combined chemotherapy and radiation therapy to the head and neck region.

Among the individual causes of dysphagia across all groups of patients with hematologic malignancies, mucositis accounts for the vast majority of reported problems (greater than 90%). The only exception to this is in with acute leukemia undergoing induction chemotherapy, where infectious complications (predominantly fungal and viral) may account for as much as 19% of the incidence (Sonis et al., 1978).

TUMOR-RELATED CAUSES OF DYSPHAGIA AND COMMUNICATION DISORDERS

Lymphadenopathy and Tumor Masses

Patients with either Hodgkin's disease or non-Hodgkin's lymphoma can have significant mediastinal and cervical lymphadenopathy. Lymph node masses are usually movable under the force exerted during normal swallowing. Therefore, enlarged lymph nodes are a rare cause of dysphagia, except in cases where lymph nodes increase to massive sizes (greater than 5 cm) or where lymphoma is shown to invade outside of the lymph node into adjacent soft tissues or to result in adherence of lymph nodes together ("matted" lymph nodes). These processes result in physical compression or fixation of the esophagus, with mechanical obstruction to swallowing.

Even less frequently encountered are patients in whom lymphoma occurs as a primary tumor mass within the upper gastrointestinal tract, larynx, or nasopharynx. Lymphomas arising in the stomach (Isaacson, Spencer, & Finn, 1986; Moss, Valentine, Carey, & Hind, 1993) often result in the patient's experiencing a sensation of fullness on eating, and may be reported to the physician as symptoms of dysphagia. Non-Hodgkin's lymphomas of the stomach are relatively rare (Azab et al., 1989), and most often are either low-grade lymphomas (mucosa-associated lymphoid tissue [MALT] type) or intermediate-grade lymphomas (diffuse large B cell type). Rarely, lymphoma can be primary to the esophagus (Taal,Van Heerde, & Somers, 1993), although fewer than 100 cases have been reported in the world's literature since 1935. As in the lymphomas of the stomach, non-Hodgkin's lymphoma of the esophagus is frequently of MALT type or diffuse large B cell type. Hodgkin's disease has also been identified in this site.

Primary non-Hodgkin's lymphomas can also occur in the larynx (Kawaida et al., 1996) or the nasopharynx (Robbins et al., 1985), where masses can directly result in difficulties with voice (dysphonia or hoarseness) or may cause speech and communication disorders as a result of their effects on the patient's ability to breathe without undue effort or obstruction to airflow.

Infiltration of Soft Tissues

Acute leukemia can occasionally cause problems by infiltration of soft tissues ("extramedullary leukemia"). Leukemic blast cells are usually infiltrative, but they may grow as tumor masses as well. In contrast to lymphomas and other solid tumors, leukemic infiltration rarely leads to obstruction of viscera or blood vessels, and it does not produce major organ dysfunction other than the bone marrow. The most common types of leukemias to infiltrate the soft tissues of the mouth and respiratory tract are acute leukemias showing monocytic differentiation (acute monoblastic leukemia and acute myelomonocytic leukemia), chronic myelomonocytic leukemia, or occasionally CML. Infiltration is seen at diagnosis or can be indicative of relapse, and usually, but not always, correlates with the number of circulating leukemic blast cells. It is reversible if the patient responds to chemotherapy, and generally does not result in long-term morbidity or sequelae such as soft tissue scarring or permanent organ dysfunction.

As was mentioned earlier, malignant lymphomas, both Hodgkin's and non-Hodgkin's types, can occasionally invade the soft tissues of the head and neck region by direct extension from enlarged and involved lymph nodes. This infiltration is often associated with an inflammatory or reparative tissue response, and may result in some degree of long-term scarring of the tissues if a response to therapy is obtained. Tumor masses such as lymphoma may also show considerable necrosis, with secondary scarring after the healing process has ensued.

Paraneoplastic Syndromes and Neurotoxicity

Unlike solid tumors, paraneoplastic syndromes with neuromuscular abnormalities are extremely rare with either leukemia or lymphoma. When these occur, dysphagia or dysphonia is generally seen as part of generalized muscle weakness, with autoantibody production by low-grade non-Hodgkin's lymphomas.

Other neurological problems may result from leukemic or lymphomatous infiltration of the central nervous system, with meningeal involvement and cranial nerve palsies. These syndromes are most frequently associated with acute leukemias showing monocytic differentiation, with patients who have extremely high white blood cell counts consisting predominantly of leukemic blast cells, or with certain subtypes of aggressive non-Hodgkin's lymphomas.

Central nervous system toxicity can be a consequence of the therapy of leukemia. The sequelae of radiation therapy to the brain are more significant and more frequently reported than those of intrathecal chemotherapy. They are discussed in the following sections of this chapter.

DYSPHAGIA AND COMMUNICATION DISORDERS SECONDARY TO CHEMOTHERAPY

Chemotherapy rarely causes problems with speech. When speech abnormalities occur, they are usually a consequence of the neurotoxicity associated with individual chemotherapeutic drugs—vincristine and cytosine arabinoside being the ones most frequently encountered. Even in this setting, neurotoxicity associated with chemotherapeutic drugs uncommonly causes problems with esophageal, laryngeal, or respiratory functions. Intrathecal chemotherapy has been reported to be associated with central nervous system abnormalities in children, but more pronounced effects are seen after radiation therapy of the brain.

Dysphagia, on the other hand, is a frequently encountered problem in association with chemotherapy. The vast majority of patients with hematologic malignancies who develop dysphagia will do so as a consequence of chemotherapy-induced toxicity. Complications occur through one of two major mechanisms: They may be a direct effect of the drug on the oral mucosa (direct toxicity), or they may be indirectly caused by myelosuppression and result in infection (indirect toxicity). Not all patients appear to be at equal risk of developing oral problems associated with any specific chemotherapeutic regimen. Factors that influence frequency and severity of complications are those related to the patient as well as the particular drug regimen. Patient factors include the type and site of malignant involvement, the age of the patient, and the oral and overall health of the individual before and during therapy (Sonis, 1985).

Therapy-related variables influence the frequency and severity with which patients will develop problems. The most important single factor is the choice of drug. Although oral toxicity is a common side effect of many forms of chemotherapy, drugs will differ in the extent of the toxicity that ensues. It may be dose related or affected by the timing or duration of the regimen. Sometimes the toxicity can be reduced or ameliorated by delivering chemotherapy in divided doses or as a continuous infusion, rather than as a single bolus. Many of the cancer chemotherapeutic drugs used to treat hematologic malignancies cause direct toxicity (Table 9–3).

Mucositis as a form of direct toxicity is the consequence of the nonspecific effects of a chemotherapeutic drug on cells of the oral and upper digestive tract epithelium, which are undergoing mitosis. Cells in the mouth and other nonkeratinized epithelia undergo rapid renewal over a 7- to 14-day period. Chemotherapy can de-

TABLE 9–3. Chemotherapeutic Agents Used to Treat Hematologic Malignancies

Bleomycin
Cytosine arabinoside*
Daunorubicin*
Doxorubicin*
Etoposide*
Hydroxyurea
Mercaptopurine
Methotrexate*
Procarbazine hydrochloride
Thioguanine
Vinblastine sulfate
Vincristine sulfate

Note. The most common drugs to be associated with clinical problems are identified by *.

crease the rate of renewal of the basal epithelium and result in mucosal atrophy (Lockhart & Sonis, 1981). This effect may be compounded by a diminished nutritional intake, which can occur secondary to the mucositis itself. A diminished intake can cause increased mucosal atrophy because cell renewal is further decreased during starvation or protein deprivation. The buccal, labial, and soft palate mucosa, along with the ventral surfaces of the tongue and floor of the mouth, are the most commonly affected sites. Mucositis as a direct toxicity is usually observed within 5–7 days after administration of chemotherapy. Mucositis usually begins as erythema, or reddening, of the soft palate and buccal mucosa, followed frequently by desquamation and swelling. Ulceration may occur from serration by a patient's natural teeth or the presence of oral or prosthodontic prostheses. As the mucosa is extremely fragile at this time, spicy or hard foodstuffs can also aggrevate the problem. Good oral care and a soft diet are often recommended (Carl, 1995).

In addition to the aforementioned direct toxicity on the mucosa of the mouth and upper digestive tract, chemotherapy can also have multiple indirect toxicities. Indirect oral toxicities include neurotoxicity and alterations of taste sensation, such that patients are unwilling to eat or undesirous of eating. Administration of the plant alkaloid vincristine can result in complaints of intermittent odontogenic pain in one or more mandibular teeth. This complaint is generally transient and does not appear to cause any long-term compromise of the patient's teeth.

Loss of appetite and complaints of decrease in taste sensation may also occur, secondary to the patient's general state of debilitation during therapy. Patients with extensive involvement at multiple lymph node sites by malignant lymphoma may also complain of general malaise and/or fevers, which can decrease the patient's ability or desire to eat. These effects must be separated from the dysphagia, which is secondary to actual organ pathology or dysfunction (Sonis, 1983).

DYSPHAGIA AND DISORDERS OF COMMUNICATION ASSOCIATED WITH RADIATION THERAPY

The complications of radiation therapy that occur with leukemia and lymphoma are similar to, but generally less severe than, the effects seen with other head and neck solid tumors. This is because the doses of radiation generally used to treat lymphoma are significantly less than those used to treat solid tumors. The acute oral mucosal response to radiation therapy is a result of mitotic death of the epithelial cells. Because the cell-cycle time of epithelium is approximately 4 days and the epithelium is at least three or four cell layers thick, radiation changes generally begin to appear at approximately 12–15 days after the start of therapy. Initially, the oral mucosa may turn a whitish color, which is then followed by the appearance of reddening and then a few days later by a patchy fibrinous exudate. If higher doses of radiation are given, ulceration may occur. The simultaneous use of chemotherapy and radiation therapy, or of radiation therapy and tobacco products, can result in an even more severe and prolonged mucositis and ulceration.

Probably more important than production of mucositis are the late effects of treatment, predominantly the appearance of xerostomia (dry mouth). This complication is a direct result of radiation to the salivary glands, and a decrease in salivary flow. Xerostomia is universally noted from high doses of radiation, and as little as 20 Gy has been reported to cause permanent cessation of salivary flow when given as a single dose (Scully & Epstein, 1996). Radiation therapy given to the nasopharynx will damage all major and minor salivary glands and typically causes the most severe and permanent xerostomia. The presence of dry mouth may lead the patient to complain of oral discomfort, loss of taste, and diminished appetite, and may additionally lead to an increased risk of oral infections (such as candidiasis and dental caries).

Radiation therapy can also cause disturbances or loss of taste sensation unrelated to xerostomia. Although the mechanism for this loss of taste has not been well elucidated, it fortunately slowly recovers within a few months of the end of radiation therapy.

More severe problems resulting from radiation therapy to the head and neck, such as fibrosis and resultant trismus or osteoradionecrosis, are extremely rare in treatment for hematologic malignancies. This is because of the relatively low doses of radiation therapy used in these tumors.

Several late effects of radiation therapy appear peculiar to patients with hematologic malignancies. Young children who have received cranial irradiation (and to a lesser extent intrathecal chemotherapy) may experience late neurological toxicity resulting from damage to the brain. If combined cranial irradiation and intrathecal chemotherapy are given, greater toxicity is observed. Many studies have attempted to correlate the timing and dose of radiation therapy to the appearance of learning disorders, including language deficits (Brown & Madan-Swain, 1993; Mulhern, Ochs, & Fairlough, 1992), but the results appear controversial. It is certain that some decrement in cognitive function occurs after radiation of the brain during early childhood, but the actual extent and severity of the abnormalities are as yet unclear. Some of this inability to determine an exact incidence and severity of dysfunction is secondary to lack of definitive baseline cognitive, speech, and language measures on young children. Any evaluation must additionally be related to their functional status prior to therapy. Approximately 50% of children who received cranial irradiation in early childhood have abnormal computed tomography scans with intracranial calcification, cerebral hypodensities, and atrophy (Winter & Prendergast, 1995). These abnormalities can result in neuronal loss and directly cause communication and speech disorders. Rarely, it has been reported that these abnormalities result in specific pathological foci within the brain and cause protracted seizures (Winter & Prendergast, 1995). These seizure disorders may present as abnormalities of speech, including aphasia.

TABLE 9–4. Most Common Infections Causing Dysphagia for Patients With Hematologic Malignancies Receiving Chemotherapy

I. Bacteria
Mycobacteria (including *M. avium* complex)
Other gram-negative organisms[a]

II. Fungi
Candida species (especially *C. albicans*)

III. Viruses
Cytomegalovirus
Herpes simplex
Varicella zoster

[a]Gram-negative bacteria are frequent colonizers of the oral mucosa of patients receiving chemotherapy or on antibiotics. These organisms more commonly directly invade the bloodstream, resulting in sepsis. However, rarely they result in local infections as well.

INFECTIOUS COMPLICATIONS FROM NEUTROPENIA CAN RESULT IN DYSPHAGIA

Another form of indirect oral toxicity due to the effects of chemotherapy is that of infectious mucositis. In general, the degree and duration of the neutropenia are the major determinant of the incidence and severity of the infection. The normal mouth flora is responsible for the majority of infections seen during periods of myelosuppression. At this point, oral flora changes to become predominantly anaerobes and gram-negative organisms such as *Klebsiella, Serratia, Enterobacter, Escherichia coli, Pseudomonas,* and *Proteus* (Dreizen & Brown, 1983). Most fungal infections are caused by a yeast, *Candida albicans.* Viral infections tend to be due to herpes simplex or cytomegalovirus (Table 9–4).

Bacterial infections generally affect three sites in the mouth: the gingiva, the oral mucosa, and the teeth. They generally start at a time when the patient's white count reaches its lowest point, usually within 12–14 days after the beginning of chemotherapy. Infections in the mouth are more frequent with preexisting periodontal disease or poor oral hygiene. They frequently present as a necrotizing gingivitis, which can spread and cause ulceration not only within the mouth but also in the esophagus and remaining gastrointestinal tract. The inflammation is frequently associated with fever and moderate to severe pain. This pain can be severe enough to require intravenous analgesics.

The identification of an infectious cause of mucositis relies on the visual identification or culture of the offending organisms. In the mouth, tissue biopsies are usually not obtained, and cultures form the basis of most diagnoses. In the esophagus, however, tissue biopsies are commonly obtained for diagnosis. Viruses can often be seen as intracellular inclusions when the vesicles, ulcers, or lesions are scraped onto slides and stained for evaluation under a microscope. Bacteria can be seen as colonies on Gram stain of a lesion, with final identification upon culture. The ulcer or lesion itself can be cultured. With low white counts, the infection frequently becomes systemic, at which point the organism can be identified in the blood. Fungi are also cultured, but can be identified on staining of the lesion when the fungal hyphae or yeast bodies are noted to invade the adjacent tissue. It may be important to obtain a deep biopsy for culture, as a superficial erosion or ulcer can be colonized or "superinfected" by other mouth flora.

RELATIONSHIP OF THROMBOCYTOPENIA TO HEMORRHAGE AND SYMPTOMS OF DYSPHAGIA OR DYSPHONIA

Chemotherapy can result in other types of indirect oral toxicity, in addition to mucositis. The intense therapy that is given to patients with acute leukemia, in combination with their already poorly functioning bone marrow, can result in significant decreases in platelet count as well as white blood cell count. These decreases in platelet count can be responsible for spontaneous bruising, as well as small and large areas of hemorrhage and hematoma formation. In general, hemorrhage does not occur spontaneously unless the platelet count reaches very low levels (generally less than 5,000/μl). However, almost any level of thrombocytopenia can predispose to mucosal bleeding when the area is provoked by trauma or there is a preexisting lesion (ulcerated tumor, infection, or periodontal disease). Hematomas can cause mechanical obstruction by the formation of a mass, or they can cause vocal fold dysfunction or elevation of the tongue with consequent compromise of respiration, speech, and swallowing.

MANAGEMENT OF DYSPHAGIA

General Management

Management requires the identification of the specific etiology for the swallowing or speech problem. When the individual cause is identified (infection, direct toxicity, tissue infiltration) by biopsy, culture, or physical examination, a specific course of management can be initiated. The general management of these individual disorders is not unique to patients with hematologic malignancies, and is well covered in other sections of this book. It will not be further elaborated on here. Prevention forms a major part of the strategy. Identification of a patient at risk, and the delineation of the time frame for risk, is of paramount importance. A general summary of the

causes and treatment of these disorders is given in Table 9–5.

UNIQUE THERAPIES WITH LEUKEMIA AND LYMPHOMA

Probably the most significant factor that sets apart patients with hematologic malignancies is the degree of bone marrow compromise that occurs from the disease as well as the subsequent therapy. This bone marrow compromise results in patients' having very low white blood cell counts and platelet counts in contrast to the majority of patients with solid tumors. Local therapies such as radiation may be used as adjuvants with certain types of lymphoma, but are less commonly employed than in other types of malignancies. Radiation doses and duration of therapy are also quite different. The chemotherapeutic regimens used to treat hematologic malignancies employ marrow-suppressive drugs at relatively high doses, thus these drugs can potentially have serious consequences. The complications of chemotherapy with leukemias and lymphoma are intermediate between those seen with the therapy of solid tumors and those seen with bone marrow transplantation.

Patients with hematologic malignancies tend to have more frequent and more serious problems, with oral and mucosal bleeding, infection, and mucositis from the toxicity of chemotherapy. Mucosal bleeding can occasionally be controlled with topical thrombin or local therapies. Platelet transfusions are often required. Infections are best treated from a primary preventive mode, and prophylactic antibiotics or antifungals are commonly employed. Hydration and maintenance of good nutrition, good mouth care, and continued vigilant observation are required.

CONCLUSIONS

The number of newly diagnosed patients with malignant diseases appears to be rising annually (Sonis, 1983). The prognosis for these individuals depends on the response

TABLE 9–5. General Strategies for the Diagnosis And Treatment of Oral Complications of Hematologic Malignancies

Problem	Diagnostic Strategy	Treatment
Tumor Growth		
Bulky lymphadenopathy	Physical examination, CT, or other radiological imaging technique	Tumor-directed (may include local radiation therapy and/or systemic chemotherapy)
Tissue infiltration	CT, MRI, or other radiological imaging technique Tissue biopsy	Tumor-directed (may include local radiation therapy and/or systemic chemotherapy; surgical resection of large obstructing masses or infected or perforating tumors is occasionally required)
Tumor Therapy		
Mucositis	Physical examination and clinical history (timing of chemotherapy or local radiation)	Local palliation: may include application of cold (ice chips or cold beverages), local anesthetics (Xylocaine Viscous, Dyclone, or oral benzocaine ointments), or systemic pain medication in severe cases
Xerostomia	Physical examination and clinical history (timing of chemotherapy or local radiation)	Saliva substitutes or mouth moisturizers
Local bleeding	Physical examination and clinical history (timing of chemotherapy or local radiation)	Platelet or clotting factor transfusions when responsible for hemorrhage; topical thrombin solutions for gingival bleeding; may require application of pressure or use of microfilbrillar collagen
Infections		
Oral candidiasis	Physical examination Direct smear Culture and species identification	Oral nystatin or clotrimazole; oral fluconazole or itraconazole for prophylaxis or established infections
Oral herpetic mucositis	Physical examination Direct smear Culture	Oral acyclovir
Bacterial infections	Culture and species identification	Systemic antibiotics directed against the specific organism identified
Neurological Problems		
Toxicity of therapy or result of previous tumor involvement	Clinical history	Many neurological toxicities resolve or improve gradually with time; chronic or long-term sequelae may require psychosocial, language, cognitive, and/or specialized learning interventions

Note. CT = computed tomography; MRI = magnetic resonance imaging.

of the tumor to treatment. As more and more different modalities of chemotherapy combined with radiation are used with hematologic malignancies, caretakers and health care personnel must be able to deal with an increasing number of complications from these treatments. Oral complications of chemotherapy can be significant, with pain, dysfunction, weight loss, bleeding, and infection occurring.

It appears probable that both the number and severity of cancer chemotherapy-related complications will increase as new, more potent, drugs and higher doses are used in an attempt to cure these tumors. Therefore, a good understanding of these complications and their prevention and therapy is needed. Clearly, as new modalities develop, more knowledge regarding treatment and care of these patients is needed.

REFERENCES

Azab, M. B., Henry-Amar, M., Rougier, P., et al. (1989). Prognostic factors in primary gastro-intestinal non-Hodgkin's lymphoma: A multi-variate analysis, report of 106 cases and review of the literature. *Cancer, 64*, 1208–1217.

Baraket, N. J., Toto, P. D., & Choukas, N. C. (1969). Aging and cell renewal of oral epithelium. *Journal of Periodontology, 40*, 599–602.

Brown, R. T., & Madan-Swain, A. (1993). Cognitive, neuropsychological, and academic sequelae in children with leukemia. *Journal of Learning Disabilities 26*, 74–90.

Carl, W. (1995). Oral complications of local and systemic cancer treatment. *Current Opinion in Oncology, 7*, 320–324.

Dreizen, S., & Brown, L. R. (1983). Oral microbial changes and infections during cancer chemotherapy. In D. E. Peterson & S. T. Sonis (Eds.), *Oral complications of cancer chemotherapy.* (pp. 41–47). Boston: Martinus Nijhoff.

Harris, N. L., Jaffe, E. S., Stein, H., Banks, P. M., Chan, J. K. C., Cleary, M. L., Delsol, G., De Wolf-Peeters, C., Falini, B., Gatter, K. C., Grogan, T. M., Isaacson, P. G., Knowles, D. M., Mason, D. Y., Muller-Hermelink, H. K., Pileri, S. A., Piris, M. A., Ralfkiaer, E., & Warnke, R. A. (1994). A revised European-American classification of lymphoid neoplasms: A proposal from the International Lymphoma Study Group. *Blood, 84*, 1361–1392.

Hoffbrand, A. V., & Pettit, J. E. (Eds.). (1993). *Essential haematology* (3rd ed.). Oxford, England: Blackwell Scientific.

Isaacson, P. G., Spencer, J., & Finn, T. (1986). Primary B cell gastric lymphoma. *Human Pathology, 17*, 72–82.

Kawaida, M., Fukuda, H., Shiotani, A., Nakagawa, H., Kohno, N., & Nakamura, A. (1996). Isolated non-Hodgkin's malignant lymphoma of the larynx presenting as a large pedunculated tumor.

ORL: Journal of Oto-Rhino-Laryngology and Its Related Specialties, 58, 171–174.

Lockhart, P. B., & Sonis, S. T. (1979). Relationship of oral complications to peripheral blood leukocyte and platelet counts receiving cancer chemotherapy. *Oral Surgery, 48*, 21–28.

Lockhart, P. B., & Sonis, S. T. (1981). Alterations in the oral mucosa caused by chemotherapeutic agents. *Journal of Dermatologic Surgery and Oncology, 7*, 1019–1025.

Moss, S., Valentine, C. B., Carey, P. B., & Hind, C. R. K. (1993). Dysphagia in an HIV-positive man. *Postgraduate Medical Journal, 71*, 247–248.

Mulhern, R. K., Ochs, J., & Fairclough, D. (1992). Deterioration of intellect among children surviving leukemia: IQ test changes modify estimates of treatment toxicity. *Journal of Consulting and Clinical Psychology, 60*, 477–480.

Ramirez-Amador, V., Esquivel-Pedraza, L., Mohar, A., Reynoso-Gomez, E., Volkow-Fernandez, P., Guarner, J., & Sanchez-Mejorada, G. (1996). Chemotherapy-associated oral mucosal lesions with leukaemia or lymphoma. *Oral Oncology, 32B*, 322–327.

Robbins, K. T., Fuller, L. M., Vlasak, M., Osborne, B., Jing, B. S., Velasquez, W. S., & Sullian, J. A. (1985). Primary lymphomas of the nasal cavity and paranasal sinuses. *Cancer, 56*, 814–819.

Scully, C., & Epstein, J. B. (1996). Oral health care for the cancer patient. *Oral Oncology, 32B*, 281–292.

Sonis, S. T. (1983). Epidemiology, frequency, distribution, mechanisms, and histopathology. In D. E. Peterson & S. T. Sonis (Eds.), *Oral complications of cancer chemotherapy* (pp. 1–12). Boston: Martinus Nijhoff.

Sonis, S. T. (1985). Oral complications of cancer therapy. In V. T. DeVita, Jr., S. Hellman, & S. A. Rosenberg (Eds.), *Cancer: Principles and practice of oncology* (pp. 2014–2021). Philadelphia: J.B. Lippincott.

Sonis, S. T., Sonis, A. L., & Lieberman, A. (1978). Oral complications receiving treatment for malignancies other than of the head and neck. *Journal of the American Dental Association, 97*, 468–472.

Taal, B. G., Van Heerde, P., & Somers, R. (1993). Isolated primary oesophageal involvement by lymphoma: A rare cause of dysphagia: Two case histories and a review of other published data. *Gut, 34*, 994–998.

Winter, E., & Prendergast, M. (1995). Cured of acute lymphoblastic leukaemia but lost for words. *Neuropediatrics, 26*, 267–269.

10

Disorders of the Upper Aerodigestive Tract Associated With High-Dose Therapy and Stem Cell Transplantation

Karen K. Fields, M.D., and Deborah L. Borger, M.S.N.

High-dose therapy followed by transplantation of stem cells derived from the bone marrow or peripheral blood, a therapeutic modality widely employed for the treatment of a variety of malignant and nonmalignant disorders, is associated with a unique spectrum of complications related to the mucous membranes of the upper aerodigestive tract (Schubert, Sullivan, & Truelove, 1986). Since the first successful allogeneic bone marrow transplants were performed in the late 1960s (Thomas, Lochte, Cannon, Sahler, & Ferrebee, 1959; Thomas, Lochte, Lu, & Ferrebee, 1957), the number of patients treated with this procedure has grown exponentially, with over 5,000 allogeneic transplants performed worldwide in 1990; and continued growth in the annual number of transplants performed is projected to be about 15% per year (Horowitz, 1995). From 1970 through 1995, over 45,000 allografts were performed worldwide. Growth in the number of autologous bone marrow or peripheral blood stem cell transplants has also been dramatic. Over 10,000 transplants

were performed worldwide in 1995, and the projected growth rate is 20% annually (Horowitz, 1995). In the interval from 1980 through 1995, it was estimated that over 30,000 autografts were performed worldwide. The indications for bone marrow or peripheral blood stem cell transplantation continue to expand as well and include leukemia, lymphoma, breast cancer, and other solid tumors as well as nonmalignant disorders such as aplastic anemia, other immunodeficiency states, and a variety of inherited disorders of metabolism.

With the increased use of this procedure comes an increased need to diagnose and control associated treatment-related toxicities. Disorders of the upper aerodigestive tract are among the most frequent treatment-related toxicities seen in patients undergoing bone marrow transplantation, and, although generally reversible, may limit the use and possibly the efficacy of this therapy. Some degree of mucositis, for example, occurs in virtually all of the patients undergoing transplantation, resulting in potential discomfort, nutritional compromise, increases in infectious complications, and other possibly life-threatening side effects. Mucositis can also result in increased transplant-related costs due to protracted hospital stays.

PRINCIPLES OF HIGH-DOSE THERAPY AND STEM CELL TRANSPLANTATION

The goal of combined high-dose therapy and bone marrow or stem cell transplantation is to deliver curative doses of chemotherapy, with or without the addition of radiation therapy. For most tumors, the doses of therapy necessary to achieve potential cure would result in lethal and irreversible marrow damage. To deliver these doses of chemotherapy and radiation therapy, "stem cells" derived from the bone marrow or the peripheral blood are infused intravenously following the completion of myeloablative therapy, thus providing the patient with rescue from the primary toxicity of high-dose therapy, that of hematopoietic toxicity. The hematopoietic stem cell represents the pluripotent cell capable of self-renewal; it is responsible for repopulation of the bone marrow with progenitors that are able to differentiate into myeloid, erthyroid, or lymphoid cell lines. The delivery of high-dose therapy itself (i.e., the conditioning regimen) is the primary function of this procedure, and the secondary procedure, the stem cell transplant, allows the delivery of maximum, curative doses of therapy. The transplant process is briefly described in Figure 10–1.

The infusion of stem cells, derived from either bone marrow or peripheral blood, enables the clinician to escalate the doses of chemotherapy or radiation therapy beyond those of lethal marrow toxicity to the next level of toxicity, that of nonhematologic dose-limiting organ toxicity. As an example of dose escalation, thiotepa, a mechlorethaminelike alkylating agent active in a variety of malignancies, has been given in the nontransplant setting in doses ranging from 10 to 60 mg/m^2, with myelosuppression noted to be the major side effect. However, when stem cell rescue is provided, the maximum tolerated dose of thiotepa that has been given alone or in combination is 1,200 mg/m^2 with protracted mucositis, delayed hematopoietic recovery, and, in some reports, central nervous system toxicity constituting the main nonhematologic dose-limiting toxicities (Fields et al., 1993). Many other drugs lend themselves well to dose escalation due to limited nonhematologic toxicity even at high doses. In addition, a steep dose-response relationship has been demonstrated for many chemotherapeutic agents, in particular the alkylating agents, thus providing further rationale for dose escalation (Frei, Teicher, Holden, Cathcart, & Wang, 1988).

The underlying disease coupled with the availability (or lack of availability) of a suitable donor determines the type of transplant to be performed. The human leukocyte antigen (HLA) system determines the histocompatibility of the donor. There are three categories of stem cell transplants: a *syngeneic transplant* using stem cells obtained from a genotypically identical twin, an *allogeneic transplant* using stem cells obtained from an HLA-matched sibling or donor that is phenotypically identical (6 out of 6 antigen match) or closely HLA-matched (less than a 6-antigen match), or an *autologous transplant* using stem cells obtained from the patient prior to administration of high-dose therapy. Potential allogeneic donors include siblings and other family members, unrelated but closely HLA-matched donors identified through one of several large bone marrow donor registries, and, more recently, HLA-matched, placentally-derived stem cells identified through one of several cord blood registries.

In diseases where the bone marrow or the immune system is the primary site of disease, an allogeneic transplant is generally indicated, although autologous transplants are occasionally performed in this setting. However, in the case of solid tumors and lymphoma, where the main goal of therapy is the delivery of high-dose anticancer therapy and stem cells are used to provide rescue from the myeloablative effects of high-dose therapy, autologous transplantation is the most appropriate given the addi-

Identify Patient
  Assess disease status
  Assess functional status including vital organ function

Identify Source of Stem Cells
  Allogeneic: Assess donor suitability
  Autologous: Bone marrow versus peripheral blood

Harvest Stem Cells
  Allogeneic: Harvest stem cells from donor following completion of conditioning regimen
  Autologous: Harvest stem cells and cryopreserve for reinfusion following completion of conditioning regimen

Conditioning Regimen (3–10 days)
  Chemotherapy
  ± Radiation Therapy

Stem Cell Transplant
  Central venous infusion of fresh allogeneic or cryopreserved autologous stem cells

Supportive Care (4–6 weeks)
  Aggressive treatment of transplant-related complications

    Hematopoietic complications
      Anemia
      Thrombocytopenia
      Neutropenia and infectious complications
      Graft failure

    Nonhematopoietic complications
      Mucositis
      Enteritis
      Other gastrointestinal complications
      Pneumonitis
      Cardiac complications
      Hepatic complications
      Renal complications
      Neurological complications
      Nutritional compromise
      Psychosocial complications
      Graft-versus-host disease

Figure 10–1. The transplant process

tional morbidity and mortality seen in patients undergoing allogeneic transplant compared to autologous transplant. Table 10–1 lists diseases commonly considered potentially curable with high-dose therapy and stem cell transplantation. The incidence of associated disorders of swallowing or communication will be related to the underlying disease, the conditioning regimen indicated

for the treatment of a specific disease, and the type of transplant (syngeneic, allogeneic, or autologous).

Successful bone marrow transplantation is largely influenced by the incidence and treatment of transplant-related complications. Disorders of the upper aerodigestive tract and gastrointestinal tract account for the most frequent nonhematopoietic toxicities

TABLE 10–1. Diseases for Which Stem Cell Transplanation Is Commonly Performed

Allogeneic Transplantation

Leukemia
   Acute myelogenous leukemia
   Chronic myelogenous leukemia
   Acute lymphocytic leukemia
   Chronic lymphocytic leukemia

Lymphoma
   Non-Hodgkin's lymphoma
   Hodgkin's disease

Other Myeloproliferative or Lymphoproliferative Disorders
   Multiple myeloma

Other Hematologic Disorders
   Aplastic anemia
   Thalessemia
   Sickle cell disease
   Fanconi's anemia

Immunodeficiency States
   Severe combined immune deficiency
   Other immunodeficiency states

Inborn Errors of Metabolism
   Gaucher's disease

Autologous Transplantation

Leukemia
   Acute myelogenous leukemia
   Chronic myelogenous leukemia
   Acute lymphocytic leukemia
   Chronic lymphocytic leukemia

Lymphoma
   Non-Hodgkin's lymphoma
   Hodgkin's disease

Other Lymphoproliferative Disorders
   Multiple myeloma

Solid Tumors
   Breast cancer
   Testicular cancer
   Ovarian cancer
   Sarcoma: adult and pediatric
   Other pediatric solid tumors including neuroblastoma
   Primary brain tumors
   Selected chemosensitive tumors

seen in patients undergoing high-dose therapy and stem cell transplantation. Table 10–2 outlines the common complications related to the mucous membranes of the upper airway associated with this therapy. The following sections will address these complications as related to high-dose therapy and stem cell transplantation.

THERAPY-INDUCED MUCOSITIS

Etiology

The relationship between mucositis and cytotoxic chemotherapy is well known (Sonis & Haley, 1996). Studies have demonstrated that the basal epithelium of the mucosa is a primary target of toxicity following chemotherapy and radiation therapy (Sonis, 1983). The subsequent decreases in cell renewal of the basal epithelium result in atrophic changes and epithelial thinning of the oral mucosa. This change and the functional oral trauma commonly seen in the mouth combine to produce the lesions of ulcerative mucositis, a classic finding in therapy-induced mucositis (Sonis, 1993). The presence of normal oral flora makes these lesions particularly susceptible to superinfection, which, in the immune-compromised host, could result in bacteremia and, subsequently, systemic infections. In addition to the increased risks of systemic infection, ulcerative mucositis results in marked physical discomfort, compromises the patient's ability to maintain adequate oral nutrition, and poses a significant bleeding threat to patients with thrombocytopenia, all of which are expected complications in the early posttransplant period.

Grading Systems

Several scoring systems have been developed in an effort to quantify the lesions and symptoms seen in patients with therapy-induced mucositis. The two scales most commonly employed are the National Cancer Institute (NCI) Common Toxicity Scale (Wilson et al., 1992) and the World Health Organization (WHO) Toxicity Scale (Sonis & Costello, 1995). Although grading systems such as these are helpful in the quantification of therapy-induced mucositis, such scales are frequently limited by the inclusion of both objective and subjective criteria. For example, oral pain and the ability to

TABLE 10–2. Common Upper Aerodigestive Tract Complications Following High-Dose Therapy and Stem Cell Transplant

Etiology	Associated Complication
Therapy-induced mucositis	Risk of systemic infection
	Pain
	Dysphagia
	Bleeding
	Airway obstruction
	Aspiration
	Nutritional compromise
	Communication defects
Infectious stomatitis/esophagitis	As above
	Risk of systemic dissemination
Graft-versus-host disease	As above
	Salivary gland dysfunction
	Xerostomia
	Peridontal disease
	Risk of extensive dental caries
	Delay in eruption of permanent teeth in children

eat are end points in both the NCI and WHO grading systems, and the interpretation of these symptoms may vary widely from patient to patient or the presence of these symptoms may be related to other, compounding transplant-related complications such as nausea and vomiting or the treatment of nonoral pain. Table 10–3 describes the NCI Common Toxicity Scale criteria for grading mucositis and Table 10–4 describes the WHO grading scale for mucositis. Comparison of treatment-related toxicity among patients, conditioning regimens, and institutions is only possible when quantifiable and universally accepted criteria are available for all patients following high-dose therapy and stem cell transplant. To this end, several newer scales have been developed that attempt to improve the uniformity of reporting of this clinically important toxicity (Schubert, Williams, Lloid, Donaldson, & Chapko, 1992; Sonis & Costello, 1995).

Pretransplant Evaluation

Evaluation of the oral mucosa and assessment of the patient's dental health are essential elements of the pretransplant work-up (Carl & Higby, 1985; Seto, Kim, Wolinshy, Mito, & Champlin, 1985; Udagama, 1984). All patients are referred to a dentist prior to consideration of transplant for specific attention to factors that predispose the patient to the development of oral complications. Dental caries should be diagnosed and treated aggressively because undiagnosed or untreated dental infections in the immediate posttransplant period could result in life-threatening systemic infections. Unfortunately, extensive reparative work is often not possible in patients referred for transplant who present with chronically poor dentition given that the underlying medical illness generally necessitates urgent therapeutic intervention. Therefore, in patients with extensive dental complications presenting for consideration of transplant, it is often necessary to recommend multiple dental extractions rather than attempt to treat multiple dental caries or other problems. A thorough dental cleaning is necessary prior to transplant to decrease the presence of plaque. Vigorous dental cleaning is contraindicated in the early posttransplant period due to the risk of bacteremia or bleeding secondary to oral in-

TABLE 10–3. National Cancer Institute Toxicity Criteria for Grading Mucositis

Grade	Criteria
0	None or discomfort only with spicy/sour foods
1	Pain without ulceration; able to drink/eat most foods
2A	As for grade 3 but < 2 weeks' duration
2B	Pain with ulceration; able to drink water
3	Painful ulceration causing complete inanition and requiring narcotic analgesics for > 2 weeks (unrelated to *Candida* or herpetic infection)
4	Fatal toxicity

TABLE 10–4. World Health Organization Criteria for Oral Mucositis Grading

Grade	Criteria
0 (none)	None
1 (mild)	Soreness/erythema
2 (moderate)	Erythema, ulcers, can eat solids
3 (severe)	Ulcers, required liquid diet
4 (life-threatening)	Can't eat
5 (fatal)	Fatal toxicity

strumentation. Often, extensive dental restoration is not possible for up to 1 year following transplantation (Schubert, Sullivan, Izutsu, & Truelove, 1983). In addition, children receiving bone marrow transplantation may show a delayed or disrupted eruption of permanent teeth (Schubert et al., 1983). One of the most important components of the pretransplant dental evaluation is patient education with attention to preventive measures.

Incidence and Risk Factors

The incidence of mucositis varies greatly from regimen to regimen, although some degree of mucositis is present in virtually all patients undergoing high-dose therapy and stem cell transplantation. Longitudinal studies have reported the presence of oral ulcers (corresponding to at least a grade II toxicity on conventional mucositis grading scales) in approximately 75% of all patients undergoing bone marrow transplantation (Woo, Sonis, Monopoli, & Sonis, 1993). Table 10–5 lists the major risk factors associated with the development of therapy-induced mucositis.

The degree and incidence of therapy-induced mucositis are influenced by the dose intensity of the regimen as well as the choice of cytotoxic agents. Regimens that include total body irradiation (TBI) are generally associated with a higher incidence and severity of oral mucositis. The use of high-dose alkylating agents alone and in combination and regimens that combine alkylating agents with etoposide have been associated with a high incidence of clinically significant mucositis (Fields et al., 1995). Additionally, the method of administration of the chemotherapeutic agent may influence the development of mucositis. Continuous infusion of some drugs has been associated with significantly more mucositis than bolus administration (Herzig, 1991). Other

TABLE 10–5. Factors That Influence the Development of Therapy-Induced Mucositis

---

Conditioning regimen

    Choice of chemotherapy agents

    Combination chemotherapy

    Dose intensity

    Method of administration

    Inclusion of total body irradiation

    The use of methotrexate for graft-versus-host disease prophylaxis

Patient specific

    Age

    Poor dental hygiene

    Presence of active infections in the oral cavity

    Prior irradiation of the head and neck

    Prior surgery of the head and neck

    Connective tissue diseases associated with salivary gland dysfunction

    Nutritional status

---

concomitant therapy administered with the conditioning regimen may also influence the development of mucositis. In the allogeneic transplant setting, for example, the use of methotrexate in the early posttransplant period for the prophylaxis of graft-versus-host disease (GVHD) is frequently associated with severe mucositis, which may necessitate reductions in the total dose of methotrexate, resulting in an increased risk of developing GVHD (Schubert et al., 1983). Thus, presence of mucositis, itself, may limit the effectiveness of the transplant.

As previously noted, the underlying dental health and the conditioning regimen constitute major risk factors for the development of therapy-induced mucositis following transplant. Another important risk factor is age. Based on animal data, it has been suggested that there is a more rapid turnover of the basal epithelium in younger patients than in older patients, predisposing the younger patient to an increased incidence of therapy-induced mucositis (O'Brien, Muska, Van Vugt, Sonis, & Haley, 1994). However, due to the slower rate of turnover of basal epithelium in the older patient, the duration of mucositis may be increased in the older patient compared to the younger patient. This has been observed clinically; one study evaluating the effect of age on transplant-related complications demonstrated an increase in the severity and duration of mucositis in patients over 55 years of age compared to patients younger than 55 years of age following autologous bone marrow transplantation, although these differences were not associated with an increased risk in transplant-related mortality or a lengthening of the hospital stay in the older patients (Partyka et al., 1996). Other risk factors associated with an increase in the incidence and severity of therapy-induced mucositis include prior irradiation of the head and neck, which can be associated with salivary gland dysfunction (Carl, 1995). For the same reasons, underlying connective tissue disorders associated with salivary gland dysfunction could also predispose the patient to the development of mucositis.

Clinical Course

The clinical course of therapy-induced mucositis is variable depending on the type of transplant, the conditioning regimen, pre-existing conditions, concomitant therapies such as the use of GVHD prophylaxis, and the development of GVHD. In general, the onset of mucositis is within 1 week of completion of the conditioning regimen and peaks within 7–14 days following transplant (Armstrong, 1994). Severe symptoms may persist for as long as 20 to 30 days following transplant, although improvement is usually observed earlier in the clinical course. One study evaluated the incidence, time of onset, duration, and severity of therapy-induced mucositis among 47 patients undergoing either allogeneic or autologous bone marrow transplantation (Mcquire et al., 1993). Patients were evaluated daily beginning 9 days prior to bone marrow transplant and continuing through day 21 following transplant. Forty-two patients (89%) developed mucositis, which began an average of 3 days following transplant, lasted an average of 9.5 days, and resolved by an average of 12.6 days posttransplant. The course of associated mucosal pain mirrored that of the clinical observations of mucositis. Thirty-six patients (86%) reported pain, which began an average of 4.5 days after transplant, lasted an average of 6.5 days, and resolved an average of 11 days following transplant.

The role of total body irradiation (TBI) in the clinical course of therapy-induced mucositis has also been evaluated. One study compared the clinical course of patients receiving a TBI-containing regimen to patients receiving a non-TBI-containing regimen (Zerbe, Parkerson, Ortlieb, & Spitzer, 1992). These investigators noted that mucositis began an average of 2 days prior to transplant and peaked an average of 8 days following transplant. Patients receiving the TBI-containing regimen had a trend toward higher oral mucositis scores during the 1st week following transplant. Additionally, these patients required twice the number of days of intravenous analgesic administration and 6 more days of total parenteral nutrition than the patients that received the non-TBI-containing regimen. Other investigators comparing a TBI-containing regimen to a non-TBI-containing regimen in 28 children undergoing autologous transplantation for the treatment of a variety of solid tumors saw a statistically significant increase in the severity and duration of mucositis in the patients receiving TBI (Borgmann et al., 1994). The median duration of mucositis was 8 days (range 0–28) in the TBI-treated patients compared to 0 days (range 0–7) in the non-TBI-treated patients ($p = .01$). Long-term follow-up of these patients revealed no improvement in survival in the children treated with TBI, prompting these authors to conclude that the increased toxicity of TBI may not be justifiable in certain diseases.

Differential Diagnosis

The differential diagnosis of therapy-induced mucositis primarily includes infections or, in the case of allogeneic transplantation, GVHD. Infectious complications of the upper aerodigestive tract, including the diagnosis and management of these complications, as seen in the patient with cancer, are discussed in detail in Chapters 11 and 14. The two most common oral infections following both allogeneic and autologous stem cell transplantation include herpes simplex virus (HSV; Schubert, Peterson, Flourneoy, Meyers, & Truelove, 1990) and *Candida* species (McDonald, Sharma, Hackman, Meyers, & Thomas, 1985). Indeed, these infections are so common in the patient undergoing transplant that prophylaxis for both HSV and *Candida albicans* is the routine in most, if not all, bone marrow transplant units.

HSV can be cultured from 37–68% of oral ulcers present in patients receiving chemotherapy or undergoing stem cell transplantation (Redding, 1990). In this patient population, HSV-positive lesions usually present in an atypical fashion, frequently involving the perioral and intraoral surfaces. With the routine use of prophylactic acyclovir in the peritransplant period, HSV rarely accounts for oral ulceration in the immediate posttransplant period. In one study, 60 patients undergoing autologous or allogenic transplants were followed for 30 days posttransplant for the presence of culturable HSV (Woo, Sonis, & Sonis, 1990). Fifty-nine patients received prophylactic acyclovir in the peritransplant period. Forty-six patients developed ulcerative lesions, and in 45 of these patients the lesions were culture-negative for HSV. In this study, neither the type of transplant (allogeneic versus autologous) nor the HSV antibody status of the patient affected the frequency of mucositis. It should be noted, however, that despite the marked decrease in reactivation of HSV in bone marrow transplant patients treated with prophylactic acyclovir, culture-positive oral HSV lesions can be seen following the discontinuation of acyclovir, and HSV should always be considered in the differential diagnosis as the etiology of the development of delayed oral ulcers.

Oral candidiasis is a common problem following both autologous and allogeneic stem cell transplantation. Such infections predispose the host to systemic candidiasis, which can have potentially fatal consequences. The mainstay for prophylaxis of oral *Candida* infections in the posttransplant patient is the use of oral nystatin or clotrimazole. A variety of other agents have been studied including miconazole, ketoconazole, fluconazole, and amphotericin B. Two controlled trials have demonstrated fluconazole to be effective in reducing the incidence of mucosal and systemic *Candida* infections when compared to placebo (Goodman, Winston, & Greenfield, 1992; Winston, Islam, Beull, & Acute Leukemia Study Group, 1991). It has also been demonstrated to be superior to oral amphotericin B and nystatin in decreasing mucosal and systemic *Candida* infections (Brammer, 1990). The optimal approach to prophylaxis of oral candidiasis will be based on trends in the supportive care of the transplant patient, with such confounding factors as the use of prophylactic systemic antibiotics, which would predispose the host to the development of *Candida* among others.

Management

The role of the transplant nurse in the management of therapy-induced mucositis is critical. Traditionally, it is the nurse who is responsible for directing the oral care of the patient undergoing high-dose therapy and stem cell transplant. This responsibility includes assessment, prevention, treatment, and education. The oral cavity is evaluated every 4 to 8 hr around the clock for those patients transplanted in the hospital. Outpatients, who usually receive chemotherapeutic regimens less toxic to the oral mucosa, are assessed daily. Assessment includes visualization of the entire oral cavity including the lips, tongue, saliva, mucous membranes, gingiva, teeth or dentures. It also includes listening to the voice for raspy sounds or difficulty talking and checking for pain and the adequacy of the airway and swallowing (Eilers, Berger, & Peterson, 1988). These findings are scored and graded as discussed above.

Oral Hygiene

Poor oral hygiene can aggravate the degree of mucositis and lead to infections of the oral mucosa following chemotherapy and radiation therapy. For these reasons, diligent mouth care is performed in the patient who is receiving high-dose therapy and stem cell transplant, for both prevention and treatment of mucositis (Burke, Wilkes, Berg, Bean, & Ingwersen, 1991). A cleansing regimen is begun with the onset of the conditioning regimen and extends past discharge until all signs of mucosal damage are resolved and the blood counts have returned to normal. All oral cleansing must be done gently with soft toothbrushes or oral swabs to minimize tissue damage, bleeding, and irritation. Such oral care regimens need to be reinstated in patients who develop GVHD of the oral cavity or in patients with other complications following transplant that involve the mouth and mucous membranes of the upper airway.

Several studies have evaluated the role of oral care regimens in decreasing the prevalence and the duration of therapy-induced mucositis, but no studies have evaluated which oral care regimen promotes the most patient comfort and compliance (Epstein, Vickars, Spinelli, & Reece, 1992; Raybould et al., 1994; Rutkauskas & Davis, 1993). Chlorhexidine gluconate rinse is used in several transplant centers for the prophylaxis of mucositis and oral infections. Randomized trials comparing chlorhexidine gluconate to various other oral care regimens have yielded conflicting results (Rutkauskas & Davis, 1993). Several authors have raised concerns that the use of chlorhexidine gluconate could result in a change in the oral bacterial flora, possibly resulting in overgrowth of gram-negative organisms that could potentially increase the risk of developing gram-negative bacteremia in the posttransplant patient (Raybould et al., 1994). However, at least one prospective, randomized trial demonstrated that, although there were no differences in the incidence or severity of mucositis, potential bacterial and fungal pathogens were less frequently identified in patients assigned to the chlorhexidine gluconate arm (Epstein et al., 1992). Experienced transplant nurses report that patients are frequently noncompliant with the use of this drug given that it can potentiate nausea, vomiting, anorexia, and oral pain. Therefore, although chlorhexidine gluconate may be part of a "standard" oral care regimen in the transplant regimen, alternative regimens promoting comfort and compliance need to be developed.

Another potential oral cleansing regimen in the transplant patient is sodium chloride solution. It has been reported to cleanse the mouth well, yet has no direct antibacterial effects (Dodd et al., 1996). Some believe that sodium chloride rinses are well tolerated, so patients are more likely to be compliant with the performance of oral care. This increased compliance appears to serve as adequate prophylaxis against infectious mucositis. Studies of sodium chloride as a mouthwash to prevent therapy-induced mucositis are ongoing and hopefully will yield a regimen that is effective at cleansing and well tolerated.

Bleeding Complications

A complication of therapy-induced mucositis in the posttransplant patient is that of mucosal bleeding. Profound thrombocytopenia is a uniform consequence of high-dose therapy. In general, routine platelet transfusions are administered to maintain an adequate platelet count in the immediate posttransplant period. Yet, despite frequent platelet transfusions, bleeding from the oral mucosa is relatively common. The amount of bleeding is generally mild and usually occurs after oral care or eating. Interventions are not always necessary, but brisk bleeding may require urgent intervention, including increasing the frequency and the threshold for platelet transfusions. Epistaxis can also occur in the posttransplant patient and should be managed with appropriate local measures as well as with platelet transfusions as necessary. Rarely, compromise of the airway secondary to bleeding can occur, requiring emergent intervention.

Communication

Commonly, patients experience difficulty in speech and breathing during periods of a severe oral breakdown. Edema can occur in the tissues of both the oral mucosa and the pharynx. The nurse and/or speech-language pathologist must assist the patient with communication. This is done with informal sign language, picture boards, and written communication. The transplant nurse must also be alert to any possible airway obstruction. Although a rare complication of transplant, upper airway obstruction due to tissue edema, aspiration, copious secretions, desquamation of the upper oral mucosa, or bleeding can necessitate urgent intratracheal intubation to protect the airway. Acute symptoms such as stridor, shortness of breath, and the inability to speak should prompt immediate evaluation of the upper airway to ensure adequate ventilation in these patients.

Pain Management

Pain is a frequent component of therapy-induced mucositis and is commonly cited by patients as the most difficult complication in the early posttransplant setting. Patients are monitored closely by nursing assessment for pain. Narcotic analgesics are the mainstay of treatment for pain associated with therapy-induced mucositis. In the immediate posttransplant period, acetaminophen is generally avoided as an agent for the control of pain because it may interfere with the patient's ability to mount a fever, one of the early signs of a serious systemic infection, which would require aggressive intervention in the immune-compromised host. Additionally, continuous administration of acetaminophen to achieve adequate pain control could result in hepatotoxicity in a patient already at risk for hepatic damage secondary to the toxic effects of high-dose chemotherapy or radiation therapy. The use of nonsteroidal anti-inflammatories, another class of medication commonly used for analgesia, is contraindicated posttransplant due to the antiplatelet effects seen with these drugs as well as the potential for gastrointestinal irritation.

When a patient is unable to swallow oral pain medications, intravenous pain medications should be administered for comfort. These generally consist of narcotics such as morphine or hydromorphone administered continuously via a patient-controlled administration (PCA) pump to accomplish the goal of adequate analgesia without excessive sedation. One study demonstrated that posttransplant patients using a PCA device for the treatment of oral pain used 50% less morphine than patients treated with continuous infusions of morphine yet received equivalent pain control (Mackie & Hill, 1989). Variations on patient-administered intravenous analgesics have confirmed the superiority of pain control with these techniques with fewer untoward, narcotic-induced side effects (Hill, Mackie, Coda, Iverson, & Chapman, 1991).

Nutrition

Therapy-induced mucositis is often associated with nutritional compromise in the posttransplant patient. Aggressive monitoring of nutritional status with daily assessments of caloric intake is needed to allow early nutritional intervention, if necessary. The use of liquid protein supplements may suffice in some patients with mild to moderate mucositis; however, total parenteral nutrition is frequently required, especially in patients expected to have a protracted clinical course. It must also be noted that dysphagia and odynophasia could predispose the patient to aspiration and pneumonitis, which would have dire consequences in an immune-compromised host.

Education

Education of the patient is one of the most important elements in the management and nursing care of the patient experiencing mucositis. The patient must be informed of the expected course prior to the development of mucositis. The importance of oral hygiene and its relationship to the healing process need to be stressed. The patient needs to be educated concerning symptoms to report and to understand potential comfort measures. Future directions for the management of mucositis experienced by patients receiving high-dose therapy and stem cell transplantation will include the refinement of cleansing regimens, continued collaboration with the entire transplant team in controlling pain, and improved methods of prevention.

Future Directions In Prevention And Management

Several new agents have the potential to attenuate or prevent therapy-induced mucositis. The hematopoietic growth factors, granulocyte and granulocyte-macrophage colony-stimulating factor (G-CSF and GM-CSF), have both been evaluated as agents that could decrease the frequency and/or duration of therapy-induced mucositis by shortening the period of aplasia posttransplant. One study comparing the number of neutrophils present in the mouth rinse obtained from patients undergoing autologous bone marrow transplantation with and without the administration of G-CSF demonstrated a significant decrease in the cumulative and the maximum daily mucositis scores in patients treated with G-CSF (Lieschke et al., 1992). Another study demonstrated a trend toward reduction in mucositis in patients receiving G-CSF following autologous bone marrow transplant, but this was not statistically significant (Rosenthal, Grigg, & Sheridan, 1994). Others have studied the role of GM-CSF in the development of mucositis (Gordon, Spadinger, Hodges, & Coccia, 1993). A study of patients undergoing autologous bone marrow transplantation with or without the administration of GM-CSF in the posttransplant period demonstrated that patients treated with GM-CSF had a significant decrease in the duration of mucositis but not in the severity of mucositis.

Transforming growth factor– (TGF–) has been demonstrated to reversibly inhibit epithelial cell cycling and may play a role in ameliorating therapy-induced mucositis. In preclinical trials of topical TGF– in hamster cheek pouch mucosa, it has been shown to decrease the intensity and duration of mucositis associated with 5-fluorouracil administration (Sonis et al., 1994). Trials evaluating the role of oral TGF– in decreasing mucositis in patients undergoing autologous bone marrow transplantation are ongoing.

Several investigators have evaluated the role of the helium-neon laser in preventing or treating therapy-induced mucositis. In one study, 10 patients undergoing bone marrow transplantation had daily laser applications to either the left or the right oral mucosa, the opposite side serving as a control, beginning the day after completion of the conditioning regimen and continuing for 5 days (Barasch et al., 1994). The laser-treated side demonstrated significantly less pain and less mucosal change than the untreated side, suggesting that the helium-neon laser could be an effective therapy for decreasing the incidence and severity of therapy-induced mucositis. Other investigators have demonstrated a significant decrease in the incidence, severity, and duration of therapy-induced mucositis with such lasers, compared to placebo, in a group of patients undergoing autologous bone marrow transplantation (Franquin, Tardius, Schubert, Hamdi, & Cowen, 1994). Although promising, this therapy may prove to be impractical to administer to large groups of patients undergoing high-dose therapy and stem cell transplantation. However, it could play a role in therapy for high-risk patients.

GRAFT-VERSUS-HOST DISEASE

GVHD frequently involves the gastrointestinal tract in both the acute GVHD phase and the chronic GVHD phase. Lymphocytic infiltration and cytotoxic changes in the mucosal epithelium occur, resulting in mucosal edema and effacement with the development of ulceration (Sale, Shulman, McDonald, & Thoma, 1979). The oral mucosa is rarely involved in acute GVHD, although esophageal involvement and involvement of the stomach and duodenum frequently can be seen. Not only does acute GVHD of the upper gastrointestinal tract pose a diagnostic dilemma, with a variety of fungal, viral, and occasionally bacterial infections included in the differential diagnosis, acute GVHD also predisposes the host to a variety of superinfections, which may have serious systemic consequences.

In chronic GVHD, the oral mucosa can be involved in up to 80% of patients (Clark et al., 1987; Sullivan et al., 1981). Oral dryness and increased oral pain and sensitivity occurring beyond 100 days following allogeneic bone marrow transplant suggest the development of chronic GVHD (Gratwhol et al., 1977; Schubert & Sullivan, 1990). A prospective study of allogeneic transplant patients demonstrated that the presence of oral atrophy, erythema, and lichenoid lesions of the buccal and labial mucosa was significantly associated with the development of chronic GVHD (Schubert et al., 1984). Of long-term survivors who develop chronic GVHD, 25–40% have persistent stomatitis and xerostomia (Schubert et al., 1983). A decrease in salivary immunoglobulin A levels is unique to transplant recipients with a diagnosis of chronic GVHD, which suggests that the mucosal immune system may be impaired (Schubert et al., 1983).

Therapy for GVHD of the upper gastrointestinal tract should be based on the overall grade and stage of systemic involvement and whether the GVHD is acute or chronic (Sullivan, 1994). The mainstay of therapy includes the use of immunosuppressants such as steroids, cyclosporine A, and azathioprine among others. As noted, it is important to consider other infectious etiologies in the differential diagnosis prior to initiating therapy. Additionally, prophylaxis for oral candidiasis and herpes simplex must be considered given the frequency of super-infection or reactivation of these infections during active GVHD. The lichenoid lesions of chronic GVHD should not be confused with oral candidiasis. Management of other complications is similar to that described for therapy-induced mucositis.

CONCLUSIONS

The upper aerodigestive tract is a frequent site for the development of a variety of complications in the patient undergoing high-dose therapy and stem cell rescue. Several factors have been demonstrated to increase the risk of developing such complications. Early recognition is critical to limiting the morbidity and potential mortality associated with these lesions. The therapy of these complications is based on multiple factors, including the systemic complications arising from the transplant itself. The approach is multidisciplinary, involving health care providers from many areas of expertise. Future strategies should include the development of therapies aimed at prevention.

REFERENCES

Armstrong, T. S. (1994). Stomatitis in the bone marrow transplant patient. An overview and proposed oral care protocol. *Cancer Nursing, 17,* 403–410.

Barasch, A., Peterson, D., Clive, J., D'Ambriosio, J., Nuki, K., & Shubert, M. (1994, June). *Laser effects on BMT conditioning-induced oral mucositis. Cancer Therapies for the 21st Century.* Presented at the 9th annual meeting of the International Society for Oral Oncology, Bethesda, MD.

Borgmann, A., Emminger, W., Emminger-Schmidmeier, W., Peters, C., Gatterer-Menz, I., Henze, G., & Gadner, H. (1994). Influence of fractionated total body irradiation on mucosal toxicity in intensified conditioning regimens for autologous bone marrow transplantation in pediatric cancer patients. *Klinische Pädiatrie, 206,* 299–302.

Brammer, K. W. (1990). Management of fungal infections in neutropenic patients with fluconazole. *Hematologie und Bluttransfusion, 33,* 546–550.

Burke, M., Wilkes, G., Berg, D., Bean, C., & Ingwersen, K. (1991). In M. B. Burke, G. M. Wilkes, & D. Berg (Eds.), *Cancer chemotherapy: A nursing process approach* (pp. 67–74). Boston: Jones & Bartlett.

Carl, W. (1995). Oral complications of local and systemic cancer treatment. *Current Opinion in Oncology, 7,* 320–324.

Carl, W., & Higby, D. J. (1985). Oral manifestations of bone marrow transplantation. *American Journal of Clinical Oncology, 8,* 81–87.

Clark, J. G., Schwartz, D. A., Flournoy, N., Sullivan, K. M., Crowford, S. W., & Thomas, E. D. (1987). Risk factors for airflow obstruction in recipients of bone marrow transplants. *Annals of Internal Medicine, 107,* 648–656.

Dodd, M. J., Larson, P. J., Dibble, S. L., Miaskowski, C., Greenspan, D., MacPhail, L., Hauck, W. W., Paul, S. M., Ignoffo, R., & Shiba, G. (1996). Randomized clinical trial of chlorhexidine versus placebo for prevention of oral mucositis in patients receiving chemotherapy. *Oncology Nursing Forum, 23,* 921–927.

Eilers, G., Berger, A., & Peterson, M. (1988). Development, testing, and application of the oral assessment guide. *Oncology Nursing Forum, 15,* 325–330.

Epstein, J. B., Vickars, L., Spinelli, J., & Reece, D. (1992). Efficacy of chlorhexidine and nystatin rinses in prevention of oral complications in leukemia and bone marrow transplantation. *Oral Surgery, Oral Medicine, Oral Pathology, 73,* 682–689.

Fields, K. K., Elfenbein, G. J., Lazarus, H. M., Cooper, B. C., Perkins, J. B., Creger, R. J., Ballester, O. F., Hiemenz, J. W., Janssen, W. E., & Zorsky, P.E. (1995). Maximum tolerated doses of ifosfamide, carboplatin, and etoposide given over six days followed by autologous stem cell rescue: Toxicity profile. *Journal of Clinical Oncology, 13,* 323–332.

Fields, K. K., Elfenbein, G. J., Perkins, J. B., Hiemenz, J. W., Janssen, W. E., Zorsky, P. E., Ballester, O. F., Kronish, L. E., & Roudy, M. C. (1993). Two novel high-dose treatment regimens for metastatic breast cancer—Ifosfamide, carboplatin, plus etoposide and mitoxantrone plus thiotepa: Outcomes and toxicities. *Seminars in Oncology, 20* (Suppl. 6), 59–66.

Franquin, J. C., Tardius, C., Schubert, M., Hamdi, M., & Cowen, D. (1994, June). *Phase III study of He-Ne laser prevention in BMT conditioning induced oral mucositis. Cancer Therapies for the 21st Century.* Presented at the 9th annual meeting of the International Society for Oral Oncology, Bethesda, MD.

Frei, E., Teicher, B. A., Holden, S. A., Cathcart, K. N., & Wang, Y. Y. (1988). Preclinical studies and clinical correlation of the effect of alkylating dose. *Cancer Research, 48,* 6417–6423.

Goodman, J. L., Winston, D. J., & Greenfield, R. A. (1992). A controlled trial of fluconazole to prevent fungal infections in patients undergoing bone marrow transplantation. *New England Journal of Medicine, 326,* 845–851.

Gordon, B., Spadinger, A., Hodges, E., & Coccia, P. (1993). Effect of granulocyte-macrophage colony-stimulating factor (GMCSF) on oral mucositis (OM) after autologous bone marrow transplantation (ABMT). *Proceedings, Annual Meeting of the American Society of Clinical Oncology, 12,* A1489.

Gratwhol, A. A., Moutsopoulous, H. M., Chused, T. M., Akizuki, M., Wolf, R. O., Sweet, J. B., & Deisseroth, A. B. (1977). Sjogren-type syndrome after allogeneic bone-marrow transplantation. *Annals of Internal Medicine, 87,* 703–706.

Herzig, R. H. (1991). High-dose etoposide and marrow transplantation. *Cancer, 67,* 292–298.

Hill, H. F., Mackie, A. M., Coda, B. A., Iverson, K., & Chapman, C. R. (1991). Patient-controlled analgesic administration. A comparison of steady-state morphine infusions with bolus doses. *Cancer, 67,* 873–882.

Horowitz, M. M. (1995). New IBMTR/ABMTR slides summarize current use and outcome of allogeneic and autologous transplants. *IBMTR Newsletter, 2,* 1–8.

Lieschke, G. J., Ramenghi, U., O'Connor, M. P., Sheridan, W., Szer, J., & Morsteyn, G. (1992). Studies of oral neutrophil levels in patients receiving G-CSF after autologous marrow transplantation. *British Journal of Haematology, 82,* 589–595.

Mackie, A. M., & Hill, H. F. (1989). Patient controlled (PCA) vs continuous infusion (CI) morphine for chemoradiotherapy induced oropharyngitis in adolescents during bone marrow transplantation. *Journal of Pain and Symptom Management, 4,* S11.

McDonald, G. B., Sharma, P., Hackman, R. C., Meyers, J. D., & Thomas, E. D. (1985). Esophageal infections in immunosuppressed patients after marrow transplantation. *Gastroenterology, 88,* 1111–1117.

Mcquire, D. B., Altomonte, V., Perterson, F., Wingard, J., Jones, R., & Grachow, L. (1993). Patterns of mucositis and pain in patients receiving preparative chemotherapy and bone marrow transplantation. *Oncology Nursing Forum, 20,* 1493–1501.

O'Brien, J. P., Muska, A. D., Van Vugt, A. G., Sonis, S. T., & Haley, J. D. (1994). Parameters effecting the course of ulcerative mucositis in hamsters. *Journal of Dental Research, 73,* 109.

Partyka, J. S., Fields, K. K., Perkins, J. B., Kronish, L. E., Lazarus, H. M., Cooper, B. W., & Elfenbein, G. I. (1996). The effects of age on tolerance of high dose ifosfamide, carboplatin and etoposide and autologous stem cell rescue: Morbidity and mortality. *Proceedings of the American Society of Clinical Oncology, 15,* 506.

Raybould, T. P., Carpenter, A. D., Ferretti, G. A., Brown, A. T., Lillich, T. T., & Henslee, J. (1994). Emergence of gram-negative bacilli in the mouths of bone marrow transplant recipients using chlorhexidine mouthrinse. *Oncology Nursing Forum, 21,* 691–696.

Redding, S. W. (1990). Role of herpes simplex virus reactivation in chemotherapy-induced oral mucositis. *National Cancer Institute Monographs, 9,* 103–105.

Rosenthal, M. A., Grigg, A. P., & Sheridan, W. P. (1994). High dose busulphan/cyclophosphamide for autologous bone marrow transplantation is associated with minimal non-hematopoietic toxicity. *Leukemia and Lymphoma, 14,* 279–283.

Rutkauskas, J. S., & Davis, J. W. (1993). Effects of chlorhexidine during immunosuppressive chemotherapy. A preliminary report. *Oral Surgery, Oral Medicine, Oral Pathology, 76,* 441–448.

Sale, G. E., Shulman, H. M., McDonald, G. B.,& Thoma, E. D. (1979). Gastrointestinal graft-versus-host disease in man. A clinicopathologic study of the rectal biopsy. *American Journal of Surgical Pathology, 3,* 291–299.

Schubert, M. M., Peterson, D. E., Flourneoy, N., Meyers, J., & Truelove, E. L. (1990). Oral and pharyngeal infection following bone marrow transplantation: Analysis of factors associated with infection. *Oral Surgery, Oral Medicine, Oral Pathology, 70,* 286–293.

Schubert, M. M., & Sullivan, K. M. (1990). Recognition, incidence and management of oral graft-versus-host disease. *National Cancer Institute Monographs, 9,* 135–143.

Schubert, M. M., Sullivan, K. M., Izutsu, K. T., & Truelove, E. L. (1983). Oral complications of cancer chemotherapy: Oral complications of bone marrow transplantation. *Developmental Oncology, 12,* 93–112.

Schubert, M. M., Sullivan, K. M., Morton, T. H., Izutsu, K. T., Peterson, D. E., Flournoy, N., Truelove, E. L., Sale, G. E., Buckner, C. D., Storb, R., et al. (1984). Oral manifestations of chronic graft-v-host disease. *Archives of Internal Medicine, 1444,* 1591–1595.

Schubert, M. M., Sullivan, K. M., & Truelove, E. L. (1986). Head and neck complications of bone marrow transplantation. *Developmental Oncology, 36,* 401–427.

Schubert, M. M., Williams, B. E., Lloid, M. E., Donaldson, G., & Chapko, M. K. (1992). Clinical assessment scale for the rating of oral mucosal changes associated with bone marrow transplantation. Development of an oral mucositis index. *Cancer, 69,* 2469–2477.

Seto, B. G., Kim, M., Wolinshy, L., Mito, R. S., & Champlin, R. (1985). Oral mucositis in patients undergoing bone marrow transplantation. *Oral Surgery, Oral Medicine, Oral Pathology, 60,* 493–497.

Sonis, S. T. (1983). Oral complications of cancer chemotherapy: Epidemiology, frequency, distribution, mechanisms and histopathology. *Developmental Oncology, 12,* 1–12.

Sonis, S. T. (1993). Oral complications. In J. F. Holland, E. Frei, R. C. Bast, & D. L. Morton (Eds.), *Cancer medicine* (2nd ed., pp. 1381–1388). Philadelphia: Lea & Febiger.

Sonis, S. T., & Costello, K. A. (1995). A database for mucositis induced by cancer chemotherapy. *European Journal of Cancer. Part B, Oral Oncology, 31B*, 258–260.

Sonis, S. T. & Haley, J. D. (1996). Pharmacological attenuation of chemotherapy-induced oral mucositis. *Exp Opin Invest Drugs, 5*, 1155–1162.

Sonis, S. T., Lindquist, L., Van Vugt, A., Stewart, A. A., Storm, K., Qu, G. Y., Iwata, K. K., & Haley, J. D. (1994). Prevention of chemotherapy-induced ulcerative mucositis by transforming growth factor beta 3. *Cancer Research, 54*, 1135–1138.

Sullivan, K. M. (1994). Graft-versus-host disease. In S. J. Forman, K. G. Blume, & E. D. Thomas (Eds.), *Bone marrow transplantation* (pp. 339–362). Boston: Blackwell Scientific.

Sullivan, K. M., Shulman, H. M., Storb, R., Weiden, P. L., Witherspoon, R. P., McDonald, G. B., Schubert, M. M., Atkinson, K., & Thomas, E. D. (1981). Chronic graft-versus-host disease in 52 patients: Adverse natural course and successful treatment with combination immunosuppression. *Blood, 57*, 267–276.

Thomas, E. D., Lochte, H. L., Jr., Cannon, J. H., Sahler, O. D., & Ferrebee, J. W. (1959). Supralethal whole body irradiation and isologous marrow transplantation in man. *Journal of Clinical Investigation, 38*, 1709–1716.

Thomas, E. D., Lochte, H. L., Jr., Lu, W. C., & Ferrebee, J. W. (1957). Intravenous infusion of bone marrow in patients receiving radiation and chemotherapy. *New England Journal of Medicine, 257*, 491–496.

Udagama, A. (1984). Dental oncology and maxillofacial rehabilitation. In A. E. Gunn (Ed.), *Cancer rehabilitation* (pp. 47–99). New York: Raven Press.

Wilson, W. H., Jain, V., Bryant, G., Cowan, K. H., Carter, C., Cottler-Fox, M., Goldsplel, B., Steinberg, S., M., Longo, D. L., & Wittes, R. E. (1992). Phase I and II study of high-dose ifosfamide, carboplatin, and etoposide with autologous bone marrow rescue in lymphomas and solid tumors. *Journal of Clinical Oncology, 10*, 1712–1722.

Winston, D. J., Islam, Z., Beull, D. N., & Acute Leukemia Study Group. (1991). Fluconazole prophylaxis of fungal infections in acute leukemia patients: Results of a placebo-controlled double-blind, multicenter trial. *Program and Abstracts of the 31st International Conference on Antimicrobial Agents and Chemotherapy, Chicago, Sept 29–Oct 2, 1991*. Washington, DC: American Society of Microbiology.

Woo, S. B., Sonis, S. T., Monopoli, M. M., & Sonis, A. L. (1993). A longitudinal study of oral ulcerative mucositis in bone marrow transplant recipients. *Cancer, 72*, 1612–1617.

Woo, S. B., Sonis, S. T., & Sonis, A. L. (1990). The role of herpes simplex virus in the development of oral mucositis in bone marrow transplant recipients. *Cancer, 66*, 2375–2379.

Zerbe, M., Parkerson, S., Ortlieb, M., & Spitzer, T. (1992). Relationships between oral mucositis and treatment variables in bone marrow transplant patients. *Cancer Nursing, 15*, 196–205.

11

Oral Manifestations of Human Immunodeficiency Virus Disease

Eva S. Quiroz, M.D., and John N. Greene, M.D.

The last 15 years has seen some major breakthroughs in managing patients infected with human immunodeficiency virus (HIV). Most notable is the use of combination antiretroviral therapy, which has significantly decreased the development of opportunistic infections in all areas of the body, including the oropharynx. Esophageal candidiasis, the most common cause of swallowing dysfunction, has been significantly reduced with the use of prophylactic antifungal therapy. Speech dysfunction secondary to vocal fold and hypopharynx pathology remains rare. More commonly, central nervous system (CNS) infections or malignancies account for dysphonia and aphasia. The primary infections of the CNS in HIV infected patients are toxoplasmosis, cryptococcosis, tuberculosis, histoplasmosis, cytomegalovirus (CMV), HIV, and progressive multifocal leukencephalopathy. Non-Hodgkin's lymphoma is the primary malignancy. The primary focus of this chapter is to familiarize the clinician to recognize and manage the more common causes of oral and pharyngeal pathology that affect the HIV-infected patient (Table 11–1)

Proper oral hygiene in persons infected with HIV has profound implications not only on quality of life but also on prognosis.

Management requires a team approach among ancillary health professionals, physician, and dentist (American Dental Association, 1995; Weinert, Grimes & Lynch, 1996). Oral lesions were among the first documented features of the acquired immunodeficiency syndrome (AIDS) (Small et al., 1983; Weinert et al. 1996). It is estimated that more than 90% of patients infected with HIV will have at least one oral manifestation at some time during the course of the disease (Greenspan, Greenspan, & Schiodt, 1990; McCarthy, 1992; Weinert et al., 1996). Oral lesions are frequent and have infectious and noninfectious causes, including bacterial, viral, or fungal infections, related to medications or neoplasm or idiopathic (Greenspan et al., 1990; Weinert et al., 1996). Infections may be rapidly progressive, persistent, and life threatening. Severe oral pain, dysphagia, odynophagia, and loss of taste sensation may lead to anorexia and wasting syndrome (Reiter, 1996).

Poor oral health has a tremendously negative impact on nutrition, speech, social interactions, and general well-being. As further immunologic impairment develops, quality of life is affected and the risks for oral complications increase (Kirby & Munoz,

163

TABLE 11–1. Causes of Oral Pathology in Patients With HIV Infection

Fungal
Candida species
   Pseudomembranous candidiasis (thrush)
   Erythematous candidiasis
   Hyperplastic candidiasis
   Angular cheilitis
Dimorphic yeast
   Cryptococcosis
   Histoplasmosis

Viral
Herpes simplex virus (HSV)
Varicella-zoster virus (VZV)
Cytomegalovirus (CMV)
Epstein Barr virus (EBV)
Human papillomavirus (HPV)
Enteroviruses

Bacterial infections
Acute necrotizing gingivitis
Linear gingival erythema
Periodontal disease
Pharyngitis/sinusitis

Other
Mycobacterium avium intracellulare (MAI)
Mycobacterium tuberculosis (MTB)
Escherichia coli
Bartonella (Rochalimaea)/bacillary angiomatosis
Spirochetes
   Primary syphilis
   Secondary syphilis

Malignancy or tumor
Squamous cell carcinoma
Kaposi's sarcoma
Non-Hodgkin's lymphoma

Granulomatous disease
Sarcoid
Wegener's granulomatosis

Idiopathic
Esophageal strictures
Minor aphthous ulcers
Major aphthous ulcers/Sutton's disease/Mikulicz's aphthae
Herpetiform ulcers
Lichen planus

1994; Royce & Luckman, 1991). In addition, oral lesions serve as clinical markers of HIV disease progression (Glick, Muzyka, Lurie, & Salkin, 1994; Glick, Muzyka, Salkin, & Lurie, 1994). Important goals are the maintenance of good oral hygiene, appropriate nutrition, and close follow-up.

The most important step in patient care is to obtain a good clinical history and perform a thorough physical exam. A complete oral exam is essential and includes careful inspection and palpation of the oral cavity. The oral exam can be performed within minutes (Greenspan & Greenspan, 1992; Katz et al., 1992; Weinert et al. 1996). See Table 11–2 for components of a brief oral examination and Table 11–3 for presenting signs and symptoms of oral disease.

It is important to include a detailed history of dysphagia symptoms such as duration, sensation of bolus sticking, and location. Ask if any maneuvers "dislodge" the bolus, and if there is presence of chronic cough or weight loss. Look for signs and symptoms of eating disorders and symptoms that might indicate neurological problems: nasal regurgitation, diplopia, ptosis, dysphonia and/or dysarthria, diffuse muscle weakness, and reflux esophagitis.

The most common complaints encountered are nasal congestion, postnasal drip, dry mouth, oral thrush, loss of taste, loss of appetite, nausea, inability to swallow and tolerate some medications, poor dentition, and gingivitis. These directly affect senses of taste and smell, which may lead to malnourishment and poor adherence to the prescribed medical regimen. Most recently, with the advent of highly active antiretroviral therapy (HAART), including combinations of protease inhibitors, opportunistic pathogens are significantly decreasing, most notably oropharyngeal and esophageal candidiasis.

FUNGAL INFECTIONS

Oral Candidiasis

Prior to HAART, the prevalence of oral mycosis in HIV infection had steadily increased, with *Candida* species the most common (Samaranayake, 1992; Schiodt, Greenspan, & Greenspan, 1996a). Candida species are commensal intraoral flora found in 20% to 50% of healthy persons (Samaranayake, 1989). During immunosuppression, *Candida* overgrowth leads to invasive disease and is difficult to eradicate. *Can-*

TABLE 11–2. Brief Oral Examination

1. Inspect the lips and corners of the mouth.
2. Examine the gingiva and oral mucosa.
   A. Evert the upper and lower lips.
   B. Look for evidence of ulceration, erythema, or abscess.
3. Use a tongue blade to retract the cheeks.
   A. Visualize the buccal mucosa, teeth, and gingiva.
   B. Look for lesions or ulcerations.
4. Assess salivary function.
   A. Massage the parotid gland and observe the expression of saliva from Stensen's duct.
   B. Observe submandibular salivary function.
5. Use bidigital palpation of the oral mucosa, upper and lower vestibule, and lips.
6. Examine regional lymph nodes, including cervical lymph nodes.
7. Examine the tongue and pharyngeal region and floor of the mouth. Palpate for stones in the salivary ducts.

TABLE 11–3. Presenting Signs and Symptoms of Oral Disease

Embarrassed to smile, covers the mouth with hand to avoid showing teeth

Oral lesions

Oral pain

Poor dentition, gingivitis ("inflammation or bleeding of gums")

Loose teeth

Halitosis (bad breath)

Trouble eating or swallowing

Intolerance to hot or cold meals

Dysphagia ("Food gets stuck in my throat")

Odynophagia ("It hurts when I swallow")

Dehydration

Weight loss

dida infection is frequently an early sign of HIV infection and serves as a prognostic indicator of disease progression (McCarthy, 1992). Clinical manifestations may occur during an early period of immunosuppression with CD4 counts ranging from 400–700 cells/mm³ (Samaranayake, 1990). The incidence of oropharynegeal candidiasis in HIV seropositive females increases with CD4 counts of less than 300 cells/mm³ and esophageal candidiasis with CD4 counts of less than 100 cells/mm³ (Fahey, Taylor, & Deters, 1990; Glick, Muzyka, Lurie, & Salkin, 1994; McCarthy, Mackie, Koval, Sandhu, & Daley, 1991). Early use of antifungal therapy may delay clinical presentation until a later stage when selective or total resistance to antifungal therapy may develop (Glick, Mazyka, Lurie, & Salkin, 1994). Besides *Candida albicans*, other *Candida* species that may become pathogenic in the immunocompromised host include *C. tropicalis*, *C. parapsilosis*, *C. krusei*, *C. guillermondi*, *C. glabrata*, and others (Fotos & Lilly, 1996; Odds, 1988). These nonalbicans *Candida* species are frequently inherently resistant to the azole antifungals, making treatment more difficult. *Candida* is frequently referred to as a disease of the diseased (Odds, 1988; Phelan, Saltzman, & Friedland, 1987). Its pathogenicity depends on the severity of the underlying disease, duration of hospitalization or antibiotic exposure, and corticosteroid or immunosuppressive therapy (Budtz-Jorgensen, 1990; Greenspan & Greenspan, 1987). Other factors that predispose to oral *Candida* infection include anemia, xerostomia (absence of saliva), smoking, wearing dentures, and extremes of age (McCarthy, 1992). Xerostomia may be secondary to medications (such as tricyclic antidepressants), radiation therapy, dehydration, depression, or anxiety. Besides providing mechanical cleansing and lubrication, saliva has important antimicrobial and antifungal properties (Pollock et al., 1992). Oral candidiasis can be subdivided into four different presentations.

Pseudomembranous (Thrush)

Oral thrush usually presents as white to yellowish creamy patches overlying areas of mucosal erythema (Schiodt et al., 1996a). After easy removal of the friable patch with a tongue blade, pinpoint areas of ulceration may be seen (Greenberg, 1996). The palate, buccal or labial mucosa, and tongue are the most common sites. Extension to the pharynx and esophagus results in dysphagia and odynophagia. *Candida* esophagitis is one of the AIDS-defining conditions.

Diagnosis is made by clinical presentation and the presence of pseudohyphae on smear prepared with potassium hydroxide, Gram stain, or periodic acid-Schiff stain. Treatment includes topical or systemic antifungal therapy. Recommendations include clotrimazole oral troche 10 mg orally five times per day, nystatin oral pastille 200,000 U three to five times per day, or nystatin vaginal tablets 100,000 U to be dissolved in the mouth three times per day. Nystatin vaginal tablets are bitter in taste, which might result in poor compliance. Nystatin liquid for swish and swallow is commonly prescribed with good response to treatment; however, due to its high sugar content, it may be ineffective and cause dental caries. Systemic therapy includes fluconazole 100–200 mg orally once a day or ketoconazole at a dose of 200–400 mg orally once day for 7 days. Continuous use of these medications for frequently necessary suppressive therapy may select out resistant organisms. Fluconazole has replaced ketoconazole because of the latter's liver toxicity and poor absorption due to decreased gastric acidity in the HIV-infected patient (Greenspan & Greenspan, 1992). Recently, the use of chlorhexidine as an antimicrobial rinse has been of therapeutic benefit in the management of oropharyngeal candidiasis (Addy & Hunter, 1987; Fotos & Lilly, 1996). Systemic therapy is preferred if chronic *Candida* vaginitis is also present, for treatment of both conditions and because oral re-infection from distant body sites has been demonstrated (Brammer, 1990; Fotos & Lilly, 1996; Soll, 1988). Interestingly, a recent study found the use of nebulized pentamidine to significantly reduce intraoral concentrations of *C albicans* in HIV seropositive patients (Nolan et al., 1994). However, it is not indicated for use in the treatment of candidiasis.

Erythematous Candidiasis

Erythematous candidiasis or atrophic candidiasis is associated with the use of broad-spectrum antibiotics and corticosteroid therapy (Lehner & Ward, 1970). The mucosa is erythematous and presents on the palate and dorsum of the tongue with associated depapillation (Greenspan & Greenspan, 1992; Schiodt et al., 1996a). Prevalent in the HIV seropositive patients, erythematous candidiasis is considered a harbinger of the pseudomembranous type.

Hyperplastic Candidiasis

This form of candidiasis invades and affects deeper layers of the epithelium, resulting in parakeratosis, acanthosis, and pseudoepitheliomatous hyperplasia (Greenberg, 1996). Commonly seen in smokers, a white exudate forms on the retrocommisural areas of the buccal mucosa that is practically nonremovable or only partially removed with light abrasion. The treatment consists of long-term antifungal therapy until lesion resolution. Recurrence may occur weeks after therapy cessation.

Angular Cheilitis

Angular cheilitis presents as fissures with or without exudate in the corners of the mouth. Risk factors for the development of angular cheilitis include fungal and bacterial infections, anemia, B12 deficiency, and loose dentures (Greenberg, 1996; Schiodt et al., 1996a). Treatment consists of topical nystatin ointment applied to the lesions four times per day or a short course of oral fluconazole 100 mg orally every day for 5–7 days. Consider vitamin supplement if deficiency is suspected.

DIMORPHIC FUNGI

Oral lesions due to dimorphic fungi present as persistent ulcers, nodules, or patches of mucositis. Two of the most common infections are cryptococcosis and histoplasmosis.

Oral Cryptococcosis

Cryptococcosis is a chronic fungal disease that occurs worldwide (Samaranayake, 1989). The causative agent is the yeast *Cryptococcus neoformans* commonly found in bird droppings. Primarily the lung is affected, but the CNS, skin, and mouth may be secondarily involved (Rippon, 1982). Disseminated disease may occur in patients with leukemia, patients who require steroids, and those who have acquired HIV infection (Samaranayake, 1989). Lesions usually appear papular but may present as acneiform pustules, abscesses, ulcers, granulomas, or sinus tracts. The scalp, face, and neck are the most frequent sites of cutaneous spread. Intraoral lesions may present in the gingiva of the hard and soft palate (Figure 11–1), pharynx, buccal mucosa, and tonsillar pillars (MacFarlane & Samaranayake, 1990; Samaranayake, 1989). Diagnosis is made by scraping or biopsy of the lesion with potassium hydroxide exam under the microscope and culture of the fungus on Sabouraud's media. Serum cryptococcal antigen testing is also used for diagnosis. Treatment with amphotericin B 0.5–1.0 mg/kg per day or fluconazole 400–800 mg/day is curative. Therapy is continued well after lesion resolution (6 weeks to 1 year or more). Lumbar puncture

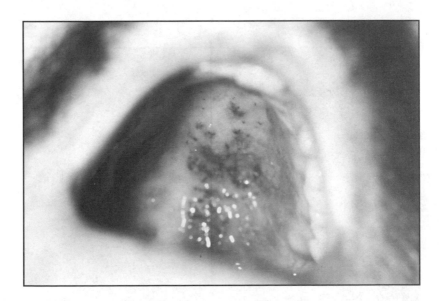

Figure 11–1. Disseminated cryptococcus involving the hard palate presented with hemorrhagic papulonodular lesions.

for cerebral spinal fluid analysis to rule out meningitis is crucial to gauge therapy dose and duration and for accurate assessment of prognosis.

Histoplasmosis

Infection caused by *Histoplasma capsulatum* frequently presents as an acute or chronic respiratory illness with or without dissemination. A chronic mucocutaneous form with ulceration of the oropharynx, including tongue, palate, and buccal mucosa, may be the initial presentation (McNally & Langlais, 1996; Samaranayake et al., 1989). Approximately 30% to 50% of patients with disseminated histoplasmosis have oral lesions (MacFarlane & Samaranayake, 1990). Diagnosis can be made by biopsy, culture, or serological testing. These tests include specific immunofluorescence test of sections or smears, a rising titer to histoplasmin antigen with complement fixation or immunodiffusion, or culture on Sabouraud's medium. A long incubation period of up to 12 weeks makes prolonged culture necessary for diagnosis. Treatment with intravenous amphotericin B 0.5–1.0 mg/kg per day or itraconazole 200 mg orally twice a day is continued until lesion resolution.

VIRAL INFECTIONS

Herpes Virus Infections

Lesions caused by herpes simplex virus (HSV) are common in the HIV-infected patient (Greenspan & Greenspan, 1992; Reichart, Gelderblom, Becker, & Kuntz, 1987; Silverman, Migliorate, Lozada, Greenspan, & Conant, 1986). New or recurrent painful oral lesions are the usual chief presentation (MacPhail, Greenspan, & Schiodt, 1989). Although lesions are found anywhere in the oral cavity, the periodontium, gingiva and palate, mucosa, and tonsillar crypts are the most common sites. In one unusual case, HSV infection presented as otalgia and hoarseness for 10 days, with soft palate paralysis on the left side. Findings on endoscopy revealed a paralyzed vocal fold in the paramedian position with a 3- to 4-mm vesicle in the area of the arytenoid cartilage. Swab culture of this lesion was positive for HSV-1 (Bachlor et al., 1996).

Initially small vesicles may develop from 1-3 mm in diameter occurring in clusters (Schiodt, Greenspan, & Greenspan, 1996c). These lesions rupture within days, leaving an ulcerated white or hemorrhagic base (Figure 11–2). Because of pain, anorexia

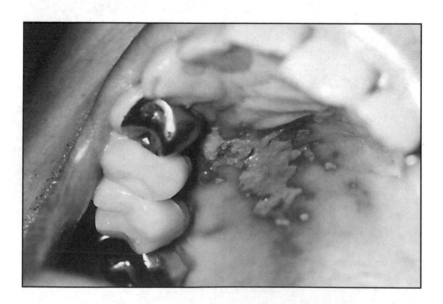

Figure 11–2. Herpes simplex infection of the hard palate presents with ulceration with a white base and red serpiginous borders.

and avoidance of brushing teeth may occur. Recurrent oral herpes is caused by reactivation of latent virus found in the trigeminal ganglion. HSV-1 is more common than HSV-2, but they present identically. Fatigue, trauma, upper respiratory tract infections, febrile illnesses, exposure to sunlight, and gastrointestinal upset may predispose to recurrent lesions. Once reactivated, the virus travels along the sensory nerve to the mucosa, similar to herpes zoster infections.

Diagnosis is made by direct fluorescent antibodies against HSV antigens in smears or by demonstrating cytopathic effect on cell culture. HSV-induced lesions may be confused with recurrent aphthous ulcers. The white ulcer base with surrounding erythema and rounded borders and buccal location usually indicates the latter. Treatment consists of acyclovir 400 mg orally three times per day for 7–10 days or famciclovir 125 mg orally twice daily for 7–10 days.

Varicella-Zoster Virus Infection

Varicella-zoster virus is in the herpesviridae family, which like HSV causes a primary infection (chickenpox), becomes latent in a ganglion cell, and can reactivate resulting in dermatomal infection (Greenberg, Friedman, & Cohen, 1987). Dermatomal herpes zoster virus is also known as shingles. Groups of vesicular lesions, usually painful, are caused by centrifugal spread of latent varicellazoster virus from sensory nerve ganglia to peripheral nerves (Irani & Johnson, 1996).

Lesions are often preceded by a prodrome of itching, tingling, or burning sensation. Within days, small blisters, or vesicles, erupt on the affected mucosa or skin and often coalesce and form larger lesions (Greenberg et al., 1987). Approximately 15-20% of the cases of herpes zoster involve the trigeminal nerve, with more than 80% of these involving the first division affecting the eyes and scalp (Greenberg et al., 1987). Externally, involvement of the second and third divisions of the trigeminal nerve results in unilateral clusters of vesicles in the maxillary or mandibular area of the face, respectively. Internally, unilateral palatal lesions can result from involvement of the second division of the trigeminal nerve. Healing usually occurs within 10–14 days, and recurrences are common. Acyclovir at higher doses than for HSV (800 mg) are required at a dosing interval of five times per day; famciclovir 500 mg three times daily is also effective with less frequent dosing. Early initiation of therapy leads to lesion resolution approximately 3 days sooner than without therapy, lessens the possibility of dissemination, and decreases the development of postherpetic neuralgia (a debilitating chronic pain syndrome of the affected area).

Cytomegalovirus

Infection with CMV is common in patients with AIDS and can result in esophagitis, colitis, several neurological disorders, and chorioretinitis. Studies indicate that 90% of patients with AIDS develop active CMV infection. During the 1996–1997 year, there was a decrease in the incidence of CMV retinitis in the United States, most likely due to HAART. CMV infection of the oral mucosa or gingiva presents as an atypical ulcer that may resemble major aphthous ulcers. A painful enlarging lesion develops on an inflamed base (Schiodt et al., 1996c). Coinfection with HSV is common (Greenberg, 1996; Greenberg, Dubin, & Stewart, 1995). CMV infection usually develops in AIDS patients with CD4 counts of less than 100 cells/mm^3, in the form of retinitis, encephalitis, esophagitis, gastroenteritis, and pneumoniae, with oral lesions rare. Recent evidence links xerostomia to the presence of CMV in saliva in patients with CD4 counts of less than 150 cells/mm^3 (Greenberg et al., 1995; Schiodt et al., 1996c). Cause and effect of this finding has not been demonstrated.

Diagnosis is made by biopsy that shows intranuclear and intracytoplasmic ("owl's eye") inclusion bodies. Isolation of the virus on shell vial cell culture usually requires 3–7 days. Viral isolation correlates with infection if histopathology demonstrates viral infection as noted above.

Treatment consists of ganciclovir, foscarnet, or both in combination. Therapy with ganciclovir or foscarnet is as follows.

1. Ganciclovir (Cytovene): 5 mg/kg intravenously (infuse at constant rate over 1 hr) every 12 hr for 14–21 days then maintenance therapy of 5 mg/kg once daily. Of note is that patients with AIDS frequently have HSV and varicella-zoster virus coinfection, which is also susceptible.
2. Foscarnet (Foscavir): 90 mg/kg intravenously every 12 hr for 14–21 days. Maintenance dosage is about 90 mg/kg in one daily infusion.

Epstein Barr Virus

Epstein Barr virus is the causative agent of oral hairy leukoplakia. First described in 1984 in San Francisco, oral hairy leukoplakia was observed in 37 homosexual men who developed AIDS (Schiodt, et al., 1987). Initially considered pathognomonic of HIV infection (Centers for Disease Control, 1986), other immunosuppressed patients secondary to organ transplantation (heart, liver, kidneys) or patients with drug-induced immunosuppression also developed the disease (Greenspan, Greenspan, & Conant, 1984; Lamster & Grbic, 1995; MacLeod, Long, Soames, & Ward, 1990; Schiodt, Norgaard, & Greenspan, 1995). The prevalence ranges from 9–25% of HIV seropositive patients and is predictive for subsequent development of AIDS (Greenspan, Greenspan, & Lennette, 1985; Schiodt et al., 1995). Lesions can be seen in patients who are asymptomatic with CD4 counts from 300–400 cells/mm^3. Epstein Barr virus replicates within the epithelial cells of the affected mucosa (Greenspan et al., 1985; Schiodt et al., 1995). The wartlike lesions are located on the lateral borders of the tongue in 95% of cases (Scuibba, 1996). Other sites include the buccal mucosa, floor of the mouth, and palate.

Diagnosis is made by clinical presentation and lack of response to antifungal treatment. Biopsy, which is rarely required, shows an epithelium with increased thickness, hyperkeratosis, hairlike keratotic projections with large balloon cells with clear cytoplasm, and pyknotic nuclei that are present in the prickle cell layer (Schiodt

et al., 1995). Treatment consists of combination therapy for the HIV infection, resulting in immune enhancement in many cases. Topical treatment with Retin-A solution applied to affected areas with a cotton swab every 1–2 weeks may be successful. With the advent of HAART, oral hairy leukoplakia has decreased substantially.

Human Papillomavirus

Human papillomavirus infection causes condyloma (warts) and focal epithelial hyperplasia (Greenspan et al., 1985; Schiodt et al., 1995). Latent infection may exist for many years, with the appearance of lesions when immunosuppression becomes significant. Extensive involvement of the oral cavity, perineum, and rectum may occur. The lesions vary from 1–3 mm in diameter to fungating lesions several centimeters in diameter. Papillary lesions of the oral cavity include (a) squamous papilloma, which is a solitary and frequently benign epithelial tumor; (b) condyloma acuminata, which often has a cauliflower appearance and is derived from genital warts; and (c) verrucae vulgaris, which demonstrates marked keratinization and is derived from common warts. Oral lesions occur most often on the labia, buccal mucosa, or gingiva (Scuibba, 1996). Lesions are sexually transmitted, with an increased risk of squamous cell carcinoma in the involved area. Close follow-up is indicated especially when rectal or cervical lesions are present. Lesions have a tendency to recur and be recalcitrant to treatment, which consists of surgical removal, laser therapy, or chemical destruction of the lesion (such as podophyllin).

BACTERIAL INFECTIONS

Bacterial infections of the oral cavity are usually polymicrobial in nature, with a predominance of anaerobic bacteria. Because of the underlying immunosuppression, patients infected with HIV may demonstrate an increase in more virulent organisms such as *Eikenella*, *Wolinella*, and *Bacteroides* species (Scuibba, 1996; Zambon, Reynolds, & Genco, 1990).

Opportunistic infection from *Mycobacterium aviumintracellulare, Mycobacterium tuberculosis,* and *Bartonella (Rochalimaea)* may also occur. In addition, periodontal disease and gingivitis are frequently found in the HIV seropositive population. Interference with swallowing may lead to wasting syndrome, and it also may predispose to aspiration pneumonia and bacteremia.

Acute Necrotizing Gingivitis

Acute necrotizing gingivitis affects approximately 10% of HIV seropositive patients (Schulten, ten Kate, & van der Waal, 1990; Scuibba, 1996; Winker, 1995). They can be asymptomatic or present with halitosis, oral pain, and friable gingiva with spontaneous or induced bleeding when the teeth are brushed. Nutrition, hydration, and social interactions may be significantly impaired by these symptoms. On physical exam there are small ulcerations of the interdental papillae. These lesions may progress to severe ulcerations of the marginal and alveolar gingiva with erosion of surrounding periodontal bone. Often the lesions demonstrate a central area of necrosis that is often gray and surrounded by fiery red gingiva (Schiodt, Greenspan, & Greenspan, 1996b). More impressive is the pronounced loss of attachment and retraction of the gingiva with exposure of the root surfaces of the teeth.

Disease progression may result in bone sequestration. This condition is also known as necrotizing stomatitis and is associated with low CD4 counts and age of over 35. Painful cervical adenopathy may be present; however, the lymph nodes are usually soft and not fixed. The differential diagnosis includes primary herpetic gingivostomatitis and erythema multiforme. Treatment includes good dental hygiene and mouth rinsing with hydrogen peroxide or 0.1–0.2% chlorhexidine. In severe cases antibiotic therapy with metronidazole 250–500 mg orally three times per day for 1 week with or without antifungal therapy may be of benefit.

Linear Gingival Erythema

Linear gingival erythema, renamed in 1993, is also known as HIV gingivitis (Schiodt et al., 1995b; Winker, 1995). It presents as a linear red band or punctate erythema of the alveolar gingiva that may bleed spontaneously. Linear gingival erythema does not progress to necrotizing gingivitis or periodontitis. Oral candidiasis is often coexistent (Grbic, Mitchell-Lewis, & Fine, 1995; Schiodt et al., 1995b). Conventional treatment that may be effective includes tooth scaling, root planing, cleaning, and mouth rinsing with 0.1–0.2% chlorhexidine. Antifungal treatment such as clotrimazole troche 10 mg five times per day, nystatin pastille 200,000 U three to five times per day, or nystatin vaginal tablets 100,000 U three times per day might be beneficial.

Periodontal Disease

Periodontal disease may present insidiously with progressive necrosis of the gingiva and surrounding soft tissue resulting in bony exposure. Once rapid progression develops, painful and destructive periodontal disease develops over a few months. Loss of alveolar crestal bone with subsequent sequestration of interseptal bone in conjunction with soft tissue necrosis may occur. The area of necrosis may extend to the vestibular mucosa or palate in a manner similar to the lesions of necrotizing stomatitis.

ORAL ULCERATION AND IATROGENIC DISEASE IN HIV INFECTION

Aphthous Ulcers

In the HIV seropositive patient aphthous ulcers are more persistent and severe than in seronegative patients. Recurrent aphthous ulcers are debilitating and may interfere with normal oral function such as eating, chewing, swallowing, and speaking. The most common symptoms are pain and weight loss (Friedman, Brenski, & Taylor, 1994). The pain may be severe enough to interfere with nutrition, hydration, and taking of medications.

Oral ulcers of bacterial, viral, fungal, and neoplastic origin may be confused with aphthous ulcers (Mandell, Bennett, & Dolin, 1995). Specific medications such as foscarnet (Gilquin, Weiss, & Kazatchkine, 1990), interferon (Penneys & Hick, 1985), and dideoxycytidine (McNeely, Yarhoan, Broder, & Lawly, 1989) can induce similar-appearing ulcerations. However, aphthous ulcers are usually culture negative unless secondarily infected. There is no known etiologic agent, and no specific microbe is implicated. However, stress, vitamin deficiency, allergies, hormonal changes, diet, trauma, viral infections, or immune dysfunction may be predisposing factors (Lindemann & Rivierte, 1985; Scully & Porter, 1989). Bacteria might play a role in disease progression, but their relationship in aphthous ulcers is not clearly defined (Rennie, Reade, & Hay, 1985). Aphthous ulcers may be categorized by size, location, and sequela into minor, major, and herpetiform (Bottomley & Rosenburg, 1990; Muzyka & Glick, 1994; Radeff, Kuffer, & Samson, 1990). See Table 11–4 for a description of various types of ulcers and their most frequently associated locations.

Any area of the gastrointestinal tract may be involved with aphthous ulcers, and lesions may not respond to therapy (Bach, Valenti, & Howell, 1988; Glick, Muzyka, 1992; Muzyka & Glick, 1994). Lesions that resemble severe recurrent aphthous ulcers have been reported to occur in the mouth, oropharynx, and esophagus of HIV seropositive patients. Other lesions have been reported in the esophagus and more distal gastrointestinal tract (Bach, Howell, & Valenti, 1990). Aphthous ulcers may even present as typhlitis or neutropenic enterocolitis in the HIV-infected patient who has resistant oral aphthae. Resolution of the lesions with administration of granulocyte colony-stimulating factor has been reported (Bach et al., 1990).

Recurrent major aphthous ulcers occur in nonkeratinized mucosa and occasionally extend to keratinized mucosa (Greenspan et al., 1990). Herpetiform and major recurrent aphthous ulcers tend to occur in locations where they interfere with eating and speaking such as the soft palate, buccal mucosa, tonsillar area, and tongue (Greenspan et al., 1990; Phelan, Eisig, & Freedman, 1991). Large solitary lesions tend to occur in patients with severely depressed immune systems, usually with CD4 counts of less than 50 cells/mm^3, and such patients have a high mortality rate (Greenspan et al., 1990; Phelan et al., 1991).

Accurate diagnosis and treatment are necessary to prevent untoward sequelae. Rare lesions that may mimic recalcitrant

TABLE 11–4. Description and Location of Ulcerations

Ulcer	Description	Number and Location
Minor aphthous	Clearly defined margins Spontaneous healing within 5–10 days Size: 2–4 mm in diameter	Number: 1–5 lesions Location: labial mucosa, buccal buccal mucosa, tongue
Major aphthous	Crateriform with deeply eroded base Persist for more than 3 weeks Spontaneous healing with associated scarring	Number: more than 1 lesion Location: any oral mucosa including heavily keratinized tissue, tonsillar area, tongue
Herpetiform	Clinically similar to ulcers caused by HSV Persist for more than 1–2 weeks	Number: 5–100 lesions Location: soft palate, tonsillar area, buccal mucosa, tongue, any region of the mouth

aphthous ulcers include histoplasmosis and non-Hodgkin's lymphoma (Greenspan et al., 1990; Laccourreye et al., 1995). Diagnosis is made on the basis of the clinical presentation and absence of other processes, and biopsy of the lesion may be necessary. Biopsy may even prompt the lesions to resolve (Sutton, 1911).

Described as early as 1911 by Richard Sutton, major recurrent aphthous ulcers constitute approximately 10% of the cases of recalcitrant aphthous ulcers (Gilman, Goodman, et al., 1985; Paterson, Georghiou, Allworth, & Kemp, 1995; Sutton, 1941) .

The differential diagnosis should include papulopruritic eruption and giant ulceration of the mouth. These lesions are small and intensely pruritic and are common in areas of high sebum of the skin, lateral neck, face and scalp, upper arms, axilla, chest, and thighs. Multiple giant ulcerations may occur in the mouth, pharynx, and esophagus. They are painful and resistant to topical therapy but may respond to thalidomide or topical corticosteroid therapy (Crawford, 1992). Treatment consists of suppression of the pathological immune reaction that causes the aphthous ulcer, treatment of any concomitant infection, relief of pain, and correction of underlying iron and vitamin deficiencies (Sutton, 1941). Topical therapy should be the first choice of treatment. This includes treatment with glucocorticoids such as fluocinonide, clobetasol, and dexamethasone elixir. The use of systemic glucocorticoids should be reserved for those patients who have several lesions that fail to respond to topical therapy or if the patient has lesions in nonoral sites such as the esophagus or colon. In these cases high-dose of prednisone is indicated at 40–60 mg orally every day for 4–7 days (Greenspan et al., 1990; Paterson et al., 1995). Steroids are given for a short course, so tapering is not necessary.

The use of topical tetracycline in oral suspension has been reported to relieve pain (Greenspan et al., 1990; Laccourreye et al., 1995; Sutton, 1911). Interestingly, the use of thalidomide for recurrent aphthous ulcers has proved to be very beneficial (McBride, 1961; Oldfield, 1994). Thalido-

mide was originally introduced as a sedative agent in the mid-1950s (McBride, 1961), and later was used as an antiemetic agent during pregnancy. It was discontinued from the market in the 1960s due to its teratogenic effects: phocomelia in the offspring of pregnant women treated with the drug (Oldfield, 1994). In 1965, the medication was used successfully to treat erythema nodosum leprosum, a complication of lepromatous leprosy (Ghigliotti, Repetto, Farris, Roy, & De March, 1993). It has been used in the treatment of chronic graft-versus-host disease following bone marrow transplant, systemic lupus erythematosus, and Behcet's disease, and as an immunosuppressant in preventing cardiac allograft rejection (McBride, 1961). It is contraindicated during pregnancy and some would avoid prescribing it to any female in her reproductive age. Another side effect of thalidomide is peripheral neuropathy, which occurs in approximately 0.5–25% of patients treated. The recommended dose is 200 mg orally every day for 14 days or until resolution of the symptoms. The mechanism of action is thought to be inhibition of tumor necrosis factor alpha. Informed consent should be obtained in patients who are treated with this medication, and, as with any medication, counseling should be provided. The use of thalidomide has been associated with a dramatic increase in weight and sense of well-being (Greenberg, 1996; Schiodt, Greenspan, & Greenspan, 1996d).

Salivary Gland Disease

Salivary gland disease often develops in HIV seropositive patients. Sialoadenitis, autoimmune-like in its presentation, is more common in children than in adults. Parotitis and changes in salivary production may cause xerostomia and dry mouth, similar to Sjögren's syndrome. This increases the risk of acquiring oral infections such as candidiasis and caries. Long-standing swelling of the gland can be associated with the development of lymphoepithelial cysts. There is a correlation between HIV-associated salivary gland pathology and extrasalivary manifestation such as hepatitis, gastritis, and the transplanta-tion-associated genetic marker, HLA-DR5.

Lichen Planus

Lichen planus is a papulosquamous disorder. The primary lesions are pruritic, flat-topped, violaceous papules. The surfaces of these papules often reveal a network of grayish lines called Whickham's striae. It commonly involves mucous membranes, especially the buccal mucosa, and presents as a netlike whitish eruption. Skin lesions occur on the wrists, shins, lower back, and genital region. This condition is often encountered in perimenopausal females. The etiology remains unclear, but it is suspected to result from an autoimmune defect. It has been linked to emotional stress. Patients with these lesions often complain of a burning sensation of the areas affected. A definite diagnosis requires biopsy of the lesion. The clinical course is variable, with occasional spontaneous remissions in 6 months to 2 years. Treatment includes topical and sublesional injection formulations of glucocorticoids.

NEOPLASMS

Squamous Cell Carcinoma

Squamous cell carcinoma continues to be the most common oral neoplasia. Its incidence increases with the use of tobacco or alcohol. Squamous cell carcinoma is also associated with nutritional deficiencies and human papillomavirus infection. The lesions may present as red or white patches (called erythroplakia or leukoplakia, respectively) in the mucosa of the tongue, oral floor, or gingiva. Many develop into exophytic masses with central ulceration. Initially the lesions are asymptomatic but eventually pain and paresthesias may develop. The differential diagnosis includes large traumatic ulcers, syphilitic chancres, and tuberculosis. The treatment consists of surgical excision, radiation, or chemotherapy.

Non-Hodgkin's Lymphoma

Non-Hodgkin's lymphoma, rarely found in the oral cavity, may present as swelling on the gingiva, palate (Figure 11–3), or retromolar area. Oral lesions may precede other

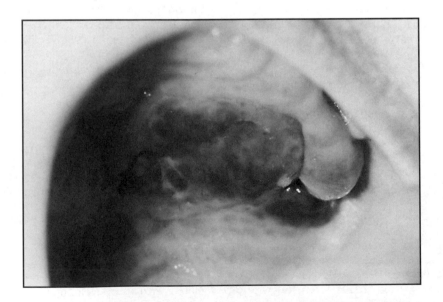

Figure 11–3. Non-Hodgkin's lymphoma recurred in this patient's hard palate, causing poorly fitting dentures.

sites of involvement or may be solitary. Lesions may present as small ulcerations and be mistaken for odontogenic infection. Oral non-Hodgkin's lymphoma may be the presenting diagnostic criteria for AIDS. Diagnosis is made by biopsy of the lesion. The treatment consists of radiation therapy or chemotherapy.

Kaposi's Sarcoma

Kaposi's sarcoma, common among homosexual men during the initial phase of the AIDS epidemic, has decreased substantially with the advent of HAART. Once Kaposi's sarcoma develops, HAART may cause lesions to regress and disappear completely. It is most commonly found in patients with low CD4 counts, which range from 150–200 cells/mm^3. It is often limited to the skin and oral mucosa, usually on the hard palate or gingiva (Figure 11–4; Greenberg, 1996). The lesions, initially flat, can subsequently become raised and tumorlike and occasionally affect the entire palate and gingiva. Superimposed infection with *Candida* in advanced stages may cause ulceration of the lesion (Schiodt et al., 1996d).

Kaposi's sarcoma may be associated with systemic illness in advanced disseminated disease. Patients may present with B symptoms of fever, chills, nausea, and weight loss as with non-Hodgkin's lymphoma. The presence of these symptoms is associated with a poor prognosis. The treatment varies depending on the extent of disease. For localized lesions, intralesional chemotherapy with vinblastine or another vinca alkaloid or cryodestruction can be used. For extensive disease, treatment modalities include systemic chemotherapy, either single agent or in combination with radiation therapy.

CONCLUSIONS

The HIV epidemic is one of the largest epidemics of this century, affecting people of all ages and social classes. The mode of transmission in our country has shifted from homosexual and injection drug abuse to predominantly heterosexual contact. HIV infection should be considered in any person who presents with recurrent oral thrush, oral lesions, or tumors such as

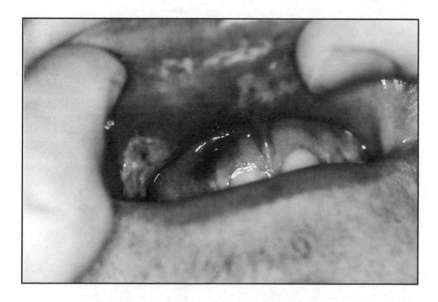

Figure 11–4. The dark-colored lesion on the gingiva above the right incisor is surrounded by radiation-induced mucositis (white ulcerative lesions on the upper lip mucosa).

Kaposi's sarcoma or lymphoma. With the advent of new antiretroviral agents and effective combination therapy, opportunistic infections, including those involving the oral cavity and esophagus, have dramatically decreased. In our experience, opportunistic infections in those patients who adhere to their medical regimen are very infrequent.

Good oral hygiene is one of the few behavior modifications that result in longer and healthier lives in the HIV-infected patient. Poor oral care may lead to malnourishment, oral infections, aspiration pneumonia, and even sepsis. The presence of dysphagia or odynophagia of any cause may lead to malnourishment, wasting syndrome, as well as poor compliance with a complicated antiretroviral regimen that may include up to 14 pills per day. Other detrimental effects include a decrease in social interactions, low self-esteem, embarrassment, and rejection.

As the HIV epidemic reaches its 3rd decade of known existence, the main causes of oropharyngeal pathology have shifted. Azole-sensitive oral candidiasis became azole resistant over a few years of prophylactic therapy. More recently, a decrease in oral candidiasis has occurred with immune function restoration with HAART.

Although cryptococcosis and histoplasmosis continue to occur mainly in those patients with CD4 counts below 100, HAART has reduced this susceptible population of patients by decreasing viral load and promoting immune reconstitution. Cases of Kaposi's sarcoma regressing while on HAART are commonplace. The success of HAART for HIV infection during the next 10 years depends on the maintenance of cellular immune function and the prevention of resistant HIV strains. Oropharyngeal disease in the HIV-infected patient will mirror this outcome.

REFERENCES

Addy, M., & Hunter, L. (1987). The effect of 0.2% chlorhexidine gluconate mouthrinse on plaque, toothstaining and *Candida* in aphthous ulcer patients. *Journal of Clinical Periodontology, 14,* 267–273.

Alexander, W. N. (1975). Venereal disease and the dentist. *Journal of the Academy of General Dentistry, 23,* 14–18.

American Dental Association. (1995). Dental management of the HIV-infected patient. *Journal of American Dental Association, 126,* 1–39.

Antoon, J. W., & Miller, R. L. (1980). Aphthous ulcers—A review of the literature on etiology, pathogenesis, diagnosis and treatment. *Journal of the American Dental Association, 101,* 803–808.

Bach, M. C., Valenti, A. J., & Howell, D. A. (1988). Odynophagia from aphthous ulcers of the pharynx and esophagus in the acquired immunodeficiency syndrome (AIDS). *Annals of Internal Medicine, 109,* 338–339.

Bach, M. C., Howell, D. A., & Valenti, A. J. (1990). Aphthous ulceration of the gastrointestinal tract in patients with the acquired immunodeficiency syndrome (AIDS). *Annals of Internal Medicine, 112,* 465–467.

Balfou, H. H., Bean, B., & Laskin, O. L. (1983). Acyclovir halts progression of herpes zoster in immunocompromised patient. *New England Journal of Medicine, 308,* 1448–1453.

Barile, M. F., Graykowski, E. A., Driscoll, E. J., & Riggs, D. B. (1963). L-form of bacteria isolated from recurrent aphthous stomatitis lesions. *Oral Surgery, Oral Medicine, and Oral Pathology, 16,* 1395–1402.

Bottomley, W. K., & Rosenburg, S. W. (Eds.). (1990). *Clinician's guide to treatment of common oral conditions* (pp. 7–8). New York: American Academy of Oral Medicine.

Boughton, C. R. (1966). Varicella-zoster in Sydney. II. Neurological complications of varicella. *Medical Journal of Australia, 2,* 444–447.

Brammer, J. R. (1990). Pharmacotherapeutics 2nd tissue penetration of fluconazole in humans. *Reviews of Infectious Disease, 12*(Suppl. 3), 5318–5326.

Budtz-Jorgensen, E. (1990). Etiology, pathogenesis, therapy and prophylaxis of yeast infections. *Acta Odontologica Scandinavica, 48,* 61–69.

Burke, B. L., Steele, R. W., & Beard, O. W. (1982). Immune responses to varicella zoster virus antigen in the aged. *Archives of Internal Medicine, 142,* 291–293.

Cauwenbergh, G. (1989). Safety aspects of ketoconazole. The most commonly used systemic antifungal. *Mycosis, 32,* 59–63.

Centers for Disease Control. (1986). Classification of HIV disease. *MMWR. Morbidity and Mortality Weekly Report, 35,* 334-339.

Crawford, C. L. (1992). Thalidomide neuropathy [Letter]. *New England Journal of Medicine, 327,* 735.

Cutter, J. E., & Glee, P. M. (1988). *Candida albicans* and *Candida stellatoidea* specific DNA fragment. *Journal of Clinical Microbiology, 269,* 1720–1724.

Dietler, R. H., & Rausher, D. B. (1989). Giant esophageal ulcer healed with steroid therapy in a patient with AIDS. *Reviews of Infectious Disease, 11,* 768–769.

Donahue, J. G., Choo, P. W., & Manson, J. E. (1995). The incidence of herpes zoster. *Archives of Internal Medicine, 155,* 1605–1609.

EC Clearinghouse on Oral Problems Related to HIV Infection and WHO Collaborating Centre on Oral Manifestations of the Immunodeficiency Virus. (1993). Classification and diagnostic criteria for oral lesions in HIV infection. *Journal of Oral Pathology and Medicine, 22,* 289–291.

Epstein, J. B. (1990). Antifungal therapy in oropharyngeal mycotic infections. *Oral Surgery, Oral Medicine, and Oral Pathology, 69,* 32–41.

Epstein, J. B., Komiyama, K., & Duncan, D. (1986). Oral topical steroids and secondary oral candidiasis. *Journal of Oral Medicine, 41,* 223–227.

Epstein, J. B., Priddy, R. W., & Sherlock, C. H. (1988). Hairy leukoplakia-like lesions in immunosuppressed patients following bone marrow transplantation. *Transplantation, 46,* 462–464.

Epstein, J. B., Sherlock, C. H., & Greenspan, J. S. (1991). Hairy leukoplakia-like lesions following bone marrow transplantation [Letter]. *AIDS, 5,* 101–102.

Fahey, J. L., Taylor, J. M., & Deters, R. (1990). The prognostic value of cellular and serologic markers in infection with human immunodeficiency virus type 1. *New England Journal of Medicine, 320,* 166–172.

Feigal, D. W., Katz, M. H., & Greenspan, D. (1991). The prevalence of oral lesions in HIV-infected homosexual and bisexual men: Three San Francisco epidemiological cohorts. *AIDS, 5,* 519–525.

Folb, P. I., & Trounce, J. R. (1970). Immunological aspects of *Candida* infection complicating steroid and immunosuppressive drug therapy. *Lancet, 2,* 1112–1114.

Fotos, P. G., & Lilly, J. P. (1996). Clinical management of oral and perioral candidosis. *Dermatologic Clinics, 14,* 273–280.

Friedman, M., Brenski, A., & Taylor, L. (1994). Treatment of aphthous ulcers in AIDS Patients. *Laryngoscope, 104,* 566–570.

Ghigliotti, G., Repetto, T., Farris, A., Roy, M. T., & De Marchi, R. (1993). Thalidomide: Treatment of choice for aphthous ulcers in patients seropositive for human immunodeficiency virus. *Journal of the American Academy of Dermatology, 28,* 271–272.

Gilman, A. G., Goodman, L. S., et al., (Eds.). (1985). *Goodman and Gilman's the pharmacological basis of therapeutics* (pp. 1463–1485). New York: Macmillan.

Gilquin, J., Weiss, L., & Kazatchkine, M. D. (1990). Genital and oral erosions induced by foscarnet. *Lancet, 335,* 287.

Glick, M., & Muzyka, B. C. (1992). Alternative therapy for major aphthous ulcers in AIDS patients. *Journal of the American Dental Association, 123,* 61–65.

Glick, M., Muzyka, B. C., Lurie, D., & Salkin, L. M. (1994). Oral manifestations associated with HIV-related disease as markers for immune suppression and AIDS. *Oral Surgery, Oral Medicine, and Oral Pathology, 77,* 344–349.

Glick, M., Muzyka, B. C., Salkin, L. M., & Lurie, D. (1994). Necrotizing ulcerative periodontitis: A marker for immune deterioration and a predictor for the diagnosis of AIDS. *Journal of Periodontology, 65,* 393–397.

Gordon, J. E. (1962). Chickenpox: An epidemiologic review. *American Journal of Medical Science, 244,* 362–389.

Gottlieb, M. S., Schroff, R., & Schranker, H. M. (1981). Pneumocystis carinii pneumonia and mucosal candidiasis in previously healthy homosexual men: Evidence of a new acquired cellular immunodeficiency. *New England Journal of Medicine, 305,* 1425–1431.

Grbic, J. T., Mitchell-Lewis, D. A., & Fine, J. B. (1995). The relationships of candidiasis to linear gingival erythema in HIV infected homosexual men and parenteral drug users. *Journal of Periodontology, 66,* 30–37.

Greenberg, M. S. (1996). HIV associated lesions. *Dermatology Clinics, 14,* 319–326.

Greenberg, M. S., Dubin, G., & Stewart, J. C. B. (1995). The relationship of oral disease to the presence of cytomegalovirus DNA in saliva of AIDS patients. *Oral Surgery, Oral Medicine, and Oral Pathology, 79,* 175.

Greenberg, M. S., Friedman, H., & Cohen, S. G. (1987). A comparative study of herpes simplex infections in renal transplant and leukemic patients. *Journal of Infectious Disease, 156,* 280–287.

Greenspan, D., & Greenspan, J. S. (1987). Oral mucosal manifestations of AIDS. *Dermatologic Clinics, 5,* 733–737.

Greenspan, J. S., & Greenspan, D. (1992). Oral lesions associated with HIV infection. In *AIDS and other manifestations of HIV infection* (2nd ed., pp. 489-498). New York: Raven Press.

Greenspan, D., Greenspan, J. S., et al. (1986). *AIDS and the dental team.* Copenhagen, Denmark: Munksgaard.

Greenspan, D., Greenspan, J. S., & Conant, M. (1984). Oral hairy leukoplakia in male homosexuals. Evidence of association with both papillomavirus and herpes-group virus. *Lancet, 2,* 831–834.

Greenspan, D., Greenspan, J. S., & De Souza, Y. G. (1989). Oral hairy leukoplakia in an HIV-negative renal transplant recipient. *Journal of Oral Pathology Medicine, 18,* 32–34.

Greenspan, D., Greenspan, J. S., & Schiodt, M. (1990). *AIDS and the mouth*. Copenhagen, Denmark: Munksgaard.

Greenspan, J. S., Greenspan, D., & Lennette, E. T. (1985). Replication of Epstein Barr virus within the epithelial cells of oral hairy leukoplakia, an AIDS-associated lesion. *New England Journal of Medicine, 313,* 1564–1571.

Hope-Simpson, R.E. (1952). Infectiousness of communicable diseases in the household (measles, chickenpox and mumps). *Lancet, 2,* 549–554.

Hope-Simpson, R. E. (1965). The nature of herpes zoster: A long term study and new hypothesis. *Proceedings of the Royal Society of Medicine, 58,* 9–20.

Horowitz, B. J., Edelstein, S. W., & Lippman, L. (1984). Sugar chromatography studies in recurrent *Candida* vulvovaginitis. *Journal of Reproduction Medicine, 29,* 441–443.

Imam, N., Carpenter, C. J., Mayer, K. H., Fisher, A., Stein, M., & Danforth, S. B. (1990). Hierarchical pattern of mucosal *Candida* infections in HIV-seropositive women. *American Journal of Medicine, 89,* 142–165.

Irani, D. N., & Johnson, R. T. (1996). New approaches to the treatment of herpes zoster and postherpetic neuralgia. *Infections in Medicine, 13,* 897–902.

Itin, P., Rufli, I., & Rudlinser, R. (1988). Oral hairy leukoplakia in an HIV-negative renal transplant patient: A marker for immune suppression. *Dermatologica, 17,* 126–128.

Katz, M. H., Greenspan, D., Westenhouse, J., Hessol, N. A., Buchbinder, S. P., & Lifson, A. R. (1992). Progression to AIDS in HIV infected homosexual and bisexual men with hairy leukoplakia and oral candidiasis: Results from 3 epidemiologic cohorts. *AIDS, 6,* 95–100.

Kirby, A. J., & Munoz, A. (1994). Thrush and fever as measures of immunocompetence in HIV-1 infected men. *Journal of Acquired Immune Deficiency Syndrome, 7,* 1242–1249.

Kolokotronis, A., Kioses, V., Antoniades, D., Mandraveli, K., Doutsos, I., & Papanayotou, P. (1994). Immunologic status in patient infected with HIV with oral candidiasis and hairy leukoplakia. *Oral Surgery, Oral Medicine, and Oral Pathology, 78,* 41–46.

Laccourreye, D., Fadlallah, J. P., Pages, J. C., Durand, H., Brasnu, D., & Lowenstein, W. (1995). Sutton's disease (periadenitis mucosa necrotica recurrens). *Annals of Otology, Rhinology and Laryngology, 104,* 301–303.

Lamster, I., & Grbic, J. T. (1995). A critical review of periodontal disease as a manifestation of HIV infection. In J. S. Greenspan & D. Greenspan (Eds.), *Oral Manifestations of HIV Infection: Proceedings of the Second International Workshop.* (pp. 246–526). Chicago: Quintessence.

Lehner, T., & Ward, R. G. (1970). Iatrogenic oral candidosis. *British Journal of Dermatology, 83,* 161–166.

Levin, M. J., Murray M., & Rotbart, H. A. (1992). Immune response of elderly individuals to a live attenuated varicella vaccine. *Journal of Infectious Disease, 166,* 253–259.

Levin, M. J., Murray, M., & Zerbe, G. O. (1994). Immune responses of elderly persons four years after receiving a live attenuated varicella vaccine. *Journal of Infectious Disease, 170,* 522–526.

Lifson, A. R., Hilton, J. F., & Westenhouse, J. L. (1994). Time from seroconversion to oral candidiasis or hairy leukoplakia among homosexual and bisexual men in three prospective cohorts. *AIDS, 8,* 73–79.

Lindemann, R. A., & Rivierte, G. R. (1985). Serum antibody responses to indigenous oral mucosa antigens and selected laboratory maintained bacteria in recurrent aphthous ulceration. *Oral Surgery, Oral Medicine, and Oral Pathology, 59,* 585–589.

Lucas, S. B., Hounou, A., Peacock, C., Beaumel, A., Djamand, G., N'Gbichi, J. M., Yeboue, K., Honde, M., Diomande, M., Giordano, C., et al. (1993). The mortality and pathology of HIV infection in a west African city. *AIDS, 7,* 1569–1579.

MacFarlane, T. W., & Samaranayake, L. P. (1990). Systemic infections. In J. H. Johns & D. K. Mason (Eds.), *Oral manifestations of systemic disease* (2nd ed., pp. 339–386). London: Balliere Tindal.

MacLeod, R. I., Long, R. Q., Soames, J. V., & Ward, M. K. (1990). Oral hairy leukoplakia in an HIV-negative renal transplant patient. *British Dental Journal, 169,* 208–209.

MacPhail, L. A., Greenspan, D., & Feigal, D. W. (1991). Recurrent aphthous ulcers in association with HIV infection: Description of ulcer types and analysis of T-lymphocyte subsets. *Oral Surgery, Oral Medicine, and Oral Pathology, 71,* 678–683.

MacPhail, L. A., Greenspan, D., & Greenspan, J. S. (1992). Recurrent aphthous ulcers in association with HIV infection: Diagnosis and treatment. *Oral Surgery, Oral Medicine, and Oral Pathology, 73,* 283–288.

MacPhail, L. A., Greenspan, D., & Schiodt, M. (1989). Acyclovir resistant, foscarnet sensitive oral herpes simplex type 2 lesion in a patient with AIDS. *Oral Surgery, Oral Medicine, and Oral Pathology, 67,* 427–432.

Maden, C., Hopkins, S. G., & Lafferty, W. E. (1994). Progression to AIDS or death following diagnosis with class IV non-AIDS disease: Utilization of a surveillance database. *Journal of Acquired Immune Deficiency Syndrome, 7,* 972–977.

Mandell, G. L., Bennett, J. E., & Dolin, R. (Eds.). (1995). Odontogenic infections. In *Mandell, Douglas, and Bennett's principles and practice of infectious diseases.* (4th ed., Vol. 1, pp. 593–602). New York: Churchill Livingstone.

Manders, S. M., Kostman, J. R., Mendez, L., & Russim, V. L. (1995). Thalidomide resistant HIV-associated aphthae successfully treated with granulocyte colony-stimulating factor. *Journal of American Academy of Dermatology, 33*, 380–382.

Mazur, M. H., & Dolin, R. (1978). Herpes zoster at the NIH: A 20-year experience. *American Journal of Medicine, 65*, 738–744.

McBride, W. G. (1961). Thalidomide and congenital abnormalities [Letter]. *Lancet, 2,* 1358.

McCarthy, G. M. (1992). Host factors associated with HIV-related oral candidiasis. A review. *Oral Surgery, Oral Medicine, and Oral Pathology, 173,* 181–186.

McCarthy, G. M., Mackie, I. D., Koval, J., Sandhu, H. S., & Daley, T. D. (1991). Factors associated with increased frequency of HIV-related oral candidiasis. *Journal of Oral Pathology and Medicine, 20,* 332–336.

McNally, M. A., & Langlais, R. P. (1996). Condition peculiar to the tongue. *Dermatologic Clinics, 14,* 257.

McNeely, M. C., Yarhoan, R., Broder, S., & Lawly, T. J. (1989). Dermatologic complications associated with administration of 2′, 3′-dideoxycytidine in patients with human immunodeficiency virus infection. *Journal of the American Academy of Dermatology, 21,* 1213–1217.

Meyer, I., & Shklar, G. (1967). The oral manifestations of acquired syphilis. *Oral Surgery, 23,* 45–47.

Muzyka, B. C., & Glick, M. (1994). Major aphthous ulcers in patients with HIV disease. *Oral Surgery, Oral Medicine, and Oral Pathology, 77,* 116–120.

Newland, J. R. (1989, May). Oral ulcers: Keys to differential and definite diagnosis. *Consultant,* 157–161.

Nielsen, H., & Bentsen, K. D. (1994). Oral candidiasis and immune status of HIV infected patients. *Journal of Oral Pathology and Medicine, 23,* 140–143.

Nolan, A., Lamey, P. J., MacFarlane, T. W., Aitchison, T. C., Shaw, J., & Sirel, J. Y. (1994). The effect of nebulized pentamidine on the concentration of intra-oral *Candida albicans* in HIV infected patients. *Journal of Medical Microbiology, 41,* 95–97.

Odds, F. C. (1988). *Candida and candidosis* (2nd ed.). Philadelphia: W. B. Saunders.

Oksala, E. (1990). Factors predisposing to oral yeast infections. *Acta Odontologica Scandinavica, 48,* 71–74.

Oldfield, E. C. (1994). Thalidomide for severe apthhous ulceration in patients with human immunodeficiency virus (HIV) infection. [Letter]. *American Journal of Gastroenterology, 89,* 2276–2277.

Paterson, D. L., Georghiou, P. R., Allworth, A. M., & Kemp, R. J. (1995). Thalidomide as treatment of refractory aphthous ulceration related to human immunodeficiency virus infection. *Clinical Infectious Diseases, 20,* 250–254.

Penneys, N. S., & Hick, B. (1985). Unusual cutaneous lesions associated with acquired immune deficiency syndrome. *Journal of the American Academy of Dermatology, 13,* 845–852.

Phelan, J. A., Eisig, S., & Fredman, P. D. (1991). Major aphthous-like ulcers in patients with AIDS. *Oral Surgery, Oral Medicine, and Oral Pathology, 71,* 68–72.

Phelan, J. A., Saltzman, B. R., & Friedland, G. H. (1987). Oral findings in patients with acquired immunodeficiency syndrome. *Oral Surgery, Oral Medicine, and Oral Pathology, 64,* 50–56.

Pollock, J. J., Santarpia, R. P., III, Heller, H. M., Xu, L., Lal, K., Fuhrer, J., Kaufman, H. W., & Steigbigel, R. T. (1992). Determination of salivary anti-candidal activities in healthy adults and patients with AIDS: A pilot study. *Journal of Acquired Immune Deficiency Syndrome, 5,* 610–617.

Radeff, B., Kuffer, R., & Samson, J. (1990). Recurrent aphthous ulcers in patient infected with human immunodeficiency virus: Successful treatment with thalidomide. *Journal of the American Academy of Dermatology, 123,* 523–525.

Ragozzino, M. W., Melton, L. J., & Kurland, L. T. (1982). Population based study of herpes zoster and its sequela. *Medicine, 61,* 310–316.

Rees, T. D., & Binnie, W. H. (1996). Recurrent aphthous stomatitits. *Dermatologic Clinics, 14,* 243–256.

Reggiani, M., & Paulizzi, P. (1990). Hairy leukoplakia in liver transplant patients. *Acta Dermatology Venerology, 70,* 87–88.

Reichart, P. A. (1992). Oral ulcerations and iatrogenic disease in HIV infection. *Oral Surgery, Oral Medicine, and Oral Pathology, 73,* 212–214.

Reichart, P. A., Gelderblom, H. R., Becker, J., & Kuntz, A. (1987). AIDS and the oral cavity: The HIV infection—Virology, etiology, origin, immunology, precautions and clinical observations in 110 patients. *International Journal of Oral and Maxillofacial Surgery, 16,* 129–153.

Reiter, G. S. (1996). The HIV wasting syndrome. *AIDS Clinical Care, 8,* 11.

Rennie, J. S., Reade, P. C., & Hay, K. D. (1985). Recurrent aphthous stomatitis. *British Dental Journal, 159,* 361–367.

Rippon, J. W. (1982). *Medical mycology* (2nd ed.). Philadelphia: W. B. Saunders.

Rogers, R. S. (1977). Recurrent aphthous stomatitis: Clinical characteristics and evidence for an immunopathogenesis. *Journal of Investigational Dermatology, 69,* 499.

Royce, R. A., & Luckmann, R. S. (1991). The natural history of HIV-1 infection: Staging classifications of disease. *AIDS, 5,* 355–364.

Samaranayake, L. P. (1989). Oral candidosis: Predisposing factors and pathogeneses. In D. D. Derrick (Ed.), *Dental annual* (pp. 219–235). Bristol, England: Wright.

Samaranayake, L. P. (1990). Host factors and oral candidosis. In L. P. Samaranayake & T. W. MacFarlane (Eds.), *Oral candidosis* (pp. 66–104). London: Wright.

Samaranayake, L. P. (1992). Oral mycoses in HIV infection. *Oral Surgery, Oral Medicine and Oral Pathology, 3,* 171–180.

Schiodt, M., Greenspan, D., & Greenspan, J. S. (1996a). HIV-related oral lesions: Fungal infections. *Journal of Respiratory Diseases, 17,* 385–390.

Schiodt, M., Greenspan, D., & Greenspan, J. S. (1996b). HIV-related oral lesions: Bacterial infections. *Journal of Respiratory Disorders, 17,* 502–504.

Schiodt, M., Greenspan, D., & Greenspan, J. S. (1996c). HIV-related oral lesions: Recognizing viral infections. *Journal of Respiratory Diseases, 17,* 580–582.

Schiodt, M., Greenspan, D., & Greenspan, J. S. (1996d). HIV-related oral lesions: Neoplasms and other lesions. *Journal of Respiratory Diseases, 17,* 653–655.

Schiodt, M., Norgaard, T., & Greenspan, J. S. (1995). Oral hairy leukoplakia in an HIV negative woman with Behcet's syndrome. *Oral Surgery, 79,* 53–56.

Schulten, E. A., ten Kate, R. W., & van der Waal, I. (1990). Oral findings in HIV-infected patients attending a department of internal medicine. The contribution of examination towards the clinical management of HIV disease. *Quarterly Journal of Medicine, 76,* 741–745.

Scuibba, J. J. (1996). Recognizing the oral manifestations of AIDS. *Oncology, 6,* 64–76.

Scully, C., Laskaris, G., Pinborg, J., Porter, S. R., & Reichart, P. (1991a). Oral manifestations of HIV infection and their management. I. More common lesions. *Oral Surgery, Oral Medicine, and Oral Pathology, 71,* 158–166.

Scully, C., Laskaris, G., Pindborg, J., Porter, S. R., & Reichart, P. (1991b). Oral manifestations of HIV infection and their management. II. Less common lesions. *Oral Surgery, Oral Medicine, and Oral Pathology, 71,* 167–171.

Scully, C., & McCarthy, G. (1992). Management of oral health in persons with HIV infection. *Oral Surgery, Oral Medicine, and Oral Pathology, 73,* 215–225.

Scully, C., & Porter, S. R. (1989). Recurrent aphthous stomatitis: Current concepts of etiology, pathogenesis and management. *Journal of Oral Pathology and Medicine, 18,* 21–27.

Shepp, D. H., Dandliker, P. S., & Meyers, J. D. (1986). Treatment of varicella zoster virus infection in severely immunocompromised patients: A randomized comparison of acyclovir and vidarabine. *New England Journal of Medicine, 314,* 208–212.

Sheskin, J. (1965). Thalidomide in the treatment of lepra reactions. *Clinical Pharmacology Therapeutics, 6,* 303–306.

Silverman, S., Migliorate, C. A., Lozada, N. F., Greenspan, D., & Conant, M. (1986). Oral finding in people with or at risk for AIDS: A study of 375 homosexual males. *Journal of the American Dental Association, 112,* 187–192.

Small, C. B., Klein, R. S., Friedland, G. H., Moll, B., Emeson, E. E., & Spigland, L. (1983). Community-acquired opportunistic infections and defective cellular immunity in heterosexual drug abusers. *America Journal of Medicine, 74,* 433–441.

Soll, D. R. (1988). High frequency switching in *Candida albicans* and its relation to vaginal candidiasis. *American Journal of Obstetric Gynecology, 158,* 997–1001.

Sutton, R. (1911). Periadenitis mucosa necrotica recurrens. *Journal of Cutaneous Disorders, 29,* 65–71.

Sutton, R. (1941). Recurrent scarring painful aphthae. *JAMA, 117,* 175–176.

Syrjanen, S., Laine, P., Happoinen, R. P., & Niemela, M. (1989). Oral hairy leukoplakia is not a specific sign of HIV infection but related to suppression in general. *Journal of Oral Pathology and Medicine, 18,* 28–31.

Vincent, S. D., & Lilly, G. E. (1992). Clinical history and therapeutic features of aphthous stomatitis. Literature review and open clinical trial employing steroids. *Oral Surgery, Oral Medicine, and Oral Pathology, 74,* 79–86.

Weinert, M., Grimes, R. M., & Lynch, D. P. (1996). Oral manifestations of HIV infection. *Annals of Internal Medicine, 125,* 485–496.

Whitley, R. J. (1991). Encephalitis caused by herpes viruses, including B virus. In W. M. Scheld, R. J. Whitley, & D. T. Durack (Eds.), *Infections of the central nervous system* (pp. 41–86). New York: Raven Press.

Winker, J. R. (1995). Pathogenesis of HIV associated periodontal disease: What's known and what isn't. In J. S. Greenspan & D. Greenspan (Eds.), *Oral Manifestations of HIV Infection: Proceedings of the Second International Workshop* (pp. 262–272). Chicago: Quintessence.

Zambon, J. J., Reynolds, H. S., & Genco, R. J. (1990). Studies of the subgingival microflora in patients with acquired immunodeficiency syndrome. *Journal of Periodontology, 61,* 699–704.

12

Nursing Management of Dysphagia

Penelope Stevens Fisher, M.S., R.N., C.O.R.L.N.

Dysphagia and its management present the clinician with multiple opportunities for creative interventions. When the etiology of the disease stems from cancer or the side effects of the cancer treatment, the complexity is increased. The approach to the patient needs to be comprehensive from all aspects of physical and psychosocial care. It is of paramount importance that the efforts of the multidisciplinary care team be coordinated to enhance positive patient outcomes. One member of the dysphagia care team who has developed team coordination and complex care skills is the specialty registered nurse.

NURSES AND NURSING CARE

Historically, nursing has been associated with care of people with illnesses. The role of the nurse has evolved through the years as education, experiences, specialization, certification, and autonomy enhanced the value and presence of nursing practice within the multidisciplinary team. Today, registered nurses serve as the patient care managers who coordinate activities for individuals seeking health care for illness or wellness. The role includes responsibility as patient advocate, knowledgeable ad-

visor, triage officer, and facilitator to access the system (Mochia, 1993). Nurses have developed innovative intrapreneurial and entrepreneurial skills and established themselves as professional caregivers and educators (Manion, 1990).

Specialization in Nursing

Specialization and certification have validated the focus of care to specific health care issues and concerns. The otorhinolaryngology (ORL) nurse generalist is a registered nurse with a minimal educational level (RN, BSN) practicing in the specialty of ORL nursing. The ORL Nurse Specialist (Advanced Practice Nurse) is a registered nurse with a graduate degree (MS, MSN) in nursing who is an expert in ORL nursing. Certification of an ORL nurse (CORLN) signifies tenure in the specialty, active practice, and successful completion of a comprehensive board-approved examination that tests knowledge regarding the life span of otorhinolaryngological disorders and assesses knowledge about patient care management (Standards Committee SOHN, 1993).

Cancer nursing is also identified as a nursing specialty. Registered nurses with experience and who pass a certification examination are credentialed by the Oncology Nursing Society. Within most nursing organizations, there are special interest groups that further delineate education for practice in specific patient populations such as those with head and neck cancer.

The specialized nurse is educationally prepared to provide leadership, coordination, and liaison activities for the interdisciplinary team serving patients with otolaryngological disorders (Fisher, 1994). Additionally, the nurse serves as a team member promoting collaborative practice among all members of the otolaryngological interdisciplinary team (Sullivan & Fisher, 1995).

Practice Settings

The challenge of caring for the patient with dysphagia is described in several chapters of this book. The complexity of patient care management dictates the need for a collaborative interdisciplinary team with the flexibility of bringing care and treatment interventions to the patient. Comprehensive services may be needed in a variety of health care settings. Nurses are educated to practice in many settings (Table 12–1).

The management of dysphagia may be required in each of these settings as care

is planned for the successful rehabilitation of patients with neurological, mechanical, or psychiatric origins of swallowing dysfunction. A defined process provides the greatest success.

THE NURSING PROCESS

The nursing process is a scientifically based problem-solving system that explores the health care concern in an organized manner. Components of the process include assessment, planning, intervention, and evaluation, which are described in Table 12–2.

TABLE 12–1. Practice Setting of the Registered Nurse

Hospitals
Extended care facilities
Community health
Clinics/ambulatory care
Home health
Physician offices
Schools
Congregate living center
Retirement homes
Hospice
Occupational health
Wellness centers
Rehabilitation facilities

TABLE 12–2. Definitions: Nursing Process

Component	Description
Assessment	Collection of client health data by interview, examination, observation, and review of health records.
	Data collection is systematic and ongoing.
	Data collection is analyzed and a diagnosis is determined.
	The nursing diagnosis is determined, validated, and used to identify individualized attainable outcomes.
Planning	A mutually formulated client care plan is developed reflecting met needs of the client, continuity of care, ORL nursing practice, and a multidisciplinary approach.
Intervention	Interventions to provide client care are implemented consistently, safely, and appropriately.
Evaluation	A systematic and ongoing review of the client's progress toward attainment of outcomes.
	Effectiveness of interventions is evaluated by the client and practioner, and needed revisions are made.

Source: Adapted from *SOHN Scope of Practice: ORL Standards of Professional Performance,* by Standards Committee SOHN, 1993, New Smyrna Beach, FL: Society of Otorhinolaryngology and Head-Neck Nurses.

Assessment of the Dysphagic Patient

The nurse may be the first health care provider to recognize signs and symptoms of dysphagia and/or odynophagia. The nurse must be knowledgeable about the symptoms, associated risk factors, possible complications, diagnostic tests, and treatment modalities. Each component requires patient education and possible nursing care interventions. Signs and symptoms have been discussed throughout this book, but those that may be detected by the nurse are listed in Table 12–3.

The nursing assessment will determine if the patient is at risk for dysphagia or associated complications such as pulmonary problems or altered nutritional status. Components of the nursing evaluation include history and medical record review, physical exam, patient interview, observations during meals, and chest and cervical airway auscultation (Sievers, 1997).

The nursing evaluation begins with a history and physical of the patient. The depth of these components will be correlated to the experience and education of the practicing nurse. Those nurses on the swallowing rehabilitation team or those working in the speciality of otorhinolaryngology will have developed enhanced skills and collaborative networking with other

TABLE 12–3. Signs and Symptoms of Dysphagia and Odynophagia

How Recognized	Sign or Symptom
Observed	Confusion
	Dysarthric speech
	Nasal air emission during speech
	Voice quality
	Weight loss and distribution
	Facial expression, function
	Mandible position
	Dental occlusion
	Drooling
	Coughing
	Choking
	Effortful chewing
	Prolongation of meals
	Nasal regurgitation
	Mouth odor
	Aspiration
	Absent gag reflex
Reported	Food sticking
	Frequency of swallowing
	Heartburn
	Gastroesophageal reflux
	Hoarseness
	Slurring/clumsy speech
	Throat discomfort/pain
	Substernal pain radiation to jaw, back, neck, left arm
	Productive cough
	Retained secretions
	Referred otalgia

Source: Adapted from "Evaluation of Swallowing Disorders," by R. M. Miller. In *Dysphagia: Diagnosis and Management*, edited by M. Groher, 1984, Stoneham, MA: Butterworth, and "Dysphagia and Odynophagia," by C. Stiernberg. In *Otolaryngology—Head and Neck Surgery*, edited by W. Meyerhoff and D. Rice, 1992, Philadelphia: W. B. Saunders.

disciplines for validation and interactions for findings. Table 12–4 explores the chief complaint. Table 12–5 lists considerations of abnormal findings to be explored as problems possibly related to dysphagia.

Planning the Care of the Dysphagic Patient

After review and collection of clinical data, the nurse approaches the patient's needs using a problem-oriented system to formu-

late a patient-focused care plan. Analysis and interpretation of the data are assimilated and shared with members of the swallowing rehabilitation team and the patient. A realistic problem-solving plan that is mutually agreed on and has attainable goals is documented and activated.

The patient's response to the health care problem must be considered during planning. Identification of the value of physical function to the patient and issues related to quality of life such as eating with

TABLE 12–4. Dysphagia: Chief Complaints

Identified Problem	Patient's Complaint	Family Member's or Examiner's Observation
Weight loss	Sudden or gradual loss Too difficult to swallow and spend energy	Won't eat what is prepared Clothing not fitting
Food management sticking or no control	At first, meats would not go down, now only can get soft foods in Liquids may cause choking	Starts a meal, does not finish Leaves table often Multiple swallows Regurgitates food/liquid Chokes during meal, gurgles Intolerant of specific food consistencies Cannot take pills
Taste	Food has no flavor and does not taste good	Avoids usual favorites Treatment modalities for neurogenic, muscular, or cancer disorders may alter taste
Coughing	Coughs/chokes when eating Cannot drink liquids Coughs/chokes when not eating/drinking	Any or certain foods and/or liquids cause coughing and/or choking Cough unrelated to meal time but could be related to dysphagia and its complications or other pulmonary disease
Copious oral secretions	Drools Constant attempt to swallow	Face, clothes wet Uses multiple tissues Lack of oral sensation
Breath odor	Bad taste in mouth Acid/bitter taste Foul-smelling belch	Halitosis Gastric reflux and inability to swallow
Activity of daily living changes	Meals take increased time Cannot eat out Tires easily Cannot eat whole meal	Fatigue due to effort/time to finish meal Coughing Eats alone Avoids going out with friends

TABLE 12–5. Data From History and Physical That May Contribute to the Etiology of Dysphagia

Review of Systems	History	Physical Examination
Oral cavity	Surgery Neurological disease Congenital anomaly Cerebrovascular accident	Wounds, ulcerations of the mucosa Infections Motor dysfunction Fasciculations Atrophy Masses Desensate tongue Defect of palate
Oropharynx hypopharynx		Tonsillar hypertrophy Ulceration or submucosal bulging Bitter taste
Larynx	Mass Polyps Hoarseness	Pooling of secretions in vallecula and/or piniform sinuses Paralyzed vocal cord Inflamed arytenoids Contact ulcer on the vocal processes
Neck	Mass Surgery Trauma	Masses Failure of suprahyoid muscle to lift larynx during swallow Absence of laryngeal click Foul taste in mouth during neck palpation
Neuro	Neurological disease (i.e., trigeminal neuralgia/tic douloureux)	Motor dysfunction Pain and/or anesthesia
	Dysfunction of cranial nerve: V (trigeminal)	Dysfunction of muscles of mastication Decreased strength of bite Anesthesia of areas of tongue, alveolar ridge
	VII (facial)	Taste alterations Two thirds of tongue and hard and soft palate Lips may not close or be pursed Nasal ala immobile on respiration Paralysis buccinator muscle: food in cheek Loss of control of oral secretions
	IX (glossopharyngeal)	Loss of taste in posterior one third of tongue Motor dysfunction of tongue Desensate pharynx Dysfunction of stylopharyngeus muscle: palate will not elevate during swallowing Alteration in gag reflex
	X (vagus)	Dysfunction with sensory components of gag reflex and cough Speech alterations due to dysfunction of intrinsic muscles of larynx, recurrent laryngeal nerve Dysfunction of palatal lifting Dysfunction of secretomotor properties of glands of the pharyngeal and laryngeal mucosa Hypersecretion of gastric acid Desensate tongue, pharynx, larynx, trachea, esophagus

(continued)

TABLE 12–5. *(continued)*

Review of Systems	History	Physical Examination
	XII (hypoglossal)	Dysfunction of intrinsic extrinsic muscles of tongue
		Alterations in taste and sensation of tongue
		Alterations in chewing, sucking, swallowing
		Deviated tongue to side of inactive muscle
Pulmonary	Aspiration	Fluid and air mixed
	Lung disease	Sounds of cervical in pulmonary airways
	Pneumonia	Rales, rhonchi, crackles rub
		Fremitus
		Productive cough
		Fever

Source: Adapted from "Dysphagia and Odynophagia," by C. Stiernberg. *In Otolaryngology—Head and Neck Surgery,* edited by W. Meyerhoff and D. Rice, 1992, Philadelphia: W. B. Saunders, and *Cranial Nerves: Anatomy and Clinical Components,* by L. Wilson-Pauwels, E. Akesson, and P. Stewart, 1988, Philadelphia: B. C. Decker.

family and friends must be explored. Additionally, the patient's method of learning, coping strategies, and belief in compliancy must be known and understood to provide the best opportunity for education and rehabilitation.

The patient's support system is paramount in achieving positive outcomes. Family support, care, and attention from informed significant others motivate the patient and enhance the success of the professional care team. The nurse often serves as the psychosocial liaison for the patient, providing assistance or referring to an available psychosocial specialist. Psychosocial aspects for care of the dysphagic patient are essential to the care plan of the patient and are discussed in Chapter 15.

Implementation of Care and Nursing Interventions

The degree of dysphagia will dictate the level of care. The spectrum can range from mild dysfunction of a specific phase of swallowing to the complete absence of the process and a tube-dependent lifestyle. In many settings it may be the nurse who assists the patient with learning and/or practicing the skills to adapt or correct the swallowing difficulty.

King (1981) has described nursing as perceiving, thinking, relating, and judging in a face-to-face encounter with a patient in an environment that requires an established relationship to cope with health states and adjust to alterations in activities of daily living. This relationship is founded in trust, communication, and transactions.

The process of human interaction involves perception, judgment, and action. Actions that are mutually explored can result in goal attainment or transactions (King, 1981). Care of the dysphagic patient will require specific transactions to achieve successful nursing interventions. The specialty skills of the nurse will be able to stimulate responses that are necessary for patient's ownership and willingness to participate in the difficult process of swallowing rehabilitation. Nursing interventions provide management of nutrition, hydration, airway maintenance, and education.

Nursing interventions become significantly more comprehensive when dysphagia is caused by cancer or is the direct result of cancer treatment. The location of the cancer and extent of the disease determine the need for surgery, radiation, chemotherapy, or combination of all. These modalities and their outcomes have been discussed throughout this book. It is important to note that care of the patient with head and neck cancer may require a nursing specialty approach centered around nutrition, airway management and acceptance of a new lifestyle involving possible disfigurement, loss of voice, and the continuous challenge of swallowing.

Nutrition and Hydration

Chapter 13 comprehensively reviews assessment, planning, interventions, and evaluation of nutritional services. The discussion in this chapter will relate to care of the devices used to provide nutrition and hydration to the patient.

Three methods of receiving nutritional supplements are oral, parenteral, and enteral feeding.

ORAL FEEDINGS. Patients with dysphagia require adequate positioning, meticulous mouth care, skill in the use of a suction machine, appropriate choice of foods, and visual monitoring of meal intakes. Tools are often used to assist with consumption or measurement of nutrition. Breck or clinician-fashioned syringe feeders, glossectomy feeding spoon, teapots, and/or calorie counter provide methods of assistance and tracking.

PARENTERAL FEEDINGS. Hydration and nutritional support can be delivered by peripheral or central venous access devices for short periods of time. Insertion, monitoring, and maintenance of a peripheral intravenous line is standard nursing care. Although monitoring and maintenance of a central venous line may be part of the registered nurse's role, usually insertion is completed by a physician or an advanced practice nurse's. Hyperalimentation is another short-term solution for nutrition. Management of hyperalimentation is best done with the team approach, using the skills of a nutritional support team and the nurse. Attentive observations and assertive nursing interventions are needed to prevent complications of parenteral feedings. Complications can include fluid overload, clotted catheter, air emboli, malpositioned catheter, arterial puncture, pneumothorax, hyperglycemia, hypoglycemia, and infections.

ENTERAL FEEDING. The decision to use enteral feedings correlates with the expected length of rehabilitation, the severity of the dysphagia, and the patient's anatomic structure. There are several types of feeding tubes. Nasogastric and nasointestinal feeding tubes are short-term approaches and usually used when there is a positive gag reflex. Percutaneous endoscopic gastrostomy tube, gastrostomy, or jejunostomy tubes may be used in the absence of the gag reflex and are initiated in long-term swallowing rehabilitation.

Cleanliness of equipment, the tubes, and the body entry point is paramount in preventing local infections. Creative anchoring of the tube with appropriate taping or commercial tube holders will prevent skin irritation and malposition of the tube. Instilling water following each medication or feeding assists in cleanliness and provides additional hydration to the patient. Additionally, this checks the tube's integrity, patency, and connecting adapters. This also assists in preventing a clogged tube. Clogged tubes can best be treated with various solutions of carbonated beverages, juice, and meat tenderizer or gentle aspiration with a syringe. Managing volume, volume rate, type of supplement, positions to avoid aspiration, abdominal distention, vomiting, cramping, dumping, and diarrhea are discussed in Chapter 13.

Airway Management

In the dysphagic patient, pooling of secretions in the pharynx creates a high risk for respiratory complications. Nursing interventions focus on safe airway management.

ASPIRATION. Aspiration can be life threatening. It is particularly morbid for the elderly who may have confounding medical problems such as lung and cardiac disorders. Symptoms of aspiration may be occult and unrecognized by the patient or caregiver (Logemann, 1986). Precautions for care are listed in Table 12–6.

ASPIRATION PNEUMONIA. Aspiration pneumonia is found in patients who are unable to protect the airway. Mechanical obstruc-

TABLE 12–6. Aspiration Precautions for Dysphagia

Oral intake

Avoid oral intake when alone or unattended
Establish and follow prescribed consistency, amount, and frequency of dietary intake
Provide quiet environment avoiding distractions
Maintain proper body alignment including head/neck as prescribed or with 90% head and neck flexion
Alert caretaker of possible need for airway suctioning, Heimlich maneuver, and/or cardiopulmonary resuscitation
Routinely monitor pulmonary status for aspiration complication: fever, rales, rhonchi

Enteral feedings

Evaluate tube placement for the correct position
Measure residuals prior to feeding
Check body positioning for safety
Monitor for reflux

Source: Adapted from "Nursing Evaluation and Care of the Dysphagic Patient," by A. Sievers. In *Dysphagia Assessment and Treatment Planning: A Team Approach,* edited by R. Leonard and K. Kendall, 1997, San Diego, CA: Singular Publishing Group.

tions or neuromuscular dysfunction such as paralysis of the vocal folds cause the most problems. Patients with gastroesophageal pharyngeal-tracheal reflux are also at risk. In the care of the dysphagic patient it is critical to continually monitor and manage the signs and symptoms of aspiration and pneumonia. Determination of pulmonary aspiration as to volume time and type is necessary. Repeated aspirations destroy pulmonary hygiene and prevent adequate function, resulting in severe confounding medical problems.

The nurse must understand the principles of gravity and anatomy to provide helpful interventions. Aspirates are most likely to enter the right lower lobe of the lung because of the tracheobronchial tree angle. If the patient is positioned in bed the dependent area will be at the higher risk for aspirated material. Due to increased solidification of secretions, abnormal increased density will change breath sounds. Noted adventitious sounds, changes in fremitus, and egophony should dictate respiratory care (Table 12–7).

ARTIFICIAL AIRWAYS. Artificial airways may be needed for a variety of health care reasons and indications including relief of upper airway obstruction, assisting mechanical ventilation, and enabling more

TABLE 12–7. Interventions for Aspiration Pneumonia

Medicate with prescribed antibiotic, antipyretics

Monitor fever, fluid hydration, respirations, amount, color, and consistency of mucus, oxygen saturation

Turn and position patient for posture and best drainage every 2–4 hours

Deep breathing every 2–4 hours

Use prescribed respiratory care devices: suction, incentive spirometry, humidity, pulse oximetry

Conserve energy (i.e., easier communication systems) but keep patient active

Monitor for airway obstruction, atelectasis, pulmonary edema, bronchospasm, and/or acute respiratory distress syndrome

efficient pulmonary toilet (Myers, Stool, & Johnson, 1985). During the acute stage of mechanical dysphagia it may be necessary to place a tracheostomy tube. Although this will improve pulmonary status, the tracheostomy tube may interfere with swallowing because the tube prevents the laryngeal lift that usually prepares the airway for protection. Additionally, the tracheostomy tube may prevent pulmonary air from clearing laryngeal obstructions (Arms, Dines, & Tinstman, 1974; Bonanno, 1971; Johnson, Reilly, & Mallory, 1985).

Management of a tracheostomy tube requires complex assessment and technical skill. Knowledge of the function and purpose of respiratory tubes (tracheostomy, endotracheal, and suction) needs to be comprehensive (Table12–8). Care of the tracheostomy is managed by a coordinat- ed, multidisciplinary team with specific defined roles of responsibility. The role of the nurse as coordinator provides consistent continuity of assessment, planning, and evaluation of the patient's responses and outcome of airway management (Sigler & Wills, 1985).

TABLE 12–8. Respiratory Tubes

Tube	Purpose and Considerations
Endotracheal	Short-term mechanical intubation
	Polyethylene tube inserted intraorally or intranasally by physician, advanced practice nurse, physician assistant, or respiratory therapist
	Sizes—newborn to 10.0 mm
	The largest internal diameter in the recommended range of sizes for the patient's age, gender, and physical status is selected for use
	Maintenance requires proper taping, cleanliness, and prescribed mechanical breathing
Tracheotomy	Long-term airway management
	Plastic or metal tubes with and/or without inner cannula, surgically placed between the third and fourth tracheal ring (adult) (temporary)
	Tracheostomy tubes range in size from interdiameter (ID) 4-5 mm (size 00.0) to ID 11 mm (size 10.0). Note: Laryngectomy stoma tubes can be larger in ID but are shorter in length
	Maintenance requires air patency, humidification, suction, and cleanliness
	Specialized Tubes
Cuffed	Cuffed balloon surrounds the outer diameter of the tracheotomy tube to seal the airway for positive pressure ventilation
	Pressure on the cuff ranges 20–30 mmHg
Cuffless	Used when the cuff is no longer needed
Fenestrated	Used for weaning and decannulation
	Short-term use due to possibility of tracheal mucosa filling the fenestration, which can create airway blockage
Talking Tracheotomy	Several tubes are designed to allow various degrees of voice
Special Sizes	Most manufacturers will provide individual sizes when the clinician provides the company engineer with specific measurements
Suction	Used to aspirate mucus secretions from the trachea, bronchus
	Polyethylene/silicone clear catheters
	Sizes 6–18 Fr
	The outside diameter of the suction tube should not exceed half the diameter of the tracheostomy tube
	Catheter insertion into the tracheostomy tube ranges from 4–6 in. and should suction on withdrawal only, not exceeding 10–15 s (adult) 5–10 s (child)
	Maintenance of suction equipment in institutions is an aseptic condition. At home clean technique is taught

In addition to managing secretions, care considerations for humidification, stoma site, communication, and airway safety require comprehensive intervention. Generically, nursing procedure manuals and texts review these nursing skills. More specifically, *Guidelines of Otorhinolaryngology Nursing Practice*, a publication of the Society of Otorhinolaryngology—Head and Neck Nurses, Inc., provides state-of-the-art practice guidelines related to defining characteristics, nursing diagnoses, outcome identification, and interventions for these patient care needs.

Comorbidity of the dysphagic patient may require multiple additional nursing skills. Patients with conditions of other anatomic systems, sensory deficits, psychosocial disorders, mobility impairments, or learning disabilities will need additional nursing care expertise and will not be presented in this chapter.

Patient Education

Informing the patient of enough appropriate data to make informed decisions about health care is the responsibility of every health care provider. Licensed health care providers practice within the parameters of the regulations established by a governing board for that discipline. Nurse Practice Acts legally charge and require registered nurses to provide health teaching and counseling of the ill, injured, or infirm, and prevention of illness of others (example quoted from Florida State Law: 1990 Nurse Practice Act).

The nurse on the dysphagia rehabilitation team, in addition to care coordination, serves as a teacher, reinforcer of other's teachings, validator of information, and facilitator to maintain the learning process. The nurse serves as a coach and by using coaching behaviors can facilitate cognitive-emotional processing to elicit patient behavioral self-care and self-management skills (Lewis & Zahlis, 1997). An example of this role may be seen in how the nurse assists the speech-language pathologist in the continued daily execution and reinforcement of the supraglottic swallow maneuver for airway protection.

The patient's learning process is explored during the initial nursing assessment. The patient's preferred learning style is documented so all members of the team can use principles of adult education to attain identified outcomes (Table 12–9).

Printed educational material is a relatively inexpensive manner to provide patients with needed information. The dysphagia interdisciplinary team can design tools with the group's individual specificity. Examples are shown in Figure 12–1. Additional forms of education can be provided. Educational videos, pamphlets, and other printed material can be obtained from professional organizations and public agencies.

Informal learning occurs through support groups. Almost every support group has some form of educational process. Groups that are attended best and perform well are those groups who have professional health care providers as advisors. Such groups are often led by a patient leader and a speech-language pathologist and/or registered nurse. The educated dysphagic patient who has experienced an individualized multidisciplinary care plan and the expertise of specialized health care providers who perform using a dynamic clinical guideline will have

TABLE 12–9. Learning Styles

Style	Description
Visual	Relies on visual cues, seeing what is to be learned; prefers videos, pictures, watching
Auditory	Depends on auditory cues, hearing what is to be understood; prefers audiotapes, listening about the situation
Demonstration-return demonstration	Prefers to follow observations of others so as to see and do
Conceptual thinker	Assimilates information with several different methods; concludes a concept and then performs the task

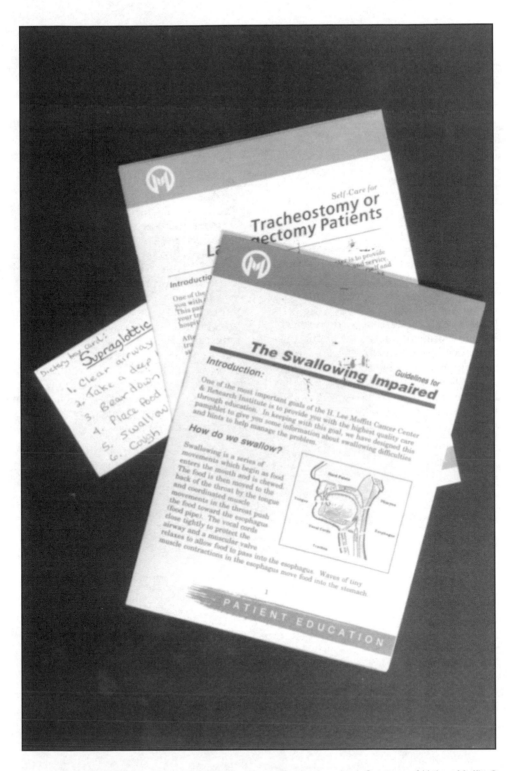

Figure 12–1. Patient education tools: guidelines for the swallowing impaired. Courtesy of H. Lee Moffitt Cancer Center and Research Institute at the University of South Florida, Tampa, Florida.

the best opportunity for successful rehabilitation outcomes.

Evaluation: Outcomes

The ultimate goal is to return the dysphagic patient to swallowing. Along the course of treatment, negotiated attainable goals are evaluated and revised to meet the changing needs of the patient. Evaluation outcomes may be measured in several ways. The patient's response can easily be evaluated at regular intervals during clinical rounds or visits. Team success can be reviewed at weekly or biweekly conferences. Algorithms and flowcharts from clinical practice guidelines can serve as a team outcomes marker and organizational time and financial cost-effectiveness measures.

Using a continuous quality improvement system, nursing management of the dysphagic patient can measure effects of nursing interventions. Brooten and Naylor (1995) have described nurse-sensitive patient outcomes as an approach to measuring nurses' effect on changing patient outcomes. Outcomes sensitive to effects of nursing actions include functional status, mental status, stress level, satisfaction with care, caregiver burden, and cost of care.

The nursing intervention of care associated with nutritional support and airway management can correlate to positive functional status. An example of a measurement tool is shown in Table 12–10.

CONCLUSIONS

The care of the dysphagic patient will always remain a challenge. It is the collaborative spirit of a motivated specialty team with a unified goal to improve the patient's quality of life that makes the difference. Nurses are proud to be a member of the swallowing rehabilitation team. Nurses believe every patient deserves a nurse (American Nurses Association, 1994). It is hoped that every team experiences the value that a nurse can bring to its care team members and to the patients whom they serve. All nurses can provide care for the ill, but it is the specialized nurse who can offer the most coordinated comprehensive approach to the patient with dysphagia.

TABLE 12–10. Example: Airway Management

Diagnosis: Dysphasia
Complication: Aspiration
Prescribed treatment: Tracheostomy
Nursing diagnosis: Airway clearance, ineffective
Plan: Patient to have tracheostomy in place for 6 weeks

Care Plan: Tracheostomy
Goal: Independent tracheostomy care in 4 days

Patient Education: Tracheostomy Modules	Mod I Initial Education	Mod II Inner Cannula	Mod III Stoma Care	Mod IV Ties	Mod V Communication
Date	2/12/98	2/12/98	2/13/98		
Nurse	Fisher	Fisher	Fisher		

Interventions	Date/Time	% Completion	Nurse	Follow-Up	% Result	Comment
Independently removes inner cannula TD: 2/13/98	2/13/98 1600	75%	Fisher	2/14/98 0800	100%	
Independently completes stoma care TD: 2/14/98	2/13/98 2300	50%	Fisher	2/14/09 0800	100%	
Independently changes trach tube ties TD: 2/14/98						
Independently able to use finger or plug trach to produce voice TD: 2/15/98						

Key: Mod - documented teaching module
       TD - target date of goal

REFERENCES

Arms, R. A., Dines, D. E., & Tinstman, T. C. (1974). Aspiration pneumonia. *Chest, 65,* 136–139.

Bates, B. (1991). *A guide to physical examination and history taking.* Philadelphia: J. B. Lippincott.

Bildstein, C. Y. (1993). Head and neck malignancies. In S. L. Groenwald, M. Frogge, M. Goodman, & C. Yarbro (Eds.), *Cancer nursing principles and practice* (pp. 1114–1148). Boston: Jones & Bartlett.

Bonanno, P. C. (1971). Swallowing dysfunction after tracheostomy. *Annals of Surgery, 174,* 29–33.

Brooten, D., & Naylor, M. (1995). Nurses' effect on changing patient outcomes. *Image, 27,* 95–99.

Bryce, J. C. (1995). Aspiration: Causes, consequences and prevention. *ORL—Head and Neck Nursing, 13,* 14–17.

Clarke, L. K. (1993). Rehabilitation for the head and neck cancer patient. *Oncology, 12,* 81–89.

Cole-Arvin, C., Notich, L., & Underhill, A. (1994). Identifying and managing dysphagia. *Nursing, 94,* 48–49.

Cutright, L. (1992). Head and neck cancer. In J. Clark & P. McGee (Eds.), *Curriculum for oncology nurses.* Philadelphia: W. B. Saunders.

Dawson, C. J., Hanrahan, K. A., Means, M. E., Reese, J. L., & Clearman, B. (1996). Development of an enteral feeding protocol. *Journal of the Society of Otorhinolaryngology and Head-Neck Nurses, 14,* 15–17.

Dilorio, C., & Price, M. (1990). Swallowing: An assessment guide. *American Journal of Nursing, 90,* 38–41.

Fisher, P. S. (1994). Nurses and the head and neck cancer team. *Cancer Control, 1,* 40–43.

Grant, M., & Rivera, L. (1995). Anorexia, cachexia, and dysphagia: The symptom experience. *Seminars in Oncology Nursing, 11,* 266–271.

Griffith, H. W. (1994). Dysphagia. In *Instructions for Patients* (p. 140). Philadelphia: W. B. Saunders.

Griggs, B. A. (1984). Nursing management of swallowing disorders. In M. E. Groher (Ed.), *Dysphagia: Diagnosis and management.* Stoneham, MA: Butterworth.

Groher, M. E. (1984). *Dysphagia: Diagnosis and management.* Stoneham, MA: Butterworth.

Harold, M. (1987). Rehabilitation of the dysphagic client following ablative surgery for laryngeal cancer. *Journal of the Society of Otolaryngology and Head-Neck Nurses, 5,* 16–18.

Johnson, J., Reilly, J., & Mallory, G. (1985). Decannulation. In E. Myers, S. Stool, & J. Johnson (Eds.), *Tracheostomy* (pp. 201–210). New York: Churchill Livingstone.

King, I. M. (1981). *A theory for nursing: Systems, concepts, process.* New York: John Wiley & Sons.

Lewis, F. M., & Zahlis, E. H. (1997). The nurse as a coach: A conceptual framework for clinical practice. *Oncology Nursing Forum, 24,* 1695–1701.

Logemann, J. A. (1986). Treatment for aspiration related dysphagia: An overview. *Dysphagia, 1,* 34–38.

Logemann, J. A. (1989). Swallowing and communication rehabilitation. *Seminars in Oncology Nursing, 5,* 205–207.

Logemann, J. A., Pauloski, B., Rademaker, A., & Colangelo, L. (1997). Speech and swallowing rehabilitation for head and neck cancer patients. *Oncology, 11,* 651–656.

Manion, J. (1990). *Change from within.* Washington, DC: American Nurses Association.

McRae-Crawford, B., & Perez, B. (1992). *Guidelines for the swallowing impaired.* Patient education pamphlet. Tampa, FL: H. Lee Moffitt Cancer Center and Research Institute.

Mochia, P. A. (1993). *Vision for nursing education.* New York: National League for Nursing,.

Myers, E., Stool, S., & Johnson, J. (1985). *Tracheotomy.* New York: Churchill Livingstone.

Ridley, M. B. (1996). Clinic practice guidelines for malignancies of the head and neck: Larynx, oropharynx, and oral cavity. *Cancer Control, 3,* 442–447.

Sievers, A. E. (1997). Nursing evaluation and care of the dysphagic patient. In R. Leonard & K. Kendall (Eds.), *Dysphagia assessment and treatment planning: A team approach.* San Diego, CA: Singular Publishing Group.

Sigler, B., & Schuring, L. (1993). *Ear, nose, and throat disorders.* St. Louis, MO: Mosby.

Sigler, B. A., & Wills, J. M. (1985). Nursing care of the patient with a tracheostomy. In E. Meyers, S. Stool, & J. Johnson (Eds.), *Tracheotomy* (pp. 211–234). New York: Churchill Livingstone.

Society of Otorhinolaryngology and Head-Neck Nursing Standards of Practice Committee. (1996). Dysphagia. In *Guidelines for otorhinolaryngology head-neck nursing practice.* New Smyrna Beach, FL: Society of Otorhinolaryngology Head and Neck Nursing.

Standards Committee SOHN. (1993). SOHN scope of practice: ORL standards of care and ORL standards of professional performance. New Smyrna Beach, FL: Society of Otorhinolaryngology and Head-Neck Nurses..

Stuart, W. (1982). Geriatric neurology for the otolaryngologist. *Otolaryngologic Clinics of North America, 15,* 345–346.

Sullivan, P. A., & Fisher, P. S. (1995). Challenges in a multidisciplinary head and neck oncology program. *Cancer Practice, 3,* 258–260.

Wood, R. P., & Northern, J. L. (1979). *Manual of otolaryngology: A symptom-oriented text.* Baltimore: Williams & Wilkins.

13

Nutrition Support of the Cancer Patient

Kathryn Allen, R.D., L.D.N., Meg Cass Kuznicki, R.N., M.S.N.,
and Jay J. Mamel, M.D.

Malnutrition occurs frequently in cancer patients. It is a significant cause of morbidity and mortality, and it can adversely affect the quality of life and interfere with cancer treatments. This chapter discusses the significant role nutritional intervention and management play in the supportive care of the cancer patient.

MALNUTRITION IN THE HOSPITALIZED PATIENT

It is estimated that 40–55% of the more than 15 million people treated in hospitals in the United States are either malnourished or at risk for malnutrition (Agradi et al., 1984; Bistrian, Blackburn, Vitale, Cochran, & Naylor, 1976; Hill et al., 1977; Messner, Stephens, Wheeler, & Hawes, 1991; Mowe & Bohmer, 1991) and up to 12% are severely malnourished (Detsky, Baker, O'Rourke, & Goel, 1987). Several researchers have demonstrated that patients with risk factors for protein-calorie malnutrition represent 30-60% of patients admitted to U.S. hospitals (Smith & Smith, 1988, 1993). Malnutrition in hospitalized patients exists independently of other medical conditions. The causes of the high prevalence of malnutri-

tion include consequences of disease or treatments, social conditions that limit ability to purchase and consume foods, and, most critical and possibly most preventable, lack of early identification of malnutrition or the absence or delay of medical nutrition intervention (Gallagher-Allred, Voss, Finn, & McCamish, 1996; Shils, 1994). In addition, malnutrition exists as a result of failure to meet nutritional requirements or as a result of decreased functional reserve combined with acute metabolic stress (Bernstein, Shaw-Stiffel, Schorow, & Brouillette, 1993). It has been reported that delayed nutritional interventions may account for the fact that as many as 75% of the patients who are well nourished on admission deteriorate during their hospital stay. This results in loss of weight and function, impaired immune response, and accelerated depletion, which ultimately lead to extended hospital stay and/or more frequent admissions.

Implications of Malnutrition

Regardless of age and diagnosis, several prospective and retrospective studies have demonstrated that, compared with well-nourished patients, malnourished patients endure longer hospital stays (Christensen,

195

1986; Reilly, Hull, Albert, Waller, & Bringardener, 1988; Robinson, Goldstein, & Levine, 1987; Weinsier, Heimburger, Samples, & Dimick, 1984), have higher costs (Christensen, 1986; Epstein, Read, & Hoefer, 1987; Reilly et al., 1988; Riffer, 1986; Robinson et al., 1987), experience slower healing (Dickhaut, DeLee, & Page, 1984; Haydock & Hill, 1986), and have more complications (Buzby, Mullen, Matthews, Hobbs, & Rosato,1980; Detsky, Smalley, & Chang, 1994; Klidjian, Archer, Foster, & Karran, 1982; Sullivan & Walls, 1994) and increased mortality rates (Reilly et al., 1988; Seltzer, Slocum, Cataldi-Betcher, Fileti, & Gerson, 1982). Specifically, it is estimated that malnourished patients have 1.5 to 3.0 times the normal length of stay for their medical condition. Researchers report incidences of likelihood of malnutrition in 59% and 48% of surgical and medical patients, respectively, who are 2.6 to 3.4 times more likely to have a predefined medical complication (Reilly et al., 1988). Protein-calorie malnutrition increases morbidity and mortality and may be associated with complications such as pneumonia, sepsis, operative site infection, delayed wound healing, or decubitus ulcers. According to two separate analyses, the total economic impact includes 35-75% higher costs per day, directly attributable to increased length of stay, complications, and use of resources for treatment (Christensen, 1986; Mears, 1994; Robinson et al., 1987). The cost of these complications and the length of stay in this population are a significant financial burden and a controllable medical liability for the health care institution (Bernstein et al., 1993).

PREVALENCE OF MALNUTRITION IN CANCER PATIENTS

It has been reported that cancer patients have the highest incidence (30–90%) of protein-calorie malnutrition (Nixon et al., 1980) seen in all hospitalized patients (Daly, Redmond, & Gallagher, 1992). Malnutrition is frequently a comorbidity in patients with esophageal cancer who present with symptoms of progressive dysphagia, anorexia,

and weight loss. According to Goodwin and Byers (1993), approximately one third of patients with advanced cancer of the head and neck are severely malnourished and another one third of these patients suffer from mild malnutrition. Consistent with these findings, Daly et al. (1992) report that significant malnutrition occurs in more than 30% of cancer patients undergoing major upper gastrointestinal procedures. Larrea and colleagues (1992) also found the highest incidence of malnutrition (78.9%) among patients with cancer of the esophagus compared to patients with other digestive and extradigestive neoplasia. Keller (1993) also reports that weight loss affects approximately two thirds of all patients with disseminated malignancy.

The impact of poor nutritional status, which commonly occurs in cancer patients, and its etiology are multidimensional. Malnutrition not only is a significant cause of morbidity and mortality but also adversely affects quality of life and may lead to delay or interruptions in cancer therapy. The degree of malnutrition in cancer patients is related to nutritional status of the patient before the development of cancer, to the tumor itself, and to the cancer therapy and its side effects. Aggressive treatment may worsen the severity of malnutrition and, without proper support and management of nutrition-related symptoms, may be a frequent cause of discontinuation of therapy and death (Robuck & Fleetwood, 1992).

BENEFITS OF NUTRITION INTERVENTION IN THE CANCER PATIENT

Proper nutrition support with early intervention and supplementation has been shown to provide for improved tolerance to therapy (Nayel, el-Ghoneimy, & el-Haddad, 1992), fewer complications, improved sense of well-being, higher response rate (Goodwin & Byers, 1993), and fewer hospitalizations (Daly & Shinkwin, 1995) in cancer patients. Perioperative nutrition support has also been found to reduce morbidity and mortality in patients undergoing surgery for malignant disease who have been identified with severe malnutrition (Heys, Park, Garlick, & Ermin, 1992; Vitello, 1994). Significant improvement in nutritional status with only 10 days of enteral hyperalimentation was observed in patients with esophageal cancer presenting with malnutrition on diagnosis (Parshad, Misra, Joshi, & Kapur, 1993).

ETIOLOGY OF MALNUTRITION IN THE CANCER PATIENT

The cause of malnutrition and nutritional deterioration in patients with cancer is multifactorial. The contributing factors and associated symptoms may be a result of the local or systemic effects of the neoplastic process (Table 13–1) or may be a result of the side effects of treatment as seen in Table 13–2. In order to properly assess the patients' needs and provide appropriate nutrition intervention, it is essential to understand the underlying causes of the derangement of nutritional status.

Localized Effects of Disease

Localized tumor effects are those that in some way physically interfere with consumption or absorption of nutrients, resulting in inadequate nutrition with or without electrolyte disturbances. Tumors that occur in the upper alimentary canal may cause dysphagia, aglutition, trismus, and odynophagia, whereas those that occur in the lower gastrointestinal tract may cause early satiety, nausea, abdominal pain, vomiting, or malabsorption. In patients with advanced metastatic disease with central nervous system involvement or primary brain tumors, food consumption and swallowing may also be impaired. Presence of disease in the medulla or pons of the brainstem may affect on the cranial nerves, which control

TABLE 13–1. Etiology of Malnutrition in Cancer Patients

Effects of Disease	Associated Symptoms
Localized	
Tumors of the upper alimentary canal	Dysphagia
	Aglutition
	Trismus
	Odynophagia
Tumors of the lower alimentary canal	Early satiety
	Nausea
	Abdominal pain
	Vomiting
	Malabsorption
Brain tumors or brain metastases	Dysphagia
	Loss of gag reflex
	Aspiration
	Hypogeusia
	Anorexia
Systemic	
Anorexia	Poor intake
	Weight loss
Cachexia	Wasting syndrome
	Poor intake
	Hypermetabolism
	Weight loss

TABLE 13–2. Treatment Effects Contributing to Malnutrition

Treatment	Associated Symptoms
Surgery	
Head and neck	Aspiration Aglutiton Dysphagia Odynophagia Hypogeusia Chyle fistula
Esophageal	Dumping syndrome Nausea Vomiting Delayed gastric emptying Early satiety Reflux Dysphagia Vitamin B12 and iron deficiencies
Small intestine	Malabsorptin Dehydration Protein-calorie malnutrition Vitamin/mineral deficiencies
Radiation therapy	
Thorax	Indigestion Esophagitis Dysphagia Early satiety
Esophageal	Dysphagia Esophagitis
Head and neck	Stomatitis Esophagitis Odynophagia Dysgeusia Hypogeusia Dysosmia Xerostomia Mucositis
Chemotherapy	Nausea Vomiting Dysgeusia Mucositis Esophagitis Anorexia Dysosmia Diarrhea Pharyngitis Constipation Learned food aversions

the act of chewing and swallowing. Impairment of the function of these nerves can also result in dysphagia due to a decrease in gag reflex, loss of sensation in the throat, loss of taste sensation, decrease in saliva production, difficulty in manipulating food in the mouth, and loss of the control of chewing and jaw movement.

Systemic Effects of Disease

Anorexia

Systemic effects of cancer, which are associated with deterioration of nutritional status, are many and vary in intensity with different disease sites and among individuals. One of the most common systemic manifestations of the disease process is anorexia (Grant & Rivera, 1995). Anorexia is defined as a loss of appetite with subsequent decrease in food intake and resultant loss of weight. Appetite is influenced by many factors including psychological and social influences; however, due to the presence of anorexia in many cases before cancer diagnosis, it has been hypothesized that primary appetite suppression occurs as a result of the secretion of substances from the tumor itself that act as anorexigenic agents. After diagnosis and during treatment, the psychological and social influences as well as toxicities of treatment compound the biological effect, making anorexia even more profound.

Cachexia

Although anorexia and weight loss may occur as separate symptoms, cancer cachexia is a syndrome characterized by loss of appetite and progressive weight loss accompanied by metabolic aberrations that may be irreversible and fatal (Mercandante, 1996; Ottery, 1994). It has been estimated that this syndrome may be present in up to 80% of cancer patients and is a significant contributor to morbidity and mortality (Albrecht & Canada, 1996). The anorexia and hypermetabolic state observed with cancer cachexia is thought by many to be due to the secretion by the tumor of cytokines that are produced from macrophages and lymphocytes (Shils, 1990). These cytokines, which include interleukin-1, interleukin-4, interleukin-6, tumor necrosis factor alpha, and interferon, can induce both appetite suppression and metabolic changes (Grant & Rivera, 1995; Keller, 1993; Laviano, Renvyle, & Yang, 1996; Shils, 1990).

These metabolic abnormalities that occur with the cachexia syndrome contribute to the rapid decline in nutritional status. They include increased metabolic rate, increased protein breakdown, increased gluconeogenesis and altered glucose metabolism, and inhibition of lipoprotein lipase (Heber & Tchekmedyian, 1992; Tayek, 1992). In contrast to simple starvation in an otherwise healthy individual in which the metabolic rate is known to decrease, in cancer patients the metabolic rate may increase in spite of decreases in energy intake. This is thought to be due to the inefficient use of energy substrate with a shift toward anaerobic glycolysis, thought to be the tumor's main energy pathway, versus normal aerobic glucose metabolism. The end product of anaerobic metabolism is lactic acid, which is also believed to contribute to anorexia (Ross, 1990). Due to an increase in gluconeogenesis and protein turnover, patients with cancer cachexia frequently show signs of protein malnutrition with muscle wasting, impaired host defense, infections, weakness, and depletion of visceral protein stores (Keller, 1993). Tumor progression is frequently observed while the host is wasting away, supporting the premise that the tumor actually competes for nutrients. Cancer cachexia is known to be a common manifestation of advanced malignant disease, progressing as the disease progresses, with a profound impact on functional status and quality of life, and increasing morbidity and mortality. The prevalence of cancer cachexia seems to depend more on the type of tumor than the size of tumor or stage of disease. For example, cachexia is more frequent in patients with carcinoma of the lung, pancreas, and stomach and less common in patients with breast cancer (Grant & Rivera, 1995; Keller, 1993).

Treatment Effects

The side effects of treatment are major contributing factors to the malnutrition and wasting syndrome commonly observed in cancer patients. It has been well established that, although nutrition support cannot be shown to directly improve survival, patients who are better nourished have improved tolerance to antineoplastic therapy. The three most common modes of therapy—surgery, radiation therapy, and chemotherapy or hormonal therapy—and their impact on swallowing and subsequent effects on nutritional status will be addressed.

Surgery

The types of cancer surgery with the most profound effect on the ability to consume adequate nutrition are tumor resections affecting the alimentary tract. Radical resection in the nasal and oropharyngeal area has obvious adverse effects on chewing and swallowing, and esophagectomy and gastrectomy may result in early satiety, gastric stasis, reflux, malabsorption, dumping syndrome, and achlorhydria. Intestinal resection may not directly interfere with food consumption; however, with major resection of the small bowel, decreased absorption of many nutrients may lead to malnutrition, loss of appetite, and decrease in performance status, which will then further impair nutrient intake. Resection of the large bowel can result in dehydration and electrolyte disturbances, which may also affect quality of life and desire to eat. Due to the significant impact on the ability to obtain adequate nourishment, the consequences of surgical treatment of head, neck, and esophageal tumors deserve special attention.

HEAD AND NECK SURGERY. Surgery is most commonly the primary mode of therapy for cancers of the head and neck. Surgery combined with radiation therapy is considered a curative modality; however, surgery-related problems can be devastating due to the physiolgial loss of function and the cosmetic deformities (Kyle, 1990).

Surgery to the head and neck area alter not only the patients' appearance but also the ability to taste, eat, drink, see, smell, and hear. Whereas a total laryngectomy eliminates the risk of aspiration due to disconnection of the trachea from the larynx, a partial or supraglottic laryngectomy, which preserves the ability to speak, increases the risk of aspiration. Both partial and total glossectomies obviously impair the oral phase of swallowing. The degree of impairment and rehabilitation depends greatly on the amount of the tongue resected. These patients often can be taught how to swallow; however, many times supplemental support with a feeding tube or a large bulb syringe is necessary until oral intake is adequate. Maxillectomy and surgery involving the mandible interfere with the patient's ability to chew and may allow regurgitation into the nasal cavity. Liquid-only and pureed diets may be tolerated with use of a prosthesis; however, many of these patients require support with tube feeding in the early postoperative period. Plastic and reconstructive surgery may minimize loss of function and deformities; however, increased needs during the postoperative period and the psychological effects of such surgery can interfere with adequate intake. Bloch (1993) provides an excellent review of nutritional management of patients with dysphagia.

CHYLE FISTULAS. Chyle fistulas or chyle leaks caused by invasion of the thoracic ducts are occasionally seen in head and neck cancer patients. These may occur as a complication of surgery or surgery combined with radiation therapy or due to progression of the tumor itself. Chyle is the result of normal synthesis of chylomicrons mixed with plasma and appears as a pale yellow liquid. Chylomicrons are formed in the intestine and contain triglycerides from dietary fat, phospholipids, cholesterol, and protein. They are formed to transport dietary glycerides via the thoracic ducts to tissues. Therefore, leakage of this chyle is a significant source of nutrient loss, containing not only calorie-dense fat but also plasma protein. Chyle fistulas are usually treated with a very low-fat diet supplemented with an elemental or semielemental formula containing medium-chain triglycerides. Medium-chain triglycerides enter the circulation without passing through the thoracic ducts, thereby decreasing lymphatic flow and providing an additional source of calories. If chyle drainage is not controlled with a fat-modified diet, it may be necessary to completely restrict oral intake and initiate total parenteral nutrition. If the fistula does not heal spontaneously after several weeks of dietary manipulation or total parenteral nutrition with nothing by mouth, surgical correction may be necessary.

ESOPHAGEAL SURGERY. Surgery is also the primary mode of therapy for localized cancer of the esophagus or gastroesophageal junction. Frequently, treatment is palliative due to the lack of obvious symptoms in the early stages and subsequent diagnosis when disease is well advanced. Common symptoms leading to diagnosis include odynophagia (painful swallowing), dysphagia (difficulty swallowing), anorexia, weight loss, gastroesophageal reflux, and choking while eating; however, 65% of the esophageal lumen must be involved before dysphagia occurs (Suarez, 1994). Protein-calorie malnutrition on initial presentation is common in this population and has been shown to increase postoperative morbidity and mortality (Goodwin & Byers, 1993). Esophagogastrectomy with gastric pull-up is used for lesions in the lower esophagus. This surgery involves tumor resection, elevation of the stomach, and reanastomosis to remaining esophagus. A change in the anatomy of the stomach from a rounded shape to a smaller reservoir from this surgery can result in dumping syndrome, nausea, vomiting, delayed gastric emptying, early satiety, reflux, dysphagia, and vitamin B12 and iron deficiencies. When insufficient esophageal tissue is available for reanastomosis, colonic or jejunal interposition may be performed. This can result in alterations in peristalsis due to the lack of normal peristaltic movements in the jejunum and dependence on gravity for the passage of food. Oral intake of nutrients may be inadequate due to the greater amount of time required for swallowing. Many of these patients will require alternative means of support with nasogastric or jejunostomy feedings, especially in the early postoperative period.

ESOPHAGEAL PROSTHESIS. As an alternative to surgery in advanced-stage esophageal cancer, an esophageal prosthesis or stent may be used as a palliative treatment for dysphagia caused by esophageal obstruction (Boyce, 1992; Nayyar, Cho, & Trotman, 1996). The esophagus is first dilated to a diameter sufficient to allow passage of food, and the tube is then placed above the gastroesophageal junction. Dietary modification consists of elimination of foods that may block the esophagus or adhere to the sides of the prosthesis (Suarez, 1994). Although this treatment is palliative and not curative, it can allow for improved food intake for 4 to 6 months after placement (Hurst, 1996). See Table 13–3 for a summary of the influences of surgery on the nutritional needs of the patient.

Radiation Therapy

Radiation therapy is also a primary treatment modality for many types of cancer and may be used as an adjunct to surgery or chemotherapy. Damaging effects of radiation on normal tissue may be acute, occurring during treatment and shortly after, or may be chronic, lasting for several weeks, months, or even years after therapy has ended. Body tissues that are most vulnerable to radiation damage are those with high turnover, rapidly dividing cells such as blood cells, hair follicles, and mucous membranes including the gastrointestinal tract (Ross, 1990). Degree of injury depends on the area irradiated, duration of treatment, and total dose of radiation (Darbinian & Coulston, 1990). The first symptoms of radiation damage from mucosal injury usually occur within 2 to 3 weeks after the start of daily therapy but may occur within the 1st week. Areas of the body with most profound adverse effects of radiation therapy on proper alimentation include the head and neck region and thorax. The adverse influences of radiation and the management of nutritional concerns are presented in Table 13–4.

THORAX. Malignancies commonly treated with irradiation of the thoracic region include esophageal cancers, lung cancers, Hodgkin's disease, and breast cancer with metastases to the internal lymph nodes. This irradiation commonly results in dys-

TABLE 13–3. Nutritional Effects of Surgery

Resected Organ	Consequences
Oral cavity	Impaired chewing and swallowing Placement of feeding tube during surgery Potential dependency on tube feedings
Esophagus	Gastric statis Decreased gastric acid production Malabsorption Fistula or stenosis necessitating long-term dependence on tube feedings
Stomach	Dumping syndrome Malabsorption Vitamin B12 deficiency
Intestine	Malabsorption; degree dependent on the extent of the resection Sodium and water imbalance with ileostomy Diarrhea Potential for abnormally high absorption of oxalates
Pancreas	Malabsorption especially fats, proteins, fat-soluble vitamins Diabetes mellitus
Liver	Transient hypoglycemia Hypoalbuminia Hyperprothrombinemia

TABLE 13–4. Nutritional Complications of Radiation

Anatomic Site	Adverse Effects During Treatment	Management
Head and neck	Anorexia	Use nutritional supplements Use nutritionally dense foods Eat with family or friends Avoid fluids at mealtime Pleasant atmosphere Serve meals attractively Small, frequent meals Assist patient in planning a well-balanced diet Administer appetite stimulants/progestational agents
	Taste alteration	Experiment with herbs and spices Experiment with high-protein and caloric foods; add fruits and sauces to desserts Increase fluid intake to 2,000–3,000 cc, unless otherwise medically contraindicated, to improve hydration of oral mucosa Use frequent oral hygiene If aversion to red meats exists, substitute high-protein foods such as cheese, casseroles, poultry, pudding, and milk shakes
	Dry mouth	Eat moist, cool, bland foods and liquids Moisten foods with gravies, broth, sauces Hard (sugar-free) candy or gum Popsicles Artificial saliva
	Stomatitis/esophagitis	Increase fluid intake to 2,000–3,000 cc unless otherwise medically contraindicated Soft, bland, cool foods Small, frequent meals Avoid acidic, spicy foods and beverages Keep lips moist Frequent mouth rinses with warm normal saline Analgesics per physician order for relief of pain Solution of 40 ml 2% viscous Xylocaine, 40 ml Benadryl (12.5 mg/5 ml), and 40 ml Maalox to relieve pain Lessen trauma to mucosa by well-aligned dentures Avoid alcohol intake
	Dysphagia	Depending on the extent, food should be soft and cooked well Sauces and gravies to moisten food Liquids high in calories and protein
	Dental caries	Pureed foods may be necessary Dental consultation Frequent fluoride treatment Good oral hygiene after each meal and at bedtime
Thorax	Esophagitis	Analgesics to relieve the discomfort Bland, soft, cool foods and liquids Foods high in protein and calories Use topical analgesic, such as Maalox, Benadryl, and Xylocaine mixture
	Indigestion	Avoid overeating Avoid spicy foods Bland diet Small, frequent meals

(continued)

TABLE 13–4. *(continued)*

Anatomic Site	Adverse Effects During Treatment	Management
Thorax *(continued)*	Fatigue	Adequate rest Rest when fatigue is experienced
Abdomen	Nausea and vomiting	Use appropriate antiemetic therapy to lessen severity of symptoms Small, frequent feedings, eaten slowly Avoid foods with strong odors Keep environment pleasant Clear liquids Carbonated beverages
	Diarrhea	Use a low-residue diet Encourage fluid intake, avoiding acidic beverages Avoid milk and milk products Encourage potassium-rich foods Avoid caffeine Antidiarrheal agents per physician's order Use skin-care measures to minimize trauma to rectal area: cleanse with mild soap; apply Desitin or Peri-cream
	Acute enteritis	Low-residue, low-fat, gluten- and milk-free liquid diet Antidiarrheal agents, steroids per physician's order
	Fistulas	Bowel rest with total parenteral nutrition Surgery

phagia due to esophagitis, with some reports of indigestion and early satiety. These side effects usually persist throughout the duration of therapy and for several weeks after completion. Whereas patients with breast cancer and those with Hodgkin's disease generally fare well throughout radiation treatments with good appetite and few side effects, those with esophageal and lung cancer are at the greatest nutritional risk.

ESOPHAGEAL CANCER. In those individuals with esophageal cancer and other mediastinal masses, dysphagia may be present before radiation therapy begins as a result of partial obstruction. Oftentimes patients have already experienced significant weight loss with inadequate intake prior to diagnosis and treatment, putting them at even greater nutritional risk. In these patients, symptoms may actually improve during treatment due to shrinkage of the tumor and alleviation of the obstruction. Concurrent high-dose radiation combined with chemotherapy has been found to provide rapid improvement of

dysphagia, with normal or near-normal long-term swallowing function (Coia, Saffen, Schultheiss, Martin, & Hanks, 1993). However, treatment effects of these combined modalities may be even more acute due to the intensity of therapy, requiring more attention to nutritional concerns.

LUNG CANCER. Nutritional status of lung cancer patients is oftentimes compromised prior to the start of treatment due to progressive weight loss, anorexia, weakness, shortness of breath, and inadequate intake. These preexisting problems combined with the dysphagia and esophagitis caused by radiation therapy present a particular challenge to the practitioner. The goal for nutrition therapy is not only for maintenance of nutritional status but also for repletion.

HEAD AND NECK CANCER. Radiation therapy is also used as primary treatment modality in early stage head and neck cancer and as an adjunct or for palliation in advanced-stage head and neck cancer. Oftentimes radiation therapy is used postoperatively or in combination with chemotherapy in head and neck cancer patients. These combined modalities present a particular challenge due to the compounded effect on nutritional risk. The most common treatment effects of radiation therapy to the head and neck region are xerostomia (dry mouth), stomatitis (inflammation of the oral cavity), esophagitis (inflammation of the esophagus), dysgeusia (taste alterations), hypogeusia (decrease in taste acuity), dysosmia (altered sense of smell), odynophagia, and ageusia (loss of taste; Darbinian & Coulston, 1990; Kyle, 1990; Ross, 1990).

Due to the sensitivity of the mouth and throat to radiation damage, esophagitis and stomatitis can occur within the 1st week of daily radiation treatments. Breakdown of the mucous membrane with ulceration can result in odynophagia, greatly impairing nutrient intake. Loss of integrity of oral mucosa due to ulceration can also increase risk of bacterial translocation and septicemia in immunocompromised patients. Alteration in taste sensation, or dysgeusia, caused by radiation-induced damage to the taste buds usually occurs during the 2nd week of therapy. These taste alterations can vary greatly among individual patients, with some experiencing a heightened sensitivity to certain types of foods and others describing a loss of sensitivity known as hypogeusia, ageusia, or "mouth blindness." A decrease in taste acuity to sweet, bitter, salty, and, to a lesser extent, sour often occurs (Darbinian & Coulston, 1990). Patients with dysgeusia commonly report aversions to meats, chocolate, and coffee due to a perception of a rancid, bitter, or metallic taste to these foods. Aversions to other high-protein foods such as eggs and dairy products also commonly occur.

Xerostomia usually begins during weeks 2 or 3 of therapy and becomes progressively more severe as treatment continues. Radiation-induced damage to the salivary glands changes not only the volume of saliva being secreted but also the consistency and pH, which further alters its protective function. Saliva changes from thin and neutral to thick and acidic. Loss of the cleansing and

protective character of saliva allows the teeth to be coated by organic material, increasing the vulnerability to bacterial damage. This can result in increased dental caries and sensitivity to temperature extremes as well as vulnerability to oral infections, which then increase oral pain. According to Ross (1990), 85% of these patients experience oropharyngeal and esophageal yeast infections, with the incidence of secondary bacterial infections approaching 100%. Xerostomia can have significant nutritional consequences due to alterations in tolerance to texture, temperature, acidity, and difficulty swallowing, with decreased salivary flow and increased salivary viscosity. A direct correlation has been found between the degree of mucositis and degree of xerostomia (Ross, 1990). Radiation therapy to the head and neck may also result in an altered sense of smell or dysosmia due to damage to the peripheral olfactory apparatus (Darbinian & Coulston, 1990). This can result in food aversions, loss of appetite, and inadequate intake due to increased sensitivity to foods with strong odors.

Chemotherapy

Treatment of malignancy with systemic antineoplastic drugs can have profound toxic effects on the gastrointestinal tract with significant negative impact on nutritional status. As with radiation therapy, the rapidly dividing cells such as those lining the gastrointestinal tract are the most vulnerable to damage from chemotherapeutic agents (Mitchell, 1996). The specific toxicities of chemotherapeutic agents and an outline of current methods of management are presented in a review article by Mitchell (1996). Common treatment effects of chemotherapy that may contribute to cachexia and malnutrition include nausea, vomiting, mucositis, esophagitis, pharyngitis, malabsorption, odynophagia, anorexia, dysosmia, diarrhea, and constipation. New advances in the development of antiemetic drugs have been very helpful in controlling nausea and vomiting; however, appetite loss, taste and smell disturbances, and dysphagia due to inflammation of mucous membranes continue to be a problem for many patients undergoing chemotherapy. Table 13–5 lists the emetic potentials of chemotherapy as they are related to the intensity and types of chemotherapeutic agents. Taste alterations and learned food aversions also commonly occur in patients undergoing chemotherapy. Some of the food most commonly reported as being avoided during chemotherapy are coffee, tea, citrus fruit, chocolate, and red meat (Holmes, 1993). Fortunately, most of these chemotherapy-related effects usually

resolve shortly after treatment has ended. Neoadjuvant therapy, which combines chemotherapy with radiation therapy, puts patients at even higher nutritional risk due to the combined effects of toxicities associated with each modality.

Immunotherapy

Severe nausea, anorexia, and flulike symptoms can result from immunotherapy with interleukin and interferon. These symp-

TABLE 13–5. Emetic Potential of Common Chemotherapeutic Agents

Potential	Agent	
Very high (> 90% incidence)	Cisplatin (>60 mg/m$_2$) Cytarabine Dacarbazine Mechlorethamine Streptozocin	
High (60–90% incidence)	Busulfan (high dose) Carmustine Carboplatin Cisplatin (<60 mg/m^2) Cyclophosphamide (>600 mg/m^2) Dactinomycin Doxorubicin (>40 mg/m^2) Ifosfamide Methotrexate (>1000 mg/m^2)	
Moderate (30–60% incidence)	Azacitidine Cyclophosphamide (<600 mg/m^2) Daunorubicin Doxorubicin (<40 mg/m^2) Idarubicin Mitomycin Mitoxantrone	
Low (10–30% incidence)	Asparaginase Bleomycin Cladrabine (<500 mg/m^2) Etoposide Floxuridine Fluorouracil Hexamethylmelamine Lomustine Melphalan Mercaptopurine	Methotrexate (<1000 mg/m^2) Paclitaxel Pentostatin Procarbazine Taxotere Teniposide Thiotepa Topotecan Vinblastine Vinorelbine
Very low (10% incidence)	Busulfan (low dose) Chlorambucil Hydroxyurea Tamoxifen 6-Thioguanine Vincristine	

toms, when they occur, are often difficult to control with antiemetic therapy and may result in significant weight loss and decline in nutritional status. It is important to maximize intake between cycles of therapy when symptoms have resolved.

NUTRITIONAL ASSESSMENT OF THE CANCER PATIENT

The prevalence of malnutrition in cancer patients and its impact on occurrence of complications and death justify the importance of early identification of risk factors, nutritional assessment, and intervention to preserve nutritional status. In order to effectively intervene in cancer patients who are at nutritional risk it is important to be able to identify those with malnutrition or likely to develop malnutrition as a result of therapy or disease.

Screening

Systematic screening and assessment of nutritional status is the first step in identification and treatment of malnutrition. Nutritional screening is defined as the process of identifying patients at nutritional risk or potential nutritional risk due to disease or medical treatment. Screening is also an effective method of prioritizing patients according to acuity or level of nutritional risk to facilitate early intervention for those with the greatest need. Screening criteria have been developed to assess for malnutrition as well as the likelihood of malnutrition (Buzby, 1990; Ottery, 1994). The patients are then classified into categories according to risk of malnutrition: high risk, moderate risk, and low risk or not compromised (Buzby, 1990). The Joint Commision on Accreditation of Healthcare Organizations (1996) now requires that all patients admitted to the hospital be screened for nutritional risk within 24 hr of admission.

Assessment

Patients who are identified as being at nutritional risk or potential risk should then be fully assessed and a nutrition care plan should be developed to provide the most appropriate intervention. Nutritional assessment involves the collection, integration, and evaluation of nutrition-related data (Nutrition Assessment of Adults, 1992). These data provide an objective basis for recommendations and for implementation of nutrition therapy if indicated. The most commonly accepted methods of assessing nutritional status include a combination of physical, biochemical, and historical data. This involves collection and evaluation of the following information: (a) anthropometric measures, (b) pertinent laboratory data, (c) diet history, (d) medical history, (e) physical exam, and (f) current treatment. Nutrient requirements can then be determined and an appropriate plan for nutrition intervention can be implemented.

Standard nutritional assessment methods, which are commonly used in hospitalized patients, are used in cancer patients as well; however, it is important to realize how cancer therapy or the disease itself can greatly affect the validity and interpretation of these parameters. The following formula is used to verify patients' weight loss or gain as a percentage of their usual body weight:

$$\% \text{ wt change} = \frac{\text{usual wt} - \text{present wt}}{\text{usual weight}} \times 100$$

Anthropometrics

Anthropometry is the measurement of the physical dimensions and composition of the body such as height, weight, body density, percent body fat, and fat free mass (Lee & Nieman, 1996). Body weight and weight history are essential components of the initial nutritonal assessment due to the significant impact of weight loss and underweight on mobidity and mortality. The patient's weight is usually obtained with an electronic or balance beam scale if the patient can stand or through use of a bed scale or chair scale if the patient is physically limited. The patient is usually weighed on admission to the hospital or as part of the routine exam in the outpatient setting. Occasionally it is difficult or impossible to obtain a patient's weight due to physical limitations from his or her medical condition, equipment attached to the patient, or lack of suitable weighing instruments. In these circumstances weight can be estimated from various other anthropometric measures such as knee height, midarm circumference, calf circumference, and subscapular skinfold thickness. Equations for using these methods to estimate body weight can be found in *Nutritional Assessment* (Lee & Nieman, 1996). Although this is not the ideal method of obtaining patient weight, it is better than having no weight at all on which to base recommendations for nutrient requirements.

Current weight is only useful as an indicator of nutritional risk or delpletion if it is evaluated in comparison to the patient's usual (premorbid) weight or ideal body weight. Weight loss must also be assessed in relation to its duration and whether it is unintentional or intended weight loss. Unintentional weight loss can be expressed as a percentage of usual body weight. Significant weight loss is defined as 1% in 1 week, 5% in 1 month, 7.5% in 3 months and 10% in 6 months, with greater than 15% weight loss indicative of severe depletion (Buzby, 1990; Nutrition Assessment of Adults, 1992). Weight of 20% or greater below ideal body weight is also indication of potential nutritional risk (Nutrition Assessment of Adults, 1992). In most cases measurement of body weight and information regarding recent weight loss are important indicators of the presence of malnutriton on initial screening and assessment; however, they have serious limitations as an outcome measure or monitoring tool. Weight of oncology patients is frequently influenced by hydration status or the presence of edema and ascites. Total weight gain or loss does not provide information regarding the composition of the weight change and does not identify protein malnutrition. For these reasons, weight and weight change must be assessed in combination with other parameters.

The most widely accepted method of estimating body composition changes is the use of standardized equipment, and procedures for measuring triceps skin fold and midarm muscle circumference. These values are then compared to a table of standard measurements based on a reference group of healthy subjects. There is still controversy regarding the validity of these measurements as part of the initial baseline assessment due to influences of inactivity and the disease process on muscle mass and due to difficulty with obtaining accurate results in the presence of edema or obesity (Frisancho, 1990). However, there is general agreement that these measurements can be useful for serial evaluation during a long course of therapy to identify large changes in body fat and lean body mass. Assessment of protein status is critical in the identification and treatment of protein-calorie malnutrition. Measurements of body composition combined with physical assessment for signs of obvious muscle wasting may help to identify significant losses in somatic protein stores; however, a more objective and sensitive measure of protein nutriture is the biochemical assessment of visceral protein stores.

Biochemical Parameters

Traditional biochemical indices of visceral protein status include serum albumin, transferrin, prealbumin, retinol binding protein, total lymphocyte count, and delayed cutaneous hypersensitivity. The appropriate laboratory tests should be selected based on their half-life or sensitivity to change, their availability within the facility, and the degree to which they are influenced by the disease process or treatment.

ALBUMIN. Serum albumin is the most commonly used and readily available biochemical parameter to assess protein status; however, it may not be a reliable indicator in the cancer population. Its relatively long half-life (14–20 days) makes it slow to respond to dietary changes, and serum concentration is influenced by hydration status. Rate of synthesis can be altered by liver involvement or renal dysfunction. Sepsis and surgery have also been shown to decrease albumin levels regardless of overall nutritional status.

TRANSFERRIN. Serum transferrin is also synthesized in the liver and therefore is influenced by liver dysfunction metastases or toxic effects of chemotherapy; however, due to its shorter half-life (8–9 days), it is more sensitive to short-term changes in nutrient intake. The limitation of using transferrin as an indicator of nutritional status in cancer patients is that serum levels will decrease in chronic infections, acute catabolic states, surgery, and renal impairment (Lee & Nieman, 1996).

PREALBUMIN. Prealbumin, also known as transthyretin and thyroxine-binding prealbumin, is also synthesized in the liver, but has a very short half-life (2–3 days), making it a much more sensitive indicator of protein status. However, as with albumin and transferrin, caution must be used when interpreting the results due to its sensitivity to other metabolic abnormalities. Prealbumin levels may be reduced with hepatic dysfunction, acute catabolic stress, sepsis, surgery, trauma, or severe enteritis or ulcers, which may result from cancer treatment or progression of disease versus inadequate intake (Lee & Nieman, 1996).

TOTAL LYMPHOCYTE COUNT AND DELAYED CUTANEOUS HYPERSENSITIVITY. Abnormalities in immune function have been associated with malnutrition. Those most frequently used in hospitalized patients are measures of total lymphocyte count and delayed cutaneous hypersensitivity reaction (Teasley-Strausburg, 1992). Although this information may be useful on initial evaluation of the newly diagnosed patient with a solid tumor, the application of these parameters during treatment is limited due to the immunosuppressive effects of steroids and many chemotherapy agents. Also, some hematologic cancers are known to cause depression of bone marrow function resulting in leukopenia.

Medical History and Physical Exam

Information regarding the patients' past diagnoses, surgeries, treatment, and physical manifestations of disease or nutrient deficit is essential to assessment of nutri-

tional status and development of a plan for nutrition therapy. Evaluation of patients' functional status and barriers to obtaining adequate nutrients are also necessary. Information to be evaluated in the review of medical history should include (a) diagnosis and stage of disease; (b) presence of complications such as infection or sepsis; (c) time since diagnosis and beginning of treatment; (d) present and past antineoplastic therapy; (e) prior surgeries (especially gastrointestinal); (f) current medications; (g) concurrent medical problems such as diabetes or inflammatory bowel disease; (h) diet order; (i) toxicities from treatment including mucositis, nausea, vomiting, diarrhea, steatorrhea, constipation, or recent unintentional weight loss; and (j) potential drug-nutrient interactions.

Social risk factors can also be identified at this time such as smoking history, alcohol or drug use, socioeconomic status, and social support system. Physical exam should include the evaluation of functional status such as the ability to chew and swallow, dental or oral problems causing odynophagia or dysphagia, signs of muscle wasting or anasarca, presence of edema, presence of skin or mouth lesion, and ability to perform instrumental activities of daily living such as cooking, shopping, and feeding self. See Appendix A for components of the physical assessment that are pertinent in the recognition of overt and potential nutritional problems.

Nutrition History

A vital component in the assessment of a patient's nutritional status is a detailed diet history and the collection of information regarding the patient's eating behavior. This is extremely important in order to identify factors that may result in diminished nutrient intake. The following information should be obtained: (a) habitual diet and any change in diet pattern, (b) frequency of meals or snacks, (c) quantity of food at meals, (d) self-imposed food restrictions, (e) ability to chew or swallow, (f) specific intolerance to texture or type of food, (g) presence of mechanical obstruction, (h) poor dentition or pain with swallowing, (i) recent or prolonged food or smell aversions, (j) taste changes, (k) early satiety, (l) nausea, (m) vomiting, (n) appetite loss, and (o) food allergies or intolerance.

Questions should be open-ended to allow for accurate recall of diet history. The patient should also be asked about cultural, religious, or ethnic differences that may affect eating habits or food choices. Information regarding level of physical activity is also important in determining nutrient requirements. After diet history is obtained, current nutrient intake should be compared to predicted requirements to determine adequacy of intake and need for intervention. Appendix B outlines relevant avenues of questioning for elaboration of the diet history.

Clinical Nutritional Assessment Using Subjective Global Assessment

A relatively new method of assessing nutritional status using a variety of historical, symptomatic and physical parameters is known as the Subjective Global Assessment (SGA; Detsky, McLaughlin, et al., 1987). This screening and assessment tool was originally developed and validated at the University of Toronto and includes the following components: weight and weight history, dietary intake compared to usual, gastrointestinal symptoms for greater than 2 weeks, performance status, metabolic demands and physical assessment of muscle, and fat and fluid status such as loss of subcutaneous fat, muscle wasting, and edema. Based on these parameters the patient is assigned an SGA rating of well nourished, moderate or suspected malnutrition, or severely malnourished. The SGA not only determines current nutritional status but also identifies patients at risk of developing malnutrition or complications of malnutrition. This tool has been validated and recognized as a cost-effective tool for nutritional screening. A modification of the SGA was recently developed for specific use in oncology patients. The modified SGA includes added nutrition- or treatment-related questions such as rate of weight loss, appetite change, dysgeusia, and dysosmia and is known as the oncology Patient-Generated Subjective Global Assessment (PG-SGA; Ottery, 1994). The adapted version of the SGA also allows the patient to complete 60% of the tool, which is why it is referred to as a "patient-generated assessment." The remaining 40% includes medical history and physical assessment by the clinician. An algorithm using the PG-SGA to provide optimal nutrition intervention has also been developed to prioritize cancer patients according to their nutritional risk (Ottery, 1994). This algorithm not only delineates appropriate intervention based on degree of malnutrition or potential for malnutrition, but also provides guidelines for appropriate reassessment based on nutritional risk and cytotoxic therapy.

Determining Nutritional Requirements

ENERGY. Basal metabolic rate (BMR) or basal energy expenditure (BEE) represents the actual measure of energy expenditure in the resting and fasting state. In healthy adults, this accounts for 65–75% of total energy expenditure. It is well accepted that many malignancies exert a metabolic effect on the host; the difficulty lies in predicting to what degree metabolic rate is affected due to the great variability in individual response as well as type of cancer and combination of therapies. Studies have measured the BEE in a variety of cancer patients. Cancer patients with pancreatic tumors, solid tumors, or liver carcinomas have been observed to be hypermetabolic (Falconer, Fearon, Plester, Ross, & Carter, 1994; Hyltander, Korner, & Lundholm, 1993; Merli et al., 1992); however, other studies have not demonstrated a similar pattern in cancers of the lung and colon, esophageal cancers, and metastatic liver cancer (Fredrix, Soeters, Rouflart, von Meyenfeldt, & Saris, 1991; Nixon et al., 1988; Thomson, Hirshberg, Haffejee, & Huizinga, 1990). Although others have demonstrated no differences in BMR between cancer patients and controls, the decrease in energy expenditure that is normally seen in starvation and weight loss in healthy men and women could not be demonstrated in weight-losing gastric or colorectal cancer patients (Fredrix et al.,

1991). The best and most accurate method of determining calorie expenditure is by measuring metabolic rate via direct or indirect calorimetry under a variety of conditions. However, this method is limited by the expense and availability of the necessary equipment and the added inconvenience in performing additional diagnostic testing on the already stressed and anxious patient. Another, simpler, method for calculating expected metabolic rate is with a formula developed by Harris and Benedict (1919). This equation, used in combination with accepted activity and stress factors, is widely used for calculating BEE in hospitalized patients. This method takes into account the patient's gender, height (H) in centimeters, weight (W) in kilograms, and age (A) in years, which are factors known to influence metabolic rate. The equation for men is BEE = 66.47 + 13.75W + 5.0H − 6.76A. The equation for women is BEE = 655.1 + 9.56W + 1.85H − 4.68A.

The accuracy of this equation has been verified in validation studies comparing actual measurements and predicted values of healthy individuals with a mean difference of only 4% (Long, 1984). Final calculations of predicted total energy expenditure are derived using the Harris-Benedict equation multiplied by an activity factor or a stress factor as seen in Table 13–6. These factors are based on data collected by Long, Schaffel, Geiger, Schiller, and Blakemore (1979) measuring the metabolic response to injury and illness.

In order to determine an estimate of energy requirements it is critical to obtain information regarding the patient's nutritional status, treatment, and any additional metabolic stresses as identified in the nutritional assessment. To determine calorie needs in the absence of surgery or infection, as is often the case with cancer patients, a factor of 1.15 × BEE can be used for weight maintenance or 1.5 × BEE for repletion and anabolism (Dempsey & Mullen, 1985). Because these calculations are an estimate and not based on actual measurement of caloric expenditure, the best indicator of adequacy is the patient's response to the nutrition regimen. Monitoring of patient progress and adjustments of calorie goals,

TABLE 13–6. Activity and Stress Factors for Calculating Total Energy Expenditure

Activity Factor	
Bedrest	1.2
Low activity	1.3
Moderate activity	1.5–1.75
Highly active	2.0
Injury Factor	
Minor surgery	1.1
Major surgery	1.2
Mild infection	1.2
Moderate infection	1.2–1.4
Sepsis	1.4–1.8
Skeletal trauma	1.2–1.4
Skeletal or head trauma (Treated with steroids)	1.6

Source: "The Energy and Protein Requirements of the Critically Ill Patient," by C. L. Long. In *Nutritional Assessment,* edited by R. A. Wright and S. B. Heymsfield, 1984, Boston: Blackwell Scientific.

as needed, are essential parts of the nutrition care plan.

PROTEIN. Injury and illness are known to produce marked losses of protein as indicated by increases in urinary nitrogen excretion (Long, 1984). Acceleration of protein turnover and derangements in protein metabolism have also been seen in cancer patients (Shike, 1996). In contrast to simple starvation where the body attempts to spare protein, the opposite is true under conditions of metabolic stress such as the cancer process itself or combined with antineoplastic therapy. The most accurate method of determining protein requirements in a hypermetabolic patient is based on urinary nitrogen loss; however, this is impractical in most settings due to the labor intensity involved in collecting 24-hr urine specimens and fecal specimens for total nitrogen output in addition to accurately calculating protein intake. The only setting in which this might be feasible is in critical care. According to the Food and Nutrition Board of the National Research Council (1989) the protein requirement for healthy adults is .8 g/kg per day. Protein requirements are typically calculated based on the patient's ideal or desirable body weight using either the Metropolitan Height-Weight Tables or by another frequently used method, which allows 100 lbs for the first 5 ft plus 5 lbs for each additional inch for females and 106 lbs for the first 5 ft plus 6 lbs for each additional inch for males (Hamwi, 1964). A desired weight range can then be created allowing for ±10% for frame size (Lee & Nieman, 1996).

The estimated protein requirement can then be determined based on the degree of protein depletion and the metabolic stress factors. For the well-nourished, mildly stressed individual the protein needs may only be .8–1.0 g/kg ideal body weight; however, with mild to moderate depletion combined with metabolic stress, 1.5–2.0 g protein/kg ideal body weight may be required to achieve positive nitrogen balance and protein repletion. Another method of estimating protein requirements is by calculating the ratio of nitrogen to nonprotein calories. It is recommended to provide 1 g nitrogen (protein in grams divided by 6.25) per 120 to 150 nonprotein calories for anabolism in the moderately to severely malnourished or stressed patient (Copeland & Ellis, 1994; Long, 1984). As with estimating calorie requirements, the best indicator of whether protein needs are being met is with monitoring and reassessment for weight gain and nitrogen retention in the malnourished patient and weight maintenance and nitrogen equilibrium in the well-nourished patient (Buzby, 1990).

NUTRITION CARE PLAN

After screening and comprehensive assessment of nutritional status and nutritional risk, appropriate intervention can be initiated. The nutrition care plan should be problem focused, identifying specific nutrition-related symptoms or educational needs. Table 13–7 addresses common nutrition symptoms associated with cancer diagnosis and therapy that may be interfering with proper alimentation and suggestions for intervention. The plan of care should also include appropriate follow-up to reassess effectiveness of intervention and modify the

plan as needed. Outcome measures or goals should be clearly defined and measurable. Expected outcome may be functional, behavioral, or clinical depending on the type of intervention (Ottery, 1994).

Low Nutritional Risk

Patients who have no nutritional symptoms and are determined to be in good nutritional status on initial assessment are given general information regarding the importance of maintenance of nutritional status. Specific education regarding how to obtain or maintain optimal nutrient intake may be provided.

Potential Nutritional Risk

Patients who have symptoms affecting their food intake but no clinical symptoms of malnutrition should receive specific education regarding recommended intervention, potential side effects of treatment, and their management. These patients who are at nutritional risk despite absence of clinical protein-calorie malnutrition will require careful monitoring and follow-up to identify need for intervention for preservation of nutritional status.

High Nutritional Risk or Malnutrition

Patients who at baseline are identified as being at high nutritional risk or diagnosed with protein-calorie malnutrition should receive specific intervention and education with a goal of repletion, preferably prior to initiation of treatment, although oftentimes this is not practical in the acute care setting. For the patient at high nutritional risk, serial assessments should be performed, including reevaluation of tolerance to oral intake, anthropometric measures, biochemical parameters, compliance to recommendations, as well as psychological and situational barriers to compliance. The patient's response to cytotoxic therapy and prognosis will also influence the nutrition care plan and intervention strategies. Ongoing communication among all members of the health care team—including the attending

TABLE 13–7. Interventions for Symptoms Associated With Cancer and/or Treatment

Symptom	Suggested Intervention
Anorexia	Encourage small, frequent meals. Encourage calorie/protein-rich meals and snacks.
	Increase caloric density of foods with added fats and sugar (National Cancer Institute,1994)
	Encourage use of liquid high-calorie/high-protein supplements (e.g., Ensure Plus, Sustacal Plus). Consider appetite stimulant such as Megace, corticosteroids, Marinol (Grant & Rivera, 1995).
Early satiety	Small, frequent calorie/protein-dense meals or supplements. Avoid drinking liquids or having broth-type soups before or with meals unless dry mouth is also a problem. Avoid carbonated beverages and high-fiber/low-calorie foods (e.g., salads); substitute with calorie-dense low-volume foods.
Dysgeusia	Identify specific food aversions or taste alterations. Provide suggestions for alternative choices with similar nutrient content, such as cheese, legumes, eggs instead of meats in case of meat aversion. Serving foods cold or at room temperature lessens the flavor intensity of most foods. Sucking on sour balls or chewing sour gum can help with increased sensitivity to sweetness, and can help to diminish metallic taste that is sometimes reported.
Hypogeusia/ageusia	Identify specific flavors that are particularly diminished so that appropriate flavor-enhancing techniques can be employed such as adding sugar, spices, or sauces. Tart foods and tart seasoning will generally enhance flavors, as will serving food warm when possible. Odor, texture, and attractive presentation can encourage taste perception, as can a pleasant atmosphere.
Trismus	Tube feeding must be administered to provide alternative means of support.
Esophageal fistula (chyle leak)	Very low-fat diet (10-20 g/day) supplemented with medium-chain triglycerides (MCT) or a semielemental formula that contains a high percentage of fat as MCT (e.g., Lipisorb, Peptamen, Vital HN). If no decrease in output is seen with modified diet, may need to withhold oral intake and administer total parenteral nutrition (TPN). If fistula does not close spontaneously, may need surgical intervention.
Dysphagia	Tolerance of consistency and texture should be determined by swallowing studies and confirmed with an evaluation by speech-language pathologist. In general thin liquids and foods that fall apart or are in small pieces should be avoided such as rice, pasta, corn or peas, dry cottage cheese, and ground or chopped meat. Also avoid foods with a fibrous or stringy consistency such as some vegetables and meats. Foods with a thick or pasty consistency such as puddings, pureed foods, casseroles, and thick liquids such as thick creamed soups are usually better tolerated. Thin liquids may also be thickened with commercial thickening agents such as Thick-it or Thicken-it. A blenderized diet consisting of all the various food groups or supplementation with a commercially prepared high calorie/high-protein formula may be necessary to meet macronutrient and micronutrient requirements (Bloch, 1993).
Dysosmia	Help patient to identify which odors are most offensive so they may be avoided. Encourage use of more cold foods or foods at room temperature, as hot or warm foods tend to be more odiferous. Encourage patient to leave the area if possible when food is being cooked to avoid strong odors given off while cooking.

(continued)

TABLE 13–7. *(continued)*

Symptom	*Suggested Intervention*
Stomatitis/ esophagitis/ odynophagia/ pharyngitis	Avoid hot, spicy, salty, or highly acidic foods. Alcohol and tobacco should be avoided.
	Avoid rough, dry or scratchy foods, which may be physically irritating. Encourage eating foods at room temperature or cold according to patient's tolerance. Icy cold foods can be soothing for some patients. Encourage use of softer, moist foods high in calorie density such as puddings, custard, mashed potatoes with gravy, scrambled eggs, milkshakes, casseroles, stews, creamy soups, cooked cereals prepared with milk. Encourage daily mouth care before and after meals and at bedtime with sterile dilute sodium bicarbonate or saline solution.
	If pain is severe, viscous lidocaine or other analgesics before meals can be very helpful.
Reflux	Encourage patient to sit up while eating and for several hours after each meal, with small, frequent meals versus fewer large meals.
	Tobacco, caffeine, alcohol, chocolate, peppermint, spearmint, and overdistention of the stomach should be avoided. Use of H2 blockers or antacid therapy may also be helpful (Fein, 1980)
Esophageal prosthesis/stent	Avoid fibrous or sticky foods such as tough fibrous meats, soft /doughy breads, pancakes, waffles, sticky noodles or rice, dried fruits, raw vegetables, or fibrous cooked vegetables.
	Encourage thorough mastication of foods to avoid large particles potentially blocking prosthesis (Division of Digestive Diseases and Nutrition, 1990).
Dental caries/ oral infections	Encourage daily mouth care and maintenance of oral hygiene. Offer foods at room temperature, avoiding temperature extremes. Avoid foods that cause dental pain (Darbinian & Coulston, 1990).
Xerostomia	Encourage daily mouth care and frequent rinsing with mild saline solution, not commercial mouthwashes. Avoid alcohol and tobacco.
	Encourage adequate liquid consumption with meals and throughout the day.
	Increase use of foods and beverages containing citric acid such as lemons, lemon juice, lemon drops, lemonade, grapefruit juice, orange juice, or orange-flavored beverages or juice bars. Use extra sauces, gravies, melted butter or margarine, oil, salad dressing, mayonnaise, broths, or cream soups to moisten foods. Sugar-free gum or candies may help to stimulate saliva flow. Soak dry foods in liquids. Consider using commercially available artificial saliva products such as Salivert, Biotene, Saligen, Mouth Kote, Glandosane.
Aspiration	In general thin liquids, sticky foods, or foods that crumble should be avoided. Commercial thickening agent such as Thick-It or Thicken-It may be used to obtain desired consistency as determined by swallowing studies and evaluation by speech-language pathologist. Patient should be sitting upright while eating or drinking and for at least 20-30 min after meals. Depending on degree and cause of aspiration as determined by speech-language pathologist, compensatory mechanisms may be employed.
Aglutition	Pureed foods may be administered with a syringe; however, supplemental tube feedings may need to be initiated until rehabilitation takes place and oral intake is adequate (Kyle, 1990).

(continued)

TABLE 13–7. *(continued)*

Symptom	Suggested Intervention
Diarrhea	Encourage increased fluid intake with the inclusion of juices and broth to replace electrolyte losses. Increasing foods containing soluble fiber such as applesauce, bananas, oat bran or use of bulk-forming supplement such as Metamucil or Citracel may help to solidify stool. Antiperistaltics such as Lomotil, Immodium, or Paregoric may also be indicated if ulceration and inflammation of the gut is not severe. Intravenous support with fluid and electrolytes may be necessary to replace losses and prevent dehydration. TPN with complete bowel rest may be necessary if diarrhea does not resolve with therapy.
Constipation	Encourage intake of high-fiber foods such as whole grain products, bran cereals, bran muffins, and a variety of fruits and vegetables. Prunes and prune juice also can have a laxative effect due to their chemical composition. At least 8 to 10 full glasses of water each day should be encouraged. Drinking hot liquids and light exercise can stimulate bowel activity. A fiber supplement in the form of a bulk-forming laxative such as Metamucil or Citracel or a store brand of psyllium is also beneficial. In severe cases that are not responsive to diet modification, a stool softener or chemical laxative may be necessary; however, overuse is not recommended due to the potential for laxative dependency.
Dumping syndrome	Postgastrectomy diet with intake of 5-6 small meals/day, avoidance of simple carbohydrate and liquids between meals rather than with meals is recommended. Encourage calorie- and protein-dense foods to compensate for limited stomach capacity.
Malabsorption	Degree and cause of malabsorption must be identified. If steatorrhea is present, fat restriction may be necessary with supplementation with semielemental formula. If malabsorption is due to pancreatic malfunction or obstruction, supplementation with pancreatic enzymes may be necessary. If due to resection or bypass of small intestine, enteral or parenteral support may be necessary depending on degree of malnutrition until remaining bowel can adapt to decreased absorptive surface. If malabsorption is due to enteritis due to chemotherapy or radiation therapy, parenteral or enteral support with an elemental or semielemental formula may be necessary until condition resolves. High-calorie, high-protein diet should be encouraged to compensate for nutrient losses unless bowel rest is indicated. Supplementation with water-soluble, water-miscible, fat-soluble vitamins and B12 injections may also be necessary if TPN is not initiated.
Delayed gastric emptying	Eating semisolid food and drinking liquids after each bite may help with facilitating passage of food and peristalsis. Staying in an upright position during meals and light activity or remaining upright after meals can also help with the use of gravity to move foods through the digestive tract. Use of medications that stimulate peristalsis and gastric emptying may be indicated.

physician, social worker, speech-language pathologist, physical therapist, dietitian, and nursing staff and the patient's family or caregiver—is essential in developing and implementing the best possible care plan for the patient. An integral part of the nutrition care plan is the establishment of short-term and long-term goals. Nutritional repletion should be the long-term goal for malnourished cancer patients who present for cancer therapy (Copeland & Ellis, 1994). Short-term behavioral or functional goals may need to be established in order to achieve this repletion.

Choosing a Method of Nutritional Support

The choice of nutritional support is dependent on the degree of function of the gastrointestinal tract, access, patient comfort and motivation, type of therapy, anticipated disease course, duration of therapy, and anticipated toxicities (Robuck & Fleetwood, 1992). The availability of caregivers, patient's performance status, and financial resources should also be considered. The preferred method of nutrition intervention, and usually the least expensive and least invasive, is a standard or modified diet plus oral supplementation (Mercandante, 1996). However, if a patient is unable to consume sufficient protein and calories for greater than 7 to 10 days, with continued decline in nutritional status (albumin < 3.4 and weight loss) due to effects of disease or treatment, alternative means of support via enteral support or total parenteral nutrition

may be indicated. Table 13–8 contains a list of criteria specific to the use of total parenteral nutrition in cancer patients.

Enteral Support

Enteral support via nasogastric tube, gastrostomy tube, or jejunostomy tube is preferred over total parenteral nutrition due to preservation of gut integrity, lower risk of infection, maintenance of immune function, and lower cost (Berg, 1992). Another indication for use of an enteral feeding tube is in the early postoperative period after major head and neck or gastrointestinal surgery when feeding will be prohibited until the surgical site is healed. Tube feeding may also be necessary for supplemental support until rehabilitation of swallowing can occur. The decision regarding which feeding tube route to use depends on the patients' condition, prognosis, anticipated duration of therapy, and comfort. A nasogastric tube is

TABLE 13–8. Criteria for Total Parenteral Nutrition

1. Inability to absorb nutrients via the gastrointestinal tract because of one or more of the following:
   A. Massive small bowel resection
   B. Radiation enteritis
   C. Intractable vomiting when adequate enteral intake is not expected for 5–7 days
   D. Severe diarrhea not expected to resolve in 5–7 days
   E. Diseases of the small intestine
   F. Bowel obstruction

2. Antineoplastic therapy
   Malnourished patients who have a reasonable chance of responding to appropriate oncologic therapy and adequate enteral intake is not expected for 7–10 days

3. Bone marrow transplant
   Patients in whom enteral intake is suboptimal and the gastrointestinal tract is not expected to function adequately within 5–7 days

4. Radiation therapy
   Malnourished patients who have a reasonable chance of responding to appropriate oncologic therapy and adequate enteral intake is not expected for 7–10 days

5. Moderate to severe pancreatitis when adequate enteral intake is not expected for 5–7 days

6. Severe malnutrition with a temporary (5–7 days) nonfunctional gastrointestinal tract

7. Severe catabolism with or without malnutrition when the gastrointestinal tract is nonfunctional for 5–7 days

8. Major surgery when adequate enteral intake is not expected to resume with 7–10 days (e.g., total pelvic exenteration)

9. Preoperative malnutrition when the gastrointestinal tract is not functional and surgery is not expected for at least 7 days

10. Enterocutaneous fistula

11. Inflammatory bowel disease when bowel rest for 2-4 weeks is indicated

the simplest and quickest route to administer feedings. If there is mechanical obstruction or surgical modification of the upper gastrointestinal tract or if it is anticipated that the tube feeding will be required long term, then a gastrostomy feeding may be preferred. The gastrostomy tube can be placed into the stomach surgically or endoscopically (Shike, 1996). Figure 13–1 demonstrates endoscopic placement of percutaneous gastrostomy. The patient with a poor gag reflex, at risk for aspiration, should have placement of the catheter in the small intestine. This may also be helpful for patients who have a normally functioning intestinal tract but are unable to consume adequate calories due to uncontrolled nausea or vomiting. A jejunostomy feeding tube is usually only placed when the patient is undergoing surgery requiring a laparotomy and it is anticipated that enteral intake will be limited for at least 7–10 days postoperatively (Sax & Souba, 1993). This allows for early postoperative feedings and preservation of gut function. Enteral feeding via gastrostomy or jejunostomy has been shown to be most effective and cost-efficient in the perioperative period (Mercer & Mungara, 1996) as well as for long-term support in patients with cancers of the head, neck, esophagus, and stomach (Shike, 1996). Table 13–9 addresses the routine nursing care for the patient receiving enteral nutrition.

Enteral Formulas

Enteral nutrition formulations for the cancer patient are essentially the same as for mildly to moderately ill patients without cancer; however, there is some evidence that formulas containing glutamine may help to restore and maintain function of the small bowel mucosa (Copeland & Ellis, 1994; Goldstein & Fuller, 1994). More than 80 different enteral formulas are available for delivery via tube feeding, with new formulations being developed on a continuous basis. A review of standard formulas and criteria for selection is presented by Bloch (1993) and Copeland and Ellis (1994). The benefit of administering total parenteral nutrition as means of support or for repletion of nutritional status remains controversial due to the lack of documentation for a favorable impact of total parenteral nutrition on response to therapy or survival (Heys et al., 1992; Shike, 1996; Shils, 1994). The decision to use total parenteral nutrition as an adjunct to therapy remains a matter of clinical judgment; however, malnourished patients who are unable to tolerate enteral feedings and show a clear response to antineoplastic treatment are usually considered candidates for parenteral support (Daly, Weintraub, et al., 1995; Shils, 1990, 1994).

Ethical Issues

The decision to use enteral tube feedings or total parenteral nutrition for patients with advanced incurable disease requires careful consideration of the goals of such support (Mercandante, 1996). It is difficult to justify expensive, aggressive, and sometimes invasive methods of nutritional support in patients who are not receiving curative antineoplastic therapy. As stated by Goldstein and Fuller (1994), "decisions regarding initiation and withdrawal of life-sustaining artificial nutrition and hydration are complex and sometimes agonizing to make" (p. 203). Conditions for which artificial feeding is refused or considered inappropriate include end-stage disease, advanced dementia, and a persistent vegetative state. The use of such support should be viewed as a palliative measure in these patients mainly to support hydration and a means of delivering necessary medications if needed. Some patients desire no support whatsoever even in the form of intravenous hydration. The decision of delivering basic support should be discussed with the family in terms of stage of cancer and prognosis, anticipated consequences of not receiving hydration or nutrition, any risks involved in administering support, and cost. In many patients the provision of enteral support via a nasogastric tube or gastrostomy tube can provide a better quality of life by restoring some degree of strength and energy and allowing patients to eat for enjoyment rather than feeling pressured to eat for repletion of nutritional status or to sustain life. Ultimately, the choice for nutritional support in the end-stage cancer patient must lie with the family and caregivers, given as much information as possible from the health care team.

PERCUTANEOUS ENDOSCOPIC GASTROSTOMY

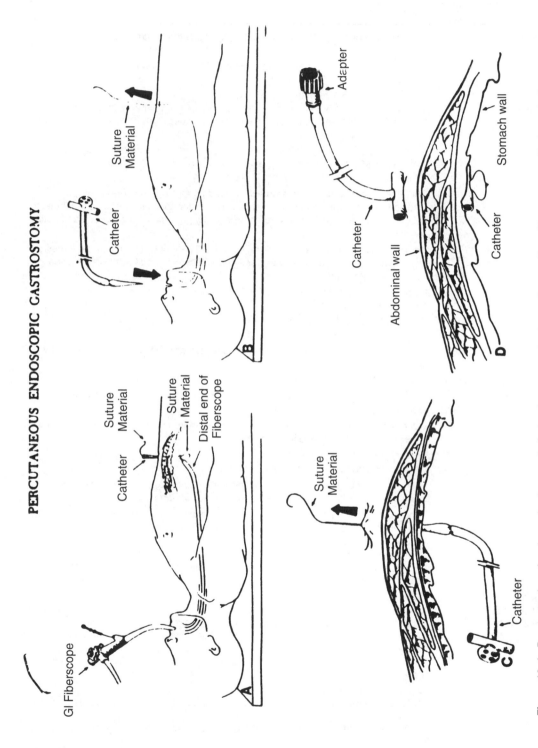

Figure 13–1. Demonstration of endoscopic placement of percutaneous gastrostomy. *Source:* From "Percutaneous Endoscopic Gastrostomy: A Review," by J. Mamel, 1987, *Nutrition in Clinical Practice, 87*, pp. 66–75. Reprinted with permission.

TABLE 13–9. Enteral Nutrition Protocol

Component	Description
Purpose	To outline the nursing care for a patient receiving enteral nutrition (tube feeding) via any feeding tube including nasogastric, gastrotomy, nasointestinal, or jejunostomy.
Supportive data	There are two methods of giving tube feeding: continuous drip or bolus. If the tip of the tube is in the intestine, it must be given by continuous drip. Below are some special instructions common to all routes.
Prevention of aspiration	Elevate head of bed 30–45 degrees during, and for 1 hr following, intermittent feedings; or at all times for continuous feedings, unless contraindicated (i.e., spinal cord injury patient).
	Keep tracheostomy cuff inflated for feeding. Do not deflate cuff for an intermittent feeding or within 1 hr afterwards. For continuous feeding, deflate cuff only as necessary to prevent tracheal complications.
	Check residuals by aspirating stomach contents prior to each intermittent gastric feeding or medication administration or every 4 hr for continuous gastric feedings. If residue greater than 100 cc or volume ordered by physician, hold feeding and notify physician.
	Do not check for residual by aspirating contents if patient has a small-bore intestinal tube. Instead, watch patient closely for signs and symptoms of retention: nausea, abdominal distention, and cramping.
	Observe all patients for volume intolerance: abdominal distention, absence of bowel sound, nausea and vomiting.
	Document and notify physician of the development of any of above findings and alter therapy as ordered.
	Discontinue feeding immediately if patient chokes or becomes cyanotic and notify physician.
Continuous feeding	Infuse continuous feeding by enteral pump to prevent runaway.
Prevention of bacterial contamination	Do not allow any feeding to exist at room temperature for longer than 4-6 hr. Give all formulas at room temperature.
	Discard any feeding after 24 hr refrigeration if prepared by food service department or if it is an opened canned formula. Date opened canned formulas.
Taping of the feeding tube	Change feeding bag and tubing every 24 hr.
	Thoroughly rinse irrigation tray and syringe or feeding bag between intermittent feedings. Label with date and time when initiated. Change every 24 hr.
	Tape nasogastric or nasointestinal tube after insertion, preferably with hypoallergenic tape to keep tube in place and to prevent accidental dislodge. Apply new tape as needed and at least every 2–3 days. Remove old tape gently and cleanse area beneath with warm water and soap before applying new tape. Hold tube securely while changing tape to prevent accidental removal.
Prevention of skin breakdown at tube entry site	Ostomies: a. Cleanse skin around site every day with saline or mild soap and water. A small gauze dressing may be applied around tube if necessary. b. Observe skin for erythema, edema, induration, excoriation, or tenderness and unusual drainage from around tube. c. Document and notify physician of development of any above findings and alter therapy as ordered.
	Nasogastric or nasointestinal tubes: a. Cleanse nares every day with warm water and then apply water-soluble lubricant if needed. b. Document and report any signs of redness, bleeding, or pressure necrosis to physician.

(continued)

TABLE 13–9. *(continued)*

Component	Description
Mouth care	Assist patients in brushing their teeth and give denture care twice a day.
Patency	Flush tube after each intermittent feeding or medication administration with 30–50 cc of cola, cranberry juice, or water with meat tenderizer dissolved in it if tube appears clogged. May try instilling pancreatic enzyme solution of one crushed viokase tablet and one sodium bicarbonate and 5 ml of tap water into tube and waiting 30 min to see if able to flush.
	Notify physician if the tube remains clogged.
Prevention of tube confusion	Always trace the origin of the tube before connecting feeding.
	Label with red tape the distal hub of the feeding tube to prevent confusion when there is an endotracheal tube with a pilot tube balloon.
Nasopharyngeal bridle care	Perform nares care every shift with NS or water, using cotton tip applicator, and then water-soluble lubricant.
	Document and report any signs of irritation to physician.
Medication administration	Flush the tube before and after the instillation of medication.
	Avoid crushed medications if possible.
	Check with pharmacist to determine if medication can be crushed. Crush well.

Alternative Nutrition Therapies

It has been estimated that in 1990, 60 million Americans used some form of alternative medicine and made more visits to alternative healers than to primary care doctors. It was also found that approximately 70% of these patients did not inform their primary physician that they were using any type of alternative therapy (Eisenberg et al., 1993). Unfortunately, cancer patients are particularly vulnerable to unproven remedies and practitioners of nutrition quackery. Those with cancers that respond poorly to conventional therapy and have a historically high mortality rate are very easily victimized by promoters of questionable and sometimes costly or dangerous methods. Cancer quackery is a multibillion-dollar industry that consists of a multitude of various therapies including herbal remedies, gadgets, metabolic therapy, purgatives, megadose vitamins, metabolic regimens, mental imagery, folk remedies, and bogus diagnostic testing. Although many of these are relatively harmless and some are inexpensive, there are numerous other risks involved. These risks include delay of conventional treatment, which may significantly affect patient survival; direct physical harm from toxicity or infection; and psychological damage caused by false hope and desperate dependence on unproven and ineffective methods. This may also rob patients of quality of life, as well as drain them of limited financial resources. Treatment that includes diet or herbal remedies can be particularly confusing in light of the recent research and publicity on the benefits of various phytochemicals in foods. Part of the popularity of herbal remedies is the general desire for a more natural cure and the misconception that "natural remedies" are more healthful or beneficial than traditional medicinals. Consumers should be reminded first of all that we have obtained some very useful but also very potent and potentially toxic drugs such as taxol, aspirin, digoxin, vincristine, and atropine from plant sources. Also, because herbs and vitamins are metabolized by the liver, as are most drugs, they can cause serious drug-drug interactions with other prescription or over-the-counter medications. Although some herbs do show promise in treatment of cancer or its symptoms, the challenge for health professionals is to determine which ones may be beneficial, which ones are useless, and which ones are potentially harmful. The next challenging task is to educate the patient about the potential risks and benefits of alternative remedies and lack of quality assurance while maintaining a positive rapport and a nonjudgmental attitude. It is important to maintain open communication with them while guiding patients toward reliable sources of information and reinforcing that they may rely on you as a resource. It is often helpful to provide a list of resources because it can be extremely time-consuming to sort through the long lists of herbs, vitamins, and other unproven treatments that patients may be considering or already using. Appendix C provides some useful resources for herbal products and Appendix D provides a recommended reading list that may help patients sort out reliable information versus quackery.

CONCLUSIONS

As discussed in this chapter, alterations in nutrition occur frequently in oncology, and nutritional support plays a role in the supportive care of cancer patients. There is little doubt that malnutrition associated with cancer has a negative prognostic effect and can contribute directly to the demise of the patient as well as increase postoperative morbidity. Nutritional therapy is an important supportive measure for the patient undergoing treatment. It increases the patient's well-being and may permit the administration of more intensive therapies.

REFERENCES

Agradi, E., Messina, V., Campanella, G., Venturini, M., Caruso, M., Moresco, A., Giacchero, A., Ferrari, N., & Ravera, E. (1984). Hospital malnutrition: Incidence and prospective evaluation of general medical patients during hospitalization. *Acta Vitaminol Enzymol, 6*, 235–242.

Albrecht, J. T., & Canada, T. W. (1996). Cachexia and anorexia in malignancy. *Hematology-Oncology Clinics of North America, 10*, 791–800.

Berg, R. D. (1992). Bacterial translocation from the gastrointestinal tract. *Journal of Medicine, 23*, 217–244.

Bernstein, L. H., Shaw-Stiffel, T. A., Schorow, M., & Brouillette, R. (1993). Financial implications of malnutrition. *Clinics in Laboratory Medicine, 13*, 491–507.

Bistrian, B. R., Blackburn, G. L., Vitale, J., Cochran, D., & Naylor, J. (1976). Prevalence of malnutrition in general medical patients. *JAMA, 235*, 1567–1570.

Bloch, A. S. (1993). Nutritional management of patients with dysphagia. *Oncology, 7* (Suppl.), 127–137.

Boyce, H. W. (1992, June). Clinical evaluation of palliative procedures. Presented at International Congress on Cancer of the Esophagus: Recent Advances in Biology, Prevention, Diagnosis and Treatment, Genoa, Italy.

Buzby, K. M. (1990). Overview: Screening, assessment and monitoring. In A. S. Bloch (Ed.), *Nutrition management of the cancer patient* (pp. 16, 18, 20). Rockville, MD: Aspen.

Buzby, G. P., Mullen, J. L., Matthews, D. C., Hobbs, C. L., & Rosato, E. F. (1980). Prognostic nutritional index in gastrointestinal surgery. *American Journal of Surgery, 139*, 160–167.

Christensen, K. S. (1986). Hospitalwide screening increases revenue under prospective payment system. *Journal of the American Dietetic Association, 86*, 1234–1235.

Coia, L. R., Soffen, E., Schultheiss, T. E., Martin, E. E., & Hanks, G. E. (1993). Swallowing function in patients with esophageal cancer treated with concurrent radiation and chemotheray. *Cancer, 71*, 281–286.

Copeland, E. M., & Ellis, L. M. (1994). Nutritional management in patients with head neck malignancis. In R. R. Million & N. J. Cassisi (Eds.), *Management of head and neck cancer: A multidisciplinary approach* (2nd ed.). Philadelphia: J. B. Lippincott.

Daly, J. M., Redmond, H. P., & Gallagher, H. (1992). Perioperative nutrition in cancer patients. *JPEN. Journal of Parenteral and Enteral Nutrition, 16*, 100S–105S.

Daly, J., & Shinkwin, M. (1995). Nutrition and the cancer patient. In G. Murphy, W. Lawrence, & R. Lenhard (Eds.), *American Cancer Society textbook of clinical oncology* (2nd ed., pp. 580–596). Atlanta, GA: American Cancer Society.

Daly, J. M., Weintraub, E. N., Shou, J., Rosato, E. E., & Lucia, M. (1995). Enteral nutrition during multimodality therapy in upper gastrointestinal cancer patients. *Annals of Surgery, 221*, 327–338.

Darbinian, J. A., & Coulston, A. M. (1990). Impact of radiation therapy on the nutrition status of the cancer patient: Acute and chronic complications. In A. S. Bloch (Ed.), *Nutrition management of the cancer patient* (pp. 181–183, 194). Rockville, MD: Aspen.

Dempsey, D. T., & Mullen, J. L. (1985). Macronutrient requirements in the malnourished cancer patient. *Cancer, 55*, 290–294.

Detsky, A. S., Baker, J. P., O'Rourke, K., & Goel, V. (1987). Perioperative parenteral nutrition: A meta-analysis. *Annals of Internal Medicine, 107*, 195–203.

Detsky, A. S., McLaughlin, J. R., Baker, J. P., et al. (1987). What is subjective global assessment of nutrition status? *JPEN. Journal of Parenteral and Enteral Nutrition, 11*, 8–13.

Detsky, A. S., Smalley, P. S., & Chang, J. (1994). Is this patient malnourished? *JAMA, 271*, 54–58.

Dickhaut, S. C., DeLee, J. C., & Page, C. P. (1984). Nutritional status: Importance in predicting wound-healing after amputation. *Journal of Bone and Joint Surgery. American Volume, 66*, 71–75.

Division of Digestive Diseases and Nutrition. (1990). *Patient information for an esophageal prosthesis.* Tampa, FL: University of South Florida College of Medicine.

Eisenberg, D. M., Kessler, R. C., Foster, C., Norlock, F. E., Calkins, D. R., & Delbanco, T. L. (1993). Unconventional medicine in the United States. *New England Journal of Medicine, 328,* 246–252.

Epstein, A. M., Read, J. L., & Hoeter, M. (1987). The relation of body weight to length of stay and charges for hospital services for patients undergoing elective surgery: A study of two procedures. *American Journal of Public Health, 77,* 993–997.

Falconer, J. S., Fearon, K. C., Plester, C. E., Ross, J. A., & Carter, D. C. (1994). Cytokines, the acute-phase response, and resting energy expenditure in cachectic patients with pancreatic cancer. *Annals of Surgery, 219,* 325–331.

Fein, J. D. (1980). Nutrition in diseases of the gastrointestinal tract. In R. S. Goodhart & M. E. Shils (Eds.), *Modern nutrition in health and disease* (p. 898). Philadelphia: Lea & Febiger.

Food and Nutrition Board of the National Research Council. (1989). *Recommended dietary allowances* (10th ed.). Washington, DC: National Academy Press.

Fredrix, E. W., Soeters, P. B., Rouflart, M. J., von Meyenfeldt, M. F., & Saris, W. H. (1991). Resting energy expenditure in patients with newly detected gastric and colorectal cancers. *American Journal of Clinical Nutrition, 53,* 1318–1322.

Frisancho, A. R. (1990). *Anthropometric standards for the assessment of growth and nutritional status.* Ann Arbor: University of Michigan Press.

Gallagher-Allred, C. R., Voss, A. C., Finn, S. C., & McCamish, M. A. (1996). Malnutrition and clinical outcomes. *Journal of the American Dietetic Association, 96,* 361–366.

Goldstein, M. K., & Fuller, J. D. (1994). Intensity of treatment in malnutrition. The ethical considerations. *Primary Care: Clinics in Office Practice, 21,* 191–206.

Goodwin, W. J., Jr., & Byers, P. M. (1993). Nutritional management of the head and neck cancer patient. *Medical Clinics of North America, 77,* 597–610.

Grant, M. M., & Rivera, L. M. (1995). Anorexia, cachexia, and dysphagia: The symptom experience. *Seminars in Oncology Nursing, 11,* 266–271.

Hamwi, G. J. (1964). Therapy: Changing dietary concepts. In T. S. Danowski (Ed.), *Diabetes mellitus: Diagnosis and treatment.* New York: American Diabetes Association.

Harris, J. A., & Benedict, F. G. (1919). Biometric studies of basal metabolism in man. Washington, DC: Carnegie Institute.

Haydock, D. A., & Hill, G. L. (1986). Impaired wound healing in surgical patients with varying degrees of malnutrition. *JPEN. Journal of Parenteral and Enteral Nutrition, 10,* 550–554.

Heber, D., & Tchekmedyian, N. S. (1992). Pathophysiology of cancer: Hormonal and metabolic abnormalities. *Oncology, 49* (Suppl. 2), 23–31.

Heymsfield, S. B., Tighe, A., & Wang, Z. M. (1994). Nutritional assessment by anthropometric and bio-chemical methods. In M. E. Shils, J. A. Olson, & M. Shike (Eds.), *Modern nutrition in health and disease* (8th ed.). Philadelphia: Lea & Febiger.

Heys, S. D., Park, K. G., Garlick, P. I., & Ermin, O. (1992). Nutrition and malignant disease: Implications for surgical practice. *British Journal of Surgery, 79,* 614–623.

Hill, G. I., Pickford, I., Young, G. A., Schorah, C. J., Blackett, R. L., Burkinshaw, L., Warren, J. V., & Morgan, D. B. (1977). Malnutrition in surgical patients: An unrecognized problem. *Lancet, 1,* 689–692.

Holmes, S. (1993). Food avoidance in patients undergoing cancer chemotherapy. *Supportive Care in Cancer, 1,* 326–330.

Hurst, J. (1996). Esophageal and gastroesophageal junction cancer. *On-Line Newsletter of the Oncology Nutrition Dietetic Practice Group, 4,* 7.

Hyltander, A., Korner, U., & Lundholm, K. G. (1993). Evaluation of mechanisms behind elevated energy in cancer patients with solid tumours. *European Journal of Clinical Investigation, 23,* 46–52.

Joint Commission of Accreditation of Healthcare Organizations. (1996). *Comprehensive accreditation manual for hospitals.* Oakbrook Terrace, IL: Author.

Keller, U. (1993, February). *Pathophysiology in cancer cachexia.* Presented at Supportive Care in Cancer, 4th International Symposium, St. Gallen, Switzerland.

Klidjian, A. M., Archer, T. J., Foster, K. J., & Karran, S. J. (1982). Detection of dangerous malnutrition. *JPEN. Journal of Parenteral and Enteral Nutrition, 6,* 119–121.

Kyle, U. G. (1990). The patient with head and neck cancer. In A. S. Bloch (Ed.), *Nutrition management of the cancer patient* (pp. 55–57). Rockville, MD: Aspen.

Larrea, I., Vega, S., Martinez, T., Torrent, J. M., Vega, B., & Nunez, B. (1992). The nutritional status and immunological situation of cancer patients. *Nutricion Hospitalaria, 7,* 178–184.

Laviano, A., Renvyle, T., & Yang, Z. J. (1996). From laboratory to bedside: New strategies in the treatment of malnutrition cancer patients. *Nutrition, 12,* 112–122.

Lee, R. D., & Nieman, D. C. (1996). *Nutritional assessment* (2nd ed., pp. 4, 303). St. Louis, MO: Mosby Year Book.

Long, C. L. (1984). Nutritional assessment of the critically ill patient. In R. A. Wright & S. B. Heymsfield (Eds.), *Nutritional assessment* (p. 168). Boston: Blackwell Scientific.

Long, C. L., Schaffel, N., Geiger, J. W., Schiller, W. R., & Blakemore, W. S. (1979). Metabolic response to injury and illness: Estimation of energy and protein needs from indirect calorimetry and nitrogen balance. *JPEN. Journal of Parenteral and Enteral Nutrition, 3,* 452–456.

Mamel, J. (1987). Percutaneous endoscopic gastrostomy: A review. *Nutrition in Clinical Practice, 87,* 66–75.

Mamel, J. (1989). Percutaneous endoscopic gastrostomy. *American Journal of Gastroenterology, 84,* 705–710.

Mears, E. (1994). Prealbumin and nutrition assessment. *Diet Currents, 21,* 1–4.

Mercandante, S. (1996). Nutrition in cancer patients. *Supportive Care in Cancer, 4,* 10–20.

Mercer, C. D., & Mungara, A. (1996). Enteral feeding in esophageal surgery. *Nutrition, 12,* 200–201.

Merli, M., Riggio, O., Servi, R., Zullo, A., DeSantis, A., Attili, A. E., & Capocaccia, L. (1992). Increased energy expenditure in cirrhotic patients with hepatocellular carcinoma. *Nutrition, 8,* 321–325.

Messner, R. L., Stephens, N., Wheeler, W. E., & Hawes, M. C. (1991). Effect of admission nutritional status on length of hospital stay. *Gastroenterology Nursing, 13,* 202–205.

Metropolitan Height and Weight Tables. (1983). *Statistical Bulletin of the Metropolitan Life Insurance Company, 64.*

Mitchell, E. P. (1996). Gastrointestinal toxicity of chemotherapeutic agents. *Seminars in Oncology, 19,* 566–579.

Mowe, M., & Bohmer, T. (1991). The prevalence of undiagnosed protein-calorie undernutrition in a population of hospitalized elderly patients. *Journal of the American Geriatrics Society, 39,* 1089–1092.

National Cancer Institute. (1994). *Eating hints for cancer patients* (NIH Publication No. 97-2079). Washington, DC: U.S. Government Printing Office.

Nayel, H., el-Ghoneimy, E., & el-Haddad, S. (1992). Impact of nutritional supplementation on treatment delay and morbidity in patients with head and neck tumors treated with irradiation. *Nutrition, 8,* 13–18.

Nayyar, S., Cho, K. D., & Trotman, B. W. (1996). Palliation of esophageal cancer with a self-expanding, silicone-covered stent and a technique for stent retrieval. *Journal of the Association for Academic Minority Physicians, 7,* 78–82.

Nixon, D. W., Heymsfield, S. B., Cohen, A., et al. (1980). Protein-calorie undernutrition in hospitalized cancer patients. *American Journal of Medicine, 68,* 683–690.

Nixon, D. W., Kutner, M., Heymsfield, S., Foltz, A. T., Carty, C., Seitz, S., Casper, K., Evans, W. K., Jeejeebhoy, K. N., Daly, J. M., et al. (1988). Resting energy expenditure in lung and colon cancer. *Metabolism: Clinical and Experimental, 37,* 1059–1064.

Nutrition Assessment of Adults. (1992). *Manual of clinical dietetics.* Chicago: American Dietetic Association.

Ottery, F. D. (1994). Cancer cachexia: Prevention, early diagnosis, and management. *Cancer Practice, 2,* 123–131.

Parshad, R., Misra, M. C., Joshi, Y. K., & Kapur, B. M. (1993). Role of entral hyperalimentation in patients of carcinoma oesophagus. *Indian Journal of Medical Research, 98,* 165–169.

Reilly, J. J., Hull, S. F., Albert, N., Waller, A., & Bringardener, S. (1988). Economic impact of malnutrition: A model system for hospitalized patients. *JPEN. Journal of Parenteral and Enteral Nutrition, 12,* 371–376.

Riffer, J. (1986). Malnourished patients feed rising costs: Study. *Hospitals, 60,* 86.

Robinson, G., Goldstein, M., & Levine, G. M. (1987). Impact of nutritional status on DRB length of stay. *JPEN. Journal of Parenteral and Enteral Nutrition, 11,* 49–51.

Robuck, J. T., & Fleetwood, J. B. (1992). Nutrition support of the patient with cancer. *Focus on Critical Care, 19,* 129–130, 132–134, 136–138.

Ross, T. R. (1990). Cancer's impact on the nutritional status of patients. In A. S. Bloch (Ed.), *Nutrition management of the cancer patient* (pp. 12, 175). Rockville, MD: Aspen.

Sax, H. C., & Souba, W. W. (1993). Enteral and parenteral feedings: Guidelines and recommendations. *Medical Clinics of North America, 77,* 863–880.

Seltzer, M. H., Slocum, B. A., Cataldi-Betcher, E. L., Fileti, C., & Gerson, N. (1982). Instant nutritional assessment: Absolute weight loss and surgical mortality. *JPEN. Journal of Parenteral and Enteral Nutrition, 6,* 218–221.

Shike, M. (1996). Nutrition therapy for the cancer patient. *Hematology/Oncology Clinics of North America, 10,* 221–234.

Shils, M. (1990). Nutrition needs of cancer patients. In A. S. Bloch (Ed.), *Nutrition management of the cancer patient* (p. 4). Rockville, MD: Aspen.

Shils, M. E. (1994). Nutrition and medical ethics: The interplay of medical decisions, patients' rights, and the judicial system. In M. E. Shils, J. A. Olson, & M. Shike (Eds.), *Modern nutrition in health and disease* (8th ed., pp. 1459–1460). Philadelphia: Lea & Febiger.

Shulkin, D. J., Kinosian, B., Glick, H., Glen-Puschett, C., Daly, J., & Eisenberg, J. M. (1993). The economic impact of infections: An analysis of hospital costs and charges in surgical patients with cancer. *Archives of Surgery, 128,* 449–452.

Smith, P. E., & Smith, A. E. (1988). *Superior nutrition care cuts hospital costs.* Tucker, GA: Nutrition Care Management Institute.

Smith, P. E., & Smith, A. E. (1993). Nutrition intervention influences the bottom line. *Health Finance Management, 47,* 34–36.

Suarez, B. (1994). Introduction to esophageal cancer. *Oncology Nutrition Dietetic Practice Group Newsletter, 2,* 4.

Sullivan, D. H., & Walls, R. C. (1994). Impact of nutritional status on morbidity in a population of geriatric rehabilitation patients. *Journal of the American Geriatrics Society, 42,* 471–477.

Tayek, J. A. (1992). A review of cancer cachexia and abnormal glucose metabolism in humans with cancer. *Journal of the American College of Nutrition, 11,* 445–456.

Thomson, S. R., Hirshberg, A., Haffejee, A. A., & Huizinga, W. K. (1990). Resting metabolic rate of esophageal carcinoma patients: A model for energy expenditure measurement in a homogenous cancer population. *JPEN. Journal of Parenteral and Enteral Nutrition, 14,* 119–121.

Vitello, J. M. (1994). Nutritional assessment and the role of preoperative parenteral nutrition in the colon cancer patient. *Seminars in Surgical Oncology, 10,* 182–194.

Weinsier, R. L., Heimberger, D. C., Samples, C. M., & Dimick, A. R. (1984). Cost containment: A contribution of aggressive nutritional support in burn patients. *American Journal of Clinical Nutrition, 39,* 673.

APPENDIX A. COMPONENTS OF THE PHYSICAL ASSESSMENT FOR MALNUTRITION

GENERAL APPEARANCE Height, weight, usual body weight, growth and development status from growth charts for infants and children, wasting obesity, edema, ascites, abnormal vital signs suggesting hypermetabolism or hypometabolism, sepsis, cardiovascular stress, dehydration, positional hypotension (orthostatic).

HEAD AND NECK Temporal wasting, change in hair color, texture distribution, sunken eyes, corneal ulceration, conjunctival suffusion or jaundice, dental and gingival disease or poorly fitting dental prosthetics, mucosal dryness, glossitis, stomatitis, cheilosis, goiter, cranial nerve palsies. Alteration in special senses (taste, smell, hearing, sight).

INTEGUMENT Thin, dry, scaling, shiny skin, pallor, or erythema. Ecchymosis or petechiae. Decubitus ulcers, poor healing of surgical wounds. Enterocutaneous fistulas. Spider angiomata, palmar erythema. Abdominal venous colateral circulation. Nail abnormalities.

MUSCULOSKELETAL Bone pain, joint swelling, peripheral edema, atrophy or wasting of muscle, strength, and range of motion.

CARDIOPULMONARY Chronic lung or heart disease characterized by dyspnea on exertion or eating, Pickwickian syndrome, abnormally distended neck veins in upright position, pulse abnormalities.

GASTROINTESTINAL Hepatosplenomegaly, ascites, scaphoid abdomen, abdominal bruits, signs of partial bowel obstruction, occult or overt gastrointestinal bleeding, chronic diarrhea, or constipation. Surgical scars from previously unmentioned surgical procedures. Succussion splash.

NEUROLOGICAL Ataxia, loss of position sense, dementia, convulsions, paralysis, motor strength fine coordination to handle eating utensils, encephalopathy.

APPENDIX B. COMPONENTS OF A DIETARY HISTORY

APPETITE	Has the individual's appetite changed lately?
	Does he or she prefer or avoid certain foods?
WEIGHT	What are the minimum, maximum, and average weights since diagnosis?
	Has weight changed recently?
	How much, over what period of time?
DIET PATTERN	Ask about the patient's typical breakfast, lunch, dinner, and snacks.
	Has the patient been asked to avoid certain foods for health or medical reasons (e.g., eggs to reduce cholesterol)?
	What are the patient's food preferences and what does he or she dislike?
EATING PATTERNS	When and where does the individual eat?
	Does the patient eat at home or in restaurant?
	Does the individual eat alone or with other people?
	Is the eating pattern regular or "when they have the time"?
	Does the patient eat snacks? What type of snacks?
	Is eating hurried or relaxed?
CHEWING AND SWALLOWING	Are chewing and swallowing impaired?
	Does the individual wear dentures?
	Do they fit well?
	Are natural teeth in good repair?
	Are gums sore?
	Does oral pain interfere with swallowing?
PHYSICAL	What activities of daily living can the individual perform?
	Does the patient exercise daily?
MEDICATION	Do any of the medications that the patient takes affect appetite or nutrient utilization?
PAST MEDICAL HISTORY	What surgeries or major illnesses occurred in the past?
	What procedures or illnesses affected the gastrointestinal tract?
SOCIOCULTURAL FACTORS	Is the individual able to afford a balanced diet?
	Who prepares meals?
	How are they prepared?
	Can food be properly stored?
	Is food often reheated?
	Where does the individual purchase food?
	How does he or she get there?
	How far away is the store?
	Do cultural habits influence the diet?
DIGESTIVE COMPLAINTS	Difficulty swallowing? Painful swallowing?
	Indigestion?
	Heartburn?
	Abdominal pain?
	Early satiety?
	Nature and frequency of bowel habits?

APPENDIX C. HELPFUL RESOURCES FOR HERBAL PRODUCTS: WEBSITES

American Botanical Council
PO Box 201660
Austin, TX 78720
512-331-8868
www.herbalgram.org/abcmission.html

Food and Drug Administration
5600 Fishers Lane
Rockville, MD 20857
800-332-0178
www.fda.gov/fdahomepage.html
Adverse reactions to herbal products should be reported to MedWatch: 200-332-1088

Herb Research Foundation
1007 Pearl Street, Suite 200
Boulder, CO 80302
303-449-2265
www.sunsite.unc.edu/herbs/

NAPALERT—Natural Products Alert Database
Program for Collaborative Research/Pharmaceutical Sciences College of Pharmacy
University of Illinois
Chicago, IL 60612
312-996-2246
www.info.cas.org/online/catalog/napralert.html

National Council Against Health Fraud (NCAHF)
P.O. Box 1276
Loma Linda, CA 92354
909-824-4690
www.primenet.com/ncahf

Office of Alternative Medicine/National Institutes of Health
9000 Rockville Pike, Mailstop 2182, Bldg 31, Room 5B-38
Bethesda, MD 20892
800-531-1794

APPENDIX D. RECOMMENDED READING LIST

Health Robbers	by Stephen Barrett, M.D. and William Jarvis, Ph.D.
Herbs of Choice	by Varro Tyler
The Honest Herbal	by Varro Tyler
Readers Guide to Alternative Health Methods	by John Zwicky, Ph.D., Arthur W. Gafner, Ph.D., Stephen Barrett, Ph.D., and William T. Jarvis, M.D.
Panic in the Pantry	by Elizabeth F.Whelan, Sc.D.M.P.H., and Frederick J. Stare, M.D., Ph.D.
The Vitamin Pushers	by Stephen Barrett, M.D., and Victor Herbert, M.D., J.D.

14

Pharmacological Considerations

Daniel E. Buffington, Pharm.D., M.B.A., Angie S. Graham, Pharm.D., and A. J. Jackson, II, Pharm.D.

Oral complications of cancer derive from numerous etiologies. Osteomyelitis, dental appliances and restorations, surgical removal of anatomic structures, and oral flora all can lead to complications. However, chemotherapeutic agents are known to worsen the effects of other causes and to damage the oral mucosa by direct and indirect mechanisms. Oral mucositis is estimated to occur in 40% of standard chemotherapy patients and 76% of bone marrow transplant patients (Berger & Kilroy, 1997). An understanding of the contributions of pharmacological agents to difficulties with swallowing and other oral functions is therefore essential; in addition, pharmacological agents are also frequently the preferred means of treatment. This chapter addresses anticancer agents and their oral toxicities, treatment agents and their benefits, and additional agents to avoid because of their deleterious effects on oral function.

ORAL COMPLICATIONS OF CANCER THERAPIES

The alkylating agents, antimetabolites, natural products, and other synthetic agents such as hydroxyurea and procarbazine hy-drochloride all cause direct stomatotoxicity. Such agents target rapidly dividing cells to interfere with cellular mitosis and halt cancer progression. Because mouth cells regenerate every 7 to 14 days, they are often injured by chemotherapy, leading to epithelial hyperplasia, collagen and glandular degeneration, and epithelial dysplasia. Symptoms are common with chemotherapy and almost inevitable with radiation therapy. Typically, the lips, inside of the cheeks, ventral surface of the tongue, soft palate, and floor of the mouth are affected (Berger & Kilroy, 1997).

Five to 7 days after treatment, the initial symptoms of stomatitis begin. Decreased mitotic activity leads to retention of superficial cells that appear white because of an increased degree of keratinization. The patient will also likely exhibit a pale, dry mucosa with dry lips. The tongue is often dry with raised papillae, the uvula is engorged and red, and the buccal mucosa along the tooth line may be scalloped or ridged. Patients typically report increased salivation and a tingling or burning sensation within the mouth. The next stage of stomatitis generally takes place between 7 to 10 days following treatment. The formerly pale, dry mucosa becomes red and wrinkled as the old cells are shed and inadequately replaced due to inhibited cellular replication. The tongue swells and develops a white coating. The practitioner may be able to visualize inflamed mucocutaneous junctions and isolated mucosal ulcers. The patient's sense of tingling or burning usually has progressed to a pain sensation with altered taste, and salivation has decreased (Holmes, 1991).

Between 10 and 14 days after therapy, the mucosa and tongue become intensely inflamed. Taste perception continues to be altered. The lips appear dry, cracked, inflamed, and swollen, and mucosal ulcerations often have run together. Pain may be sufficiently severe to require systemic analgesia. During this phase, more serious sequelae may present, such as infection or bleeding (Finley, 1991). Healing occurs 2 to 3 weeks after the drug is stopped (Berger & Kilroy, 1997). Inflammation, taste alteration, bleeding, and pain resolve. Where oral lesions are present, the practitioner may visualize granulation tissue (Finley, 1991). Recovery is seldom complete in the presence of vascular or connective tissue damage, and telangiectasis, capillary occlusion, and fibrosis may eventually ensue (Holmes, 1991). The time course of physiological response is diagrammed in Table 14–1.

Children are especially susceptible to chemotherapy- and radiotherapy-induced stomatitis. It is thought that because anticancer agents affect cells with a high mitotic index, and because children generally have a higher mucosal cell turnover rate, they experience a higher incidence of mucositis (Childers et al., 1993). The practitioner should also be aware that treatment-induced deficits in hearing and cognition may have more far-reaching effects in children by impairing their initial learning of speech and language.

Many consider methotrexate and fluorouracil the most common culprits of drug-induced mucositis (DiPiro et al., 1997). Besides its tendency to reduce the buffering capacity of saliva (Holmes, 1991), methotrexate has been shown to cause toxicity to the oral tissues when plasma concentrations exceed 5×10^{-8} for more than 42 hr. This threshold may be reached during high-dose treatment, or inadvertently in patients with renal damage, pleural effusion, or ascites. Fluorouracil is most likely to cause damage in doses of 30 mg/kg per day or more for 5 days or longer.

Prolonged courses of treatment and administration by intravenous infusion rather than boluses also increase the risk of mucositis. The adverse effects of many chemotherapeutic regimens are worsened by concomitant radiation therapy, especially radiation of the head and neck. Table 14–2 shows the anticancer drugs with the greatest potential for damage to the mouth and throat, and whether or not they are affected by radiation treatment.

Another direct toxicity is xerostomia. Damage to the salivary glands from chemotherapy or radiation creates numerous problems for the cancer patient. Swallowing and talking become painful and difficult in the absence of adequate lubrication (Holmes, 1991). Lack of wetting medium hampers the ability of the tongue's chemoreceptors to respond to stimuli. In addition, the thick, scanty, mucinous saliva that is produced tends to coat the tongue and the rest of the mouth, preventing contact between taste buds and food. Decreased appetite and weight loss rapidly ensue, and nutritional losses are aggravated by the absence of salivary enzymes to aid digestion. In the normal oral environment, saliva constantly flushes the surfaces, but this does not occur in the xerostomic patient. If the mucinous film is not mechanically removed at regular intervals, it will become a haven for bacteria. Tooth decay, gingivitis, and periodontitis are likely complications in untreated patients (Berger & Kilroy, 1997).

Finally, any chemotherapeutic agent has the potential to cause oral toxicity and complications by indirect means. Indirect toxicity frequently occurs from infection or bleeding secondary to myelosuppression or immunosuppression. A decreased platelet count exacerbates bleeding, which tends to occur at points of trauma. Also, most of the general public has some sort of underlying periodontal infection or gingivitis that can become problematic in the presence of chemotherapeutic agents. Tissue damage and bone marrow suppression offer an open

TABLE 14–1. Time Course of Stomatitis Due to Chemotherapy or Radiotherapy

Day	Signs and Symptoms
Zero	Pink, moist, intact mucosa No pain or burning No alteration in taste perception Normal salivary response
5–7	Pale, dry mucosa and lips Dry tongue with raised papillae Red, engorged uvula Scalloping or ridging of buccal mucosa along tooth line Tingling or burning sensation Increased salivation
7–10	Red, dry, wrinkled mucosa Swollen tongue with raised papillae and protective white coating Inflamed mucocutaneous junctions Mucosal ulceration presenting as isolated lesions Presentation of pain that responds to topical anesthetics Altered taste perception Decreased salivation
10–14	Intensely inflamed mucosa Intensely inflamed tongue Dry, cracked, inflamed, swollen lips Mucosal ulceration presenting as confluent lesions Presentation of pain that responds to systemic analgesia Taste alteration Infection or bleeding
14–?	Resolving inflammation of lips, tongue, and mucosa Evidence of granulation tissue at site of oral lesions Decreased pain, bleeding, and taste alteration

Source: Adapted from *Concepts in Oncology Therapeutics: A Self Instructional Course*, by R. S. Finley, 1991, Bethesda, MD: American Society of Hospital Pharmacists.

avenue for invasion by bacteria, viruses, and fungi (Finley, 1991). Reactivation of previous diseases is also a common problem. It is now recognized that patients who are seropositive for herpes simplex are good candidates for acyclovir prophylaxis when undergoing bone marrow transplantation, or in other cases of prolonged, profound myelosuppression (National Institutes of Health, 1991).

OTHER COMPLICATIONS

Anticancer drugs can affect communication through mechanisms other than stomatitis and xerostomia. Changes in hearing and cognition can also significantly affect language and speech. Cisplatin and several other agents have the potential to affect communication in ways other than direct oral toxicity.

Cisplatin can cause nerve damage in the form of ototoxicity, which can occur from both single doses (60 mg/m^2) and cumulative use (270 mg/m^2). Although 60 mg/m^2 is lower than the dose used for many solid tumors, and 270 mg/m^2 could be reached in only three or four courses of therapy, most of the hearing loss experienced with cisplatin is subclinical. A study of Finnish children treated with the "eight in one" chemotherapy protocol between 1986 and 1993 found that 17 of 30 children had normal hearing, 7 had hearing loss at high frequencies, and 6 (20%) had hearing deficits

TABLE 14–2. Anticancer Drugs That Damage the Mouth and Throat

Drug	Induces Stomatitis	Worsened by Radiation	Potential for Severe Toxicity
Bleomycin	✓		✓
Cytarabine	✓		
Dactinomycin	✓	✓	✓
Daunorubicin	✓		
Doxorubicin	✓	✓	✓
Fluorouracil	✓		✓
Hydroxyurea	✓	✓	
Methchlorethamine	✓		
Mercaptopurine	✓		
Methotrexate	✓	✓	✓
Mitomycin	✓		

Source: Adapted from *Concepts in Oncology Therapeutics: A Self Instructional Course*, by R. S. Finley, 1991, Bethesda, MD: American Society of Hospital Pharmacists.

in the speech range (Ilveskoski et al., 1996). Significant hearing loss may require alterations in the planned course of therapy. Practitioners should keep in mind that any patient at risk for negative effects on speech or language may find these effects worsened should the patient suffer hearing loss. Baseline audiograms are recommended prior to beginning treatment to document any changes (Finley, 1991).

Several drugs can cause acute encephalopathies, with mental status changes that are likely to exacerbate speech or language deficits. Intrathecal methotrexate administration results in some form of nerve tissue irritation in 50% of cases. It is even more toxic when given concomitantly with high doses of intravenous methotrexate (greater than 40 to 80 mg/m^2), with radiation treatments of more than 1,800 rads, or with cytarabine.

Fluorouracil's neurotoxicity often appears like a metastatic growth in the brain. It occurs more commonly when doses are rapidly infused or when 15 to 20 mg/kg per week or more are used. Asparaginase can also cause encephalopathy, but to a lesser extent than the other two drugs (Finley, 1991).

Other drugs can cause neurotoxicities, but these tend to cause peripheral or autonomic neurotoxicities with fewer effects on speech and language. Occasionally, neurotoxicity may take the form of a cranial neuropathy, with vocal fold paresis, facial nerve palsies, and severe jaw pain. Acute cerebellar syndromes may slur the patient's speech. These effects are of special concern for practitioners whose patients suffer from communication or swallowing disorders.

TREATMENT AND PREVENTION OF STOMATITIS

To date, there are no universal guidelines for the prevention and treatment of stomatitis in cancer patients. Common prophylaxis regimens include chlorhexidine gluconate, saline rinses, sodium bicarbonate, acyclovir, amphotericin, and ice. Treatment regimens are similarly varied and often include lidocaine or Dyclone, Maalox or Mylanta, diphenhydramine, nystatin, or sucralfate (Berger & Kilroy, 1997). Many other agents and many combinations of agents are used in clinical practice settings with the desire to deliver both preventive and palliative care. The following information is a summary of publications and research focused on both treatment and prevention of stomatitis.

Allopurinol

In animal studies, allopurinol has been shown to decrease toxicity to nonmalignant tissues during fluorouracil treatment. Studies with oral doses of allopurinol by Howell, Wung, Taetle, Hussain, and Romine (1981), Ahmann, Garewal, and Greenburg (1986), and Weiss et al. (1990) failed to find significant impact on oral mucositis from adjunctive treatment with allopurinol during fluorouracil therapy. Other researchers examined allopurinol's utility in topical form. Allopurinol mouthwash was evaluated in noncomparative trials by Clark and Slevin in 1985 with six patients, and by Tsavaris, Caragiauris, and Kosmidis in 1988 in 16 patients. These investigators observed an average reduction in mucositis of at least one grade. Later, Loprinzi et al. (1990) performed a placebo-controlled, double-blind crossover study with allopurinol mouthwash. They found a trend toward less mucositis in the placebo group, refuting earlier studies with favorable results.

More recently, a randomized, double-blind, placebo-controlled trial by Porta, Moroni, and Nastasi (1994) again obtained a positive outcome. Forty-four patients were randomized to receive either an allopurinol mouthwash or a placebo. In the 22 treated patients, stomatitis resolved in 9 and was diminished in 10. In the placebo group, stomatitis was diminished in only 3 patients, with none experiencing full resolution.

Anesthetics

Topical anesthetics such as benzocaine (Orabase, Oratect Gel) and dyclonine (Dyclone) are frequently used for stomatitis pain. Anesthetics may be used alone, but are often combined with other medications into a mouthwash or rinse. Although their use is popular, clinical studies have not established their efficacy.

Azelastine

Because of its cell membrane-stabilizing and leukocyte-suppressing actions, Osaki, Ueta, Yoneda, Hirota, and Yamamoto (1994) performed a study of azelastine's ability to prevent mucositis in oral carcinoma patients. The drug, which has been used in allergic conditions, suppresses neutrophil-reactive oxygen production through direct means and indirect mechanisms including downregulation of cytokines such as interleukin-6, tumor necrosis factor-α, and granulocyte-macrophage colony-stimulating factor. Each of 63 patients received doses of 500 mg of vitamin C, 200 IU of vitamin E, and 200 mg of glutathione daily. Thirty-seven patients were also given 2 mg of azelastine daily. In the 1st week of treatment with peplomycin, a bleomycin derivative, and 5-fluorouracil, 14 patients in the control group and 5 patients in the treatment group presented with mucosal erythema. When therapy was completed, 21 patients in the azelastine group had grade 1 or 2 mucositis, while 6 had grade 3, and 10 had grade 4 mucositis. In the control group, 2 patients persisted with grade 1 mucositis, and 3 patients persisted with grade 2, while grades 3 and 4 mucositis were induced in 6 and 15 patients, respectively. The researchers concluded that azelastine was useful for mucositis prophylaxis.

Benzydamine

Benzydamine is a nonsteroidal anti-inflammatory drug that is structurally unrelated to corticosteroids and other nonsteroidal anti-inflammatory drugs. It has analgesic, anesthetic, and antimicrobial properties in addition to its anti-inflammatory effects. The drug's actions are thought to derive from alterations in prostaglandin and thromboxane biosynthesis, which can be achieved with topical application. Benzydamine has been shown to stabilize cell membranes, and to inhibit polymorphonuclear leukocyte degranulation and platelet aggregation. Early trials showed faster pain resolution than placebo in pharyngitis, tonsillitis, and aphthous stomatitis patients, with significant topical anesthetic effect. No effects on muscular function in speech, mastication, or gag reflex were observed (Epstein, Stevenson-Moore, Jackson, Mohamed, & Spinelli, 1989).

In 1985, Sonis, Clairmont, Lockhart, and Connolly reported on a small open trial with benzydamine rinse for chemotherapy-induced mucositis. Their study found significant palliation of symptoms in seven out of nine of their patients. Kim, Chu, Lakshmi, and Houde (1986) carried out a double-blind therapeutic clinical study of benzydamine in radiation patients that found significantly reduced mouth and throat pain, and less severe mucositis. Epstein and Stevenson-Moore (1986) conducted a placebo-controlled trial of benzydamine rinse in 1986 with 29 patients. Although pain ratings steadily increased for both the placebo and the treatment groups, the treatment group's pain ratings and use of additional analgesics were lower overall.

A 1987 crossover study by Lever with four patients also presented favorable results, but with some reservations (Lever, Dupuis, & Chan, 1987). Although three of the four patients obtained pain relief from benzydamine that was equal to that of lidocaine, oral stinging was a significant problem throughout the study. Three of their original nine patients dropped out of the study due to severe oral stinging from the benzydamine rinse, and three of the final four patients elected to use the lidocaine rinse rather than the benzydamine rinse on completion of the study. Oral stinging is likely due to the content of the commercial product, which is 10% ethanol.

Epstein and Stevenson-Moore conducted a second study in 1989 with 43 patients undergoing radiation therapy (Epstein et al., 1989). Benzydamine was used as a prophylactic rinse beginning when radiation was initiated. This study demonstrated a statistically significant reduction in mucosal ulceration and inflammation.

β-Carotene

The known effects of this vitamin A precursor on cellular differentiation promoted interest in β-carotene use for adjunctive treatment in cancer patients, and in 1992 Garewal and Meyskens reported that it produced regression of oral leukoplakia lesions. With these results and the knowledge that the compound had been deemed safe by the World Health Organization in 1974, Mills (1988) initiated a study of β-carotene dietary supplementation. Ten patients receiving identical oral cancer treatment were administered 250 mg/day for the first 3 weeks and 75 mg/day for the last 5 weeks. A second group of 10 patients with identical cancer treatment served as the control. The rates of grade 1 and 2 mucositis were similar between the two groups; however, a statistically significant decrease in grade 3 and 4 mucositis was observed in the β-carotene group. Although additional study is needed to clarify the precise role of β-carotene in mucositis prevention, the results of these early studies are promising.

Capsaicin

Berger and colleagues (1995) tested a novel approach to treating the pain associated with oral mucositis. Capsaicin, the active ingredient in chili peppers, was compounded into a taffy candy and administered to 11 patients. Most subjects required 4 to 6 candies over 2 to 4 days, with all 11 reporting pain relief with continued use.

Chamomile

Asta Pharma AG in Germany produces Kamillosan Liquidum, a preparation of chamomile flowers reported to have anti-inflammatory, spasmolytic, antibacterial, and antipeptic effects. In a study of its effects on stomatitis, subjects were instructed to use 10 to 15 drops of the Kamillosan Liquidum in approximately 100 ml of warm water and irrigate the mouth at least three times a day. A total of 98 patients participated in the study, using the rinse either as prophylaxis or treatment of mucositis. The researchers concluded that the study drug was beneficial in treatment and prevention of mucositis, but their research was uncontrolled and incorporated patients with varying cancer types and treatments (Carl & Emrich, 1991).

A 1996 study of 164 patients compared the use of a chamomile mouthwash three times daily for 14 days with use of a placebo mouthwash. All patients were receiving 5-fluorouracil, and entered the study at the time of their first cycle of treatment. Statistical analysis showed no difference in stomatitis between the active drug and placebo groups (Fidler et al., 1996).

Chlorhexidine

Because oral floras are thought to contribute to stomatitis from chemotherapy and radiation treatment, many practitioners have recommended chlorhexidine oral rinses for their patients at risk for stomatitis. A 1974 study in seven children found that chlorhexidine resolved their oral candidiasis (Langslet, Olsen, Lie, & Lokken, 1974), but the next study, Sharon's 1977 trial in 18 leukemia patients, could not confirm the drug's ability to decrease *Candida* colonization (Sharon, Berdicevsky, Ben-Aryeh, & Gutman, 1977). Neither study reported whether reduced *Candida* colonization led to fewer incidences of stomatitis. The most promising investigation was carried out by Ferretti et al. (1987), which showed decreased *Candida* colonization and decreased mucositis. More trials followed, with mixed results. McGaw and Belch's study of eight patients found that chlorhexidine was useful in prophylaxis of mucositis (McGaw & Belch, 1985), but a larger study by Weisdorf et al. could not support their results (Weisdorf et al., 1989).

Weisdorf et al.'s 1989 study of chlorhexidine in 100 bone marrow transplant patients showed trends toward reduced candidiasis and plaque in patients on active drug. However, their randomized, double-blind, placebo-controlled trial found no significant differences in oral mucositis, oral pain, facilitation of oral nutrition, length of hospital stay, or rates of oral infection between patients on chlorhexidine versus placebo. A 1994 trial concurred with their results when it reported that the 27 radiation patients treated with chlorhexidine mouthwash experienced more mucositis than the 27 using placebo. The active drug group also suffered from mouthwash-induced discomfort, taste alteration, and teeth staining (Foote et al., 1994).

In 1989, Spijkervet et al. performed a randomized, double-blind, placebo-controlled study of the effectiveness of chlorhexidine in reducing mucositis. A total of 30 patients enrolled in the study, with 15 rinsing four times daily with 0.1% chlorhexidine and 15 rinsing four times daily with placebo. The patients' oral flora was cultured before and after radiation therapy to assess whether oral flora was suppressed. The study showed that mucositis occurred with similar incidence and severity in both groups. Furthermore, *Candida, Streptococcus faecalis, Staphylococci, Enterobacteriaceae, Pseudomonadaceae,* and *Acinetobacter* species were not suppressed by treatment. Only *Viridans streptococci* was reduced, and this effect occurred only after 5 weeks of treatment. The researchers concluded that chlorhexidine rinses did not accomplish the desired effect of reducing colonization and decreasing mucositis.

Additional studies by Wahlin in 1989, Samaranayake et al. in 1988, and Epstein, Vickers, Spinelli, and Reece in 1992 found no significant effect from chlorhexidine on either Candida colonization or the incidence or severity of mucositis, although Rutkauskas and Davis (1993) published a preliminary report of their randomized, placebo-controlled trial indicating that mucositis incidence and severity were decreased in bone marrow transplant patients receiving chlorhexidine. More recently, Dodd and colleagues (1996) confirmed that chlorhexidine mouth rinses were no more effective than sterile water mouth rinses in a study of 222 patients in 23 outpatient clinics and office practices in California. In the interest of costs, the researchers recommended water mouth rinses as a component of systematic oral hygiene teaching. The equivocal nature of the data on chlorhexidine's effects, and Spijkervet's observation that the drug may increase mucositis or present its own toxicity, suggest that other agents may be more reliable and therefore of greater use in practice.

Diphenhydramine

Diphenhydramine is classified as an "antihistamine" agent. It does not prevent the release of histamine, but rather competes with the circulating histamine for the H_1-receptor binding sites. This agent will competitively block the H_1-receptor sites and result in the reduction or prevention of edema and itching commonly observed in traumatized tissue. Topical administration of diphenydramine can also produce a mild anesthetic effect, possibly due to decreased permeability of nerve cell membranes, which may prevent or slow localized nerve impulses. Following repeated or prolonged administration, it is possible for patients to develop tolerance; however, the possible benefits of concomitant adminstration with other local-acting agents may support its continued use or application.

Glutamine

Animal studies pointed to beneficial effects on morbidity and mortality from chemotherapy due to glutamine administration. A randomized trial of 28 patients receiving 5-fluorouracil and folinic acid studied the effect of 16 g of glutamine daily for 8 days versus placebo. No significant differences were observed between the two groups. The authors postulated that the dose and duration of glutamine were insufficient to elicit the desired effect (Jebb et al., 1994). Another study of glutamine supplementation to total parenteral nutrition found no beneficial effects on mucositis scores (van Zaanen, van-der-Lelie, Timmer, Furst, & Sauerwein, 1994).

Skubitz and Anderson's 1996 trial included 14 patients who had experienced stomatitis after a course of chemotherapy. Patients were given 4 g of L-glutamine suspension to swish and swallow twice a day. The researchers observed decreases in the maximum grade of mucositis in 12 subjects. In addition, the total number of days of mucositis was decreased in 13 of the 14 subjects. The results of Skubitz and Anderson's study indicate that glutamine may indeed be beneficial in topical form.

Granulocyte Colony-Stimulating Factor

Granulocyte colony-stimulating factor (G-CSF) is an endogenous glycoprotein that promotes proliferation and differentiation of neutrophil precursors and enhances the effector function of mature neutrophils. The recombinant human product, r-metHuG-CSF, has been tested as an adjunct to chemotherapy in the hope that it would protect patients from neutropenia-related sequelae and allow for increased cytotoxic doses (Pettengell et al., 1992). Trials with G-CSF for prevention of neutropenia have also indicated that it may affect mucositis.

Gabrilove and colleagues (1988) tested the effects of G-CSF on absolute neutrophil count during chemotherapy, using 27 patients with transitional-cell carcinoma of the urothelium. Patients who were eligible for the trial but chose not to participate served as the control group. The open-label trial found not only an increased absolute neutrophil count, but also a significant decrease in the incidence and severity of mucositis. Only 11% of the treated patients experienced mucositis, in contrast to 44% of the patients in the nontreated group.

Another trial attempting to increase the intensity of doxorubicin treatment through the use of G-CSF also demonstrated decreased severity of mucositis, although all patients did experience mucositis (Bronchud et al., 1989). Lieschke et al.'s 1992 investigation of oral neutrophil levels in patients receiving G-CSF following autologous marrow transplantation revealed a reduced mean daily mucositis score and mean cumulative mucositis score compared to patients not receiving G-CSF. Finally, a pilot study by Kannan et al. (1997) using subcutaneous G-CSF during irradiation to the head and neck showed minimal to no mucositis, pain, and functional impairment. The authors concluded that G-CSF offered mucosal protection.

Other investigations have failed to detect beneficial effects on mucositis. In a study of G-CSF treatment following allogeneic bone marrow transplant, no differences were seen in the severity of mucositis from pretransplant chemotherapy and posttransplant methotrexate, although recovery of total white cells, neutrophils, monocytes, and lymphocytes was more rapid in comparison to the historical control group (Atkinson et al., 1991). A second study seeking to prevent neutropenia in patients with non-Hodgkin's lymphoma through the use of G-CSF observed equivalent incidences of grade 3 and 4 mucositis between the active and placebo groups, although mucositis-related treatment delays were less frequent in those on active drug (Pettengell et al., 1992).

Hydrocortisone

The acute application of hydrocortisone, a corticosteroid, is beneficial in reducing the degree of swelling and inflammatory response often observed on mucosal surfaces. The direct tissue protective benefit is thought to be due to enzyme regulation and control in areas of localized tissue damage. The primary effect of hydrocortisone is blocking a patient's ability to develop a complete inflammatory response.

Hydrogen Peroxide

In 1996, Feber performed a comparison trial of hydrogen peroxide and 0.9% saline as oral rinses in patients undergoing radical radiation therapy treatment. On average, the group receiving the saline rinse had better outcomes. The author suggested that it might be frequent mechanical cleansing of the mouth that is most helpful to patients' oral health, rather than the use of antiseptics.

Indomethacin

A 1986 study by Pillsbury, Webster, and Rosenman tested whether the prostaglandin inhibitor indomethacin would decrease the incidence of mucositis in patients with advanced head and neck cancer. Their idea came from previous works indicating positive results on gastroenteric distress from nonsteroidal anti-inflammatory drugs, identifying prostaglandins in tumors, and demonstrating the ability of prostaglandin inhibitors to reduce tumor bulk. Their randomized, double-blind, placebo-controlled trial of 20 patients found that mucositis onset was delayed and severity reduced with daily dosing of 100 mg of the drug.

Misoprostol

Misoprostol is a racemic prostaglandin E1 analogue that has been used for its protective effects on the gastric and intestinal mucosa when given before ulcerogenic compounds such as nonsteroidal anti-inflammatory drugs or ethanol. Based on this property, a study of misoprostol prophylaxis for high-dose chemotherapy-induced mucositis was undertaken. This randomized, double-blind, placebo-controlled trial enrolled nine patients in the misoprostol group and seven in the placebo group. The study was ended prematurely because an interim analysis showed significantly higher rates of mucositis in the active treatment group (Duenas-Gonzalez et al., 1996).

Nystatin

In 1977, Williams, Whitehouse, Lister, and Wrigley conducted a trial of 56 patients with acute leukemia to ascertain the effectiveness of topical nystatin suspension in preventing oral candidiasis. The study found no difference in the incidence of fungal infection between patients using nystatin suspension and patients using a placebo rinse. Degregorio, Lee, and Ries (1982) found nystatin suspension ineffective in preventing oropharyngeal candidiasis and disseminated candidiasis. The investigators concluded that nystatin should be reserved for those patients with active infection.

A later study evaluated nystatin's utility in preventing and treating *Candida* in patients with acute leukemia or lymphoma undergoing prolonged periods of intensive chemotherapy. Barrett (1984) found that nystatin eliminated *Candida* in only 1 out of 11 of their patients; its prophylactic use was also deemed of questionable value. Although clinical research with nystatin suspension has been disappointing, it is still frequently employed for *Candida* prophylaxis.

Pentoxifylline

Pentoxifylline is a xanthine-derivative hemorheologic agent that improves erythrocyte flexibility, lowers blood viscosity, and increases tissue oxygen levels (Futran, Trotti, & Gwede, 1997). In 1991, Bianco et al. reported the results of a study of pentoxifylline's impact on bone marrow transplant-related toxicity. Thirty transplant patients were given 1,200, 1,600, or 2,000 mg/day from 10 days prior to transplant to 100 days posttransplant. Their need for intravenous morphine to control oral pain was compared to that of 20 historical control patients. The treatment group required an average of 3.7 ± 1.1 days of morphine compared with 18.7 ± 1.1 in the control group. A dose-response relationship was evidenced in this trial, with patients receiving up to 1,200 mg/day of pentoxifylline requiring more intravenous morphine than patients receiving more.

In 1997, Futran et al. continued the study of pentoxifylline, using 26 patients with late radiation complications. The authors observed accelerated healing of soft tissue necrosis and fibrosis, and resolution of mucosal pain. Although information is limited on pentoxifylline's usefulness in mucositis, initial results are favorable.

Propantheline

Propantheline (Pro-Banthine) is a synthetic antimuscarinic agent. It was originally approved by the Food and Drug Administration in 1953. Propantheline competes with acetylcholine and other cholinergic agents. The degree of muscarinic receptor response may vary. The most sensitive receptors include the sweat, bronchial, and salivary glands. The clinical effects of prolonged use of propantheline include decreased sweating, decreased gastrointestinal motility, and decreased salivation (xerostomia).

Prostaglandin E_2

Dinoprostone, or prostaglandin E_2, has previously been used with success to treat gastric ulcers and leg ulcers. Although several have been suggested, the exact mechanism of action has not been determined. Early pilot studies suggested that dinoprostone's cytoprotective actions might benefit patients suffering from chemotherapy-induced mucositis (Berger & Kilroy, 1997). Kuhrer, Kuzmits, Linkesch, and Ludwig (1986) developed a pilot study of the use of topical prostaglandin E_2 in chemotherapy-induced mucosal lesions. Five patients with oral lesions were instructed to chew 0.25 mg of dinoprostone three times a day, and one patient with vaginal lesions applied a solution of 1 mg of dinoprostone in 5 ml of hydroxyethylcellulose. Four of the six patients experienced pain relief within 6 hr of treatment. The researchers also gave prophylactic topical dinoprostone to three patients; in two of these patients mucositis was successfully prevented.

In 1988, Porteder et al. reported the results of their trial of dinoprostone's effects on pain and inflammation in patients with mucositis. Participants used one 0.5-mg dinoprostone tablet four times each day. Ten patients were in the treatment group and 14 patients in the control group. Those patients receiving the drug presented with less severe stomatitis than the control group patients and reported substantially less pain. The investigators also assayed patient plasma for prostaglandin E_2's final metabolite, bicyclo-prostoglandinE_2, to learn whether systemic absorption occurred after local application. Despite the relatively large quantities of the drug used topically, no systemic absorption was evidenced. Yet another pilot study found that only 5 of 15 patients treated with 0.5 mg of dinoprostone four times a day developed an inflammatory reaction, with none of the patients developing any bullous or desquamating inflammatory lesions. The investigators assayed for the final metabolite, and their results supported those of the previous study, with no significant increase in the metabolite detected (Matejka et al., 1990).

Although the pilot studies were favorable, a more recent double-blind, placebo-controlled study of 60 bone marrow transplant patients yielded less favorable results. Labar et al. (1993) found no significant differences in the incidence, severity, or duration of mucositis between patients treated with dinoprostone and patients given placebo. The only difference uncovered in the study was an increased incidence of herpes simplex infection in patients from the prostaglandin E_2 arm of the study.

Silver Nitrate

Silver nitrate is a caustic agent that in animal studies has been shown to stimulate cell division. In 1992, Maciejewski et al. pretreated 16 head and neck cancer patients with 2% silver nitrate prior to irradiation. One side of the oral mucosa was painted with the solution three times daily for 5 days before radiation and for the first 2 days of treatment, and the other side was left unpainted to serve as a control. Mucositis severity and duration were decreased on the treated side.

A 1995 study by Dorr, Jacubek, and Kummermehr studied the effect of local conditioning of the oral mucosa with silver nitrate in 11 healthy volunteers. Silver nitrate (3%) was applied three times a day for 3 days, and then biopsies were taken and compared with those of 13 untreated volunteers. The epithelial labeling index was increased by 44%, which implies that stomatitis might be decreased by increasing the overall cell density of the oral mucosa prior to treatment.

Sodium Alginate

Previous use of sodium alginate for mucositis of the stomach and esophagus was sufficiently encouraging to prompt a study by Oshitani et al. (1990) of its benefits in oral mucositis. Sodium alginate is obtained from marine algae and used as a thickening agent in pharmaceuticals and food products. In Oshitani's placebo-controlled, randomized trial of 39 patients, those in the active treatment arm reported reduced erosions and pain.

Sucralfate

Sucralfate is a basic aluminum salt of sulfated sucrose that has been used to speed the healing of duodenal ulcers. The drug creates a protective barrier by binding to proteins at the ulcer site. Animal studies have demonstrated rapid reepithelialization of gastric mucosa following sucralfate use, and increased local production of prostaglandin E_2 (Verdi, 1993).

In 1984 and 1985, correspondence from Ferraro and Mattern relayed positive experiences with sucralfate in the treatment of chemotherapy-induced stomatitis. A pilot study with 18 patients using sucralfate suspension six times daily found that most patients reported subjective relief from pain. Of the 18, 5 could not be evaluated, 2 died before the study was completed, 2 had no clinical response, and 10 had definite responses. The results of this study prompted more in-depth research (Solomon, 1986).

Shenep et al. (1988) launched a double-blind sucralfate suspension trial in 48 children and adolescents. The subjects were randomized to receive either sucralfate or placebo every 6 hr for the first 10 weeks of intensive remission-induction chemotherapy. The study showed that patients receiving sucralfate were less likely than others to acquire colonization with potentially pathogenic organisms, and were more likely to report that they had no oral pain. However, these findings were not statistically significant, and they found no significant differences in subjective reporting of discomfort, objective scoring of mucositis severity, or maximal percent of body weight lost during therapy.

Pfeiffer's 1990 study of sucralfate suspension yielded differing results (Pfeiffer, Madsen, Hansen, & May, 199). Forty patients entered the randomized, double-blind crossover study, providing 23 evaluable subjects by the study's end. A significant reduction in objective scoring of edema, erythema, erosion, and ulceration was observed in the active treatment group. Ten patients were unable to complete the trial, because swishing either the active or the placebo suspension worsened chemotherapy-induced nausea. To overcome problems with nausea, it was suggested that the suspension have a neutral taste and that patients be instructed not to swallow after swishing. In conjunction with the trial, the researchers performed an experiment to determine the extent to which sucralfate binds to the oral mucosal lining. After swishing with 1 g of radiolabelled sucralfate, 50–100 mg were bound to the mucosa. Twenty to 30% of the original amount was still present 2½ hr after swishing.

Sucralfate suspension has been compared to diphenhydramine syrup with kaolin-pectin in a double-blind, prospective study with radiation therapy patients. Patients were instructed in oral hygiene, and told to cleanse the mouth with a baking soda and salt solution after meals and at bedtime, and to then hold 15 ml of study solution in the mouth for 3 min. Twelve patients completed the study, with six in each treatment group. No statistically significant differences were detected in the degree of mucositis, perception of pain, or perception of the mouth rinse's helpfulness. The sucralfate suspension group reported less pain overall and longer duration of pain relief from medication than the group using diphenhydramine syrup and kaolin-pectin (Barker, Loftus, Cuddy, & Barker, 1991).

Sucralfate has also been combined with fluconazole for both prevention and treatment of chemotherapy- and radiation-induced mucositis. Allison, Vongtama, Vaughan, and Shin (1995) found that the combination was effective at both treating and preventing mucositis pain and discomfort. When the combination was given prophylactically, all 20 of the patients in that arm of the study were able to achieve their prescribed radiation doses without treatment interruptions, and be maintained on a regular diet.

Epstein and Wong (1994) evaluated sucralfate suspension in high-dose radiation therapy with a double-blind, placebo-controlled, randomized, prospective trial that included 33 patients. Sixteen patients were in the active treatment arm. Although patients using sucralfate reported less pain early in treatment and required fewer analgesics later in therapy, no statistically significant reduction in mucositis was observed. Similar results were observed by Makkonen, Bostrom, and Vilja in 1994. Salivary lactoferrin and albumin, suggested markers for the degree of mucositis, were decreased, but there were no actual differences observed between the 20 subjects in the sucralfate group and the 20 subjects in the placebo group.

In contrast, Franzen, Henriksson, Littbrand, and Zackrisson (1995) obtained favorable results in their double-blind, placebo-controlled, randomized trial of 50 radiation therapy patients. They observed a lower proportion of patients with severe mucositis in the treatment group than in the placebo group. Later studies failed to confirm their results.

Meredith et al. (1997) compared sucralfate in a base consisting of antacid, diphenhydramine, and viscous lidocaine to the base alone. Their double-blind study extended over 2 years and enrolled 111 patients undergoing radiation to the head, neck, or chest sites that included the esophagus. Data were examined for treatment effects on degree of soreness, dietary changes, and objective measures of irritation or infection. Although a trend was detected toward less severe mucositis in the sucralfate group, this trend was not statistically significant. Overall, multivariate analysis did not detect treatment effects for any of the response measures.

The most recent study by Loprinzi et al. (1997), a phase III, double-blind, placebo-controlled clinical trial, tested the efficacy of sucralfate suspension in alleviating stomatitis associated with bolus 5-fluorouracil treatment. Fifty of the 131 subjects originally enrolled developed mouth tenderness. Of these, 27 were randomized to receive sucralfate and 23 were randomized to receive placebo. No differences in either the severity or duration of stomatitis were detected between the two groups. In conclusion, the literature shows varying results with sucralfate suspension.

Uridine

Uridine is another agent under investigation due to positive results in animal studies. Laboratory studies suggested that uridine rescue might allow intensification of 5-fluorouracil dosing through selective protection of host tissues. Although studies by van Groeningen, Peters, Lyva, Laurensse, and Pinedo in 1989 and by Seiter et al. in 1993 showed beneficial effects on toxicity overall, mucositis was not improved.

Vitamin E

Vitamin E's ability to treat herpetic gingivitis prompted a study of its use in mucositis. Its antioxidant activity is thought to endow vitamin E with the capacity to prevent peroxidation of membrane polyunsaturated fatty acids and stabilize membranes. In animal experiments it has inhibited tumor formation, and epidemiological data suggest that vitamin E levels are low in individuals with malignant disease.

A randomized, double-blind, placebo-controlled trial of topical vitamin E brought promising results. Patients were randomly assigned to begin using either vitamin E or placebo twice a day for 5 days as soon as mucosal lesions appeared during any cycle of chemotherapy. Patients in the active drug arm used 1 ml of vitamin E oil, or 400 mg, at each application. Among the patients using active drug, six out of nine had complete resolution of their lesions within 4 days of beginning treatment; in contrast, only one of the nine patients using placebo experienced complete resolution during the 5-day study period (Wadleigh et al., 1992). These positive results suggest the need for larger investigations of vitamin E's efficacy and determination of whether effects are due to local application or systemic absorption.

Combination Products

Rothwell and Spektor (1990) conducted a double-blind pilot study of an oral rinse consisting of hydrocortisone, nystatin, tetracycline, and diphenhydramine for control of oral mucositis in patients undergoing radiation therapy. Their 1990 report stated that the five patients in the experimental group experienced less severe mucositis with diminished incidence than the control group of seven patients. The authors tempered their results with a caution that the tetracy-

cline must be administered in a separate solution for stability reasons and that there were some confounding factors in their study, such as some participants' continued use of alcohol and tobacco during radiation therapy.

Spijkervet et al. (1991) attempted to eradicate gram-negative bacilli and fungi to reduce oral mucositis. They compared the results from 15 patients using lozenges with polymixin B 2 mg, tobramycin 1.8 mg, and amphotericin B 10 mg with results from historical controls from a previous trial. The treatment group had significantly lower mucositis scores, but because the trial was open-label and used historical controls, additional research is required.

Symonds and colleagues investigated an antibiotic pastille containing amphotericin, polymixin, and tobramycin in 1996. In this large, double-blind, placebo-controlled, randomized clinical trial, a total of 275 subjects were enrolled, with 136 in the active group. Although no statistical difference was detected between the two groups for the primary end point, development of pseudomembranes, other beneficial effects were noted. The pastilles showed a positive impact on the worst recorded mucositis grade, the severity of dysphagia, and the percentage of weight lost.

OTHER METHODS

Cryotherapy

In a 1991 study by Mahood et al., patients receiving 5-fluorouracil were instructed to place ice chips in their mouths 5 min prior to each dose of chemotherapy and continuously swish, replacing the chips as needed to keep unmelted ice in the mouth for a total of 30 min. Of the 95 patients entered into the study, 50 were randomized to receive oral cryotherapy for prevention of mucositis. Positive results were observed in physician-judged toxicity, patient-graded mucositis scores, and number of days of mucositis. Because cryotherapy is simple, inexpensive, and well tolerated, the authors now routinely recommend its use for their patients receiving 5-fluorouracil boluses. A later study by Rocke et al. (1993) examined cryotherapy for 30 mins versus 60 min. No significant differences were noted on comparison, and the authors endorsed the 30-min protocol.

Laser

Pourreau-Schneider et al. published a preliminary report in 1992 of their use of soft-laser therapy for stomatitis resulting from 5-fluorouracil chemotherapy. This technique is similar in proposed mechanism of action to that of silver nitrate. The retrospective review showed that the time to repair grade 4 mucositis was reduced from a mean of 19.3 days in control patients to 8.1 days in patients given curative laser treatments. Beneficial effects were also seen in prevention of mucositis, with a 6% incidence of mucositis during 95 cycles of chemotherapy for the treatment group versus a 43% incidence in the nontreatment group. The authors urged further study of soft-laser treatment for mucositis.

TREATMENT OPTIONS FOR XEROSTOMIA

Chemotherapy-induced xerostomia is troubling to patients, but does tend to dissipate as other symptoms of oral toxicity abate. Radiation therapy damages the parenchyma of the salivary gland, eventually causing fibrosis and secretory hypofunction. For radiation, the effect is dose-related and permanent, with many patients producing little or no saliva (Johnson et al., 1993). Although some function may return with time, it never approaches its former level (Greenspan & Daniels, 1987).

Hamlet et al. (1997) have studied the specific effects of xerostomia on mastication and swallowing in their retrospective review of 15 cancer patients with xerostomia versus 20 normal control patients. Subjects were given a liquid, a paste, and a shortbread cookie. The mean values for all measures were slightly larger in patients than in controls for the liquid and paste,

but not to an extent that was statistically significant. However, the xerostomic patients took an average of 48% longer than the controls to prepare the cookie and perform the first swallow. Xerostomic patients were found to take 46% longer for the chewing interval alone. When swallowing finally did occur, it was not significantly longer.

The change in duration of mastication is significant because it is during mastication that saliva is mixed with food. This mixing together is needed to ease the gathering together of food particles into a cohesive bolus of the necessary texture for swallowing. Because patients were instructed to chew their cookies and swallow "when ready," it is likely that they compensated for their difficulty with swallowing dry material by extending mastication and oral manipulation time. Such problems with eating, and with speaking at length or wearing dentures, prompt most caregivers to initiate treatment for their xerostomic patients before more serious sequelae such as dental caries take hold.

For patients with temporary xerostomia induced by chemotherapy alone, sugar-free gum or candies are often effective stimulants for remaining salivary function. Saliva substitutes containing carboxymethylcellulose or animal mucins are useful in some patients, although they are not always well accepted. For cost savings and convenience, patients may also elect to carry bottled water with them for frequent sipping during the day. Misting bottles of water may also be useful. However, for radiation patients with more severe, permanent dryness, first line treatment is stimulation of saliva production with a sialogogue (Epstein, Stevenson-Moore, & Scully, 1992).

Pilocarpine is a parasympathomimetic agent with muscarinic agonist and mild beta-adrenergic activity. It is an alkaloid that stimulates exocrine glands in humans, inducing diaphoresis, salivation, lacrimation, and gastric and pancreatic secretion (Johnson et al., 1993). It appears to act by direct cell stimulation rather than through the cholinesterase-acetylcholine system. Although side effects such as sweating were common, they were generally mild and manageable. Often the ophthalmic product is used intraorally, but capsules are also available (Epstein, Stevenson-Moore, & Scully, 1992). Another sialogogue, anetholetrithione or Sialor, is available in Canada. Sialogogue doses are presented in Table 14–3.

Studies by Greenspan and Daniels (1987), Fox et al. (1991), and Johnson et al. (1993) have all demonstrated increased saliva production and decreased xerostomia symptoms with oral pilocarpine. A retrospective study of patients who received pilocarpine concomitantly during radiation therapy and for 3 months after used a subjective patient questionnaire to examine effects on oral dryness and comfort, and difficulty with sleep, speech, and eating. Compared with untreated patients, the group that received pilocarpine had lower xerostomia scores in all categories (Zimmerman, Mark, Tran, & Juillard, 1997). This study suggests that pilocarpine may have a protective effect on salivary function when used during radiation therapy; however, more stringent testing is needed.

AGENTS THAT INTENSIFY ORAL COMPLICATIONS

A variety of agents can affect swallowing, voice, or speech. Most of the effects are minor in comparison to those of chemotherapeutic or radiation therapy agents; however, once a patient has developed anticancer drug-induced stomatitis or xerostomia, such drugs can significantly increase the problems the patient is experiencing. Following is a review of several classes of pharmaceuticals that may alter swallowing, voice, or speech that may be of use to practitioners in counseling their patients with oral complications of cancer therapy.

Anticholinergics

Combination antidiarrheals such as Lomotil and Donnagel contain belladonna alkaloids that have anticholinergic effects. These agents may be expected to decrease the natural secretions of the respiratory tract (Thompson, 1995). Health professionals working with cancer patients often need to prescribe antidiarrheals. The benefit of such agents must be weighed against their possible costs to the patient's oral health from dryness and irritation.

Other anticholinergic agents that may be encountered in cancer patients are benztropine and trihexyphenidyl, the anti-Parkinson's drugs. Such agents are strongly anticholinergic and must be expected to dry the oral mucosa (Thompson, 1995). Again, the benefits of these agents must be weighed against their cost to the patient's comfort.

Antihistamines

Although H_2 receptor antagonists such as ranitidine and famotidine have minimal influence outside the gastrointestinal tract, most H_1 receptor antagonists inhibit responses to acetylcholine, producing anticholinergic effects, including decreased secretions from the respiratory tract. The earliest antihistamines were ethanolamines, alkylamines, and ethylenediamines. All of the amines dry secretions. A later class, the piperazines, produces similar effects. Meclizine, which is frequently used for motion

TABLE 14–3. Sialogogues

Medication	Formulation	Dosage
Pilocarpine (various brands)	Ophthalmic drops	2–4 drops on tongue four times daily
Pilocarpine (Salagen7)	Tablets (5 mg)	5 mg three times daily
Anetholetrithione (Sialor7)	Tablets (25 mg)	1–2 tablets three times daily

sickness, and hydroxyzine, a common choice for pruritic conditions, are members of the piperazine class (Thompson, 1995).

Patients experiencing oral complications of cancer therapy should be advised of the possible ill effects of antihistamine use, and their ubiquitous presence in over-the-counter preparations. The drying action of antihistamines on the mouth, nose, and throat will not only aggravate swallowing, eating, and speaking problems for xerostomic patients, but will also exacerbate the irritation of mucositis as air passes over dried tissues. In many cases, coughing will ensue and further intensify the patient's discomfort.

If an antihistamine must be used, the practitioner would be wise to select a second-generation agent such as astemizole or loratadine. These newer piperidines are highly selective for H_1 receptors with no effect on acetylcholine, so they should have little effect on natural secretions (Thompson, 1995). Nevertheless, individual patient responses must be carefully monitored.

Antihypertensives

Loop diuretics are still commonly used to treat hypertension. Drugs included in this class are furosemide, bumetanide, and ethacrynic acid, which act to decrease blood pressure by causing loss of body water. Dryness of the vocal tract is commonly seen secondary to the loss of body water with loop diuretics and other forms of diuretics such as thiazides (Thompson, 1995). In addition, the loop diuretics have been known to result in ototoxicity. Whereas hearing losses associated with furosemide are usually transient and disappear with discontinuation of treatment, deafness from ethacrynic acid may be permanent. The duration of hearing impairment with bumetanide is unclear (Martin, 1988). Caution should be exercised in prescribing diuretics for patients with oral complications. Loop diuretics' possible negative effects on hearing can make them especially problematic in patients with speech or language difficulties.

Angiotensin-converting enzyme inhibitors are antihypertensive agents with little or no effect on the moisture content of the mouth. However, coughing is a common side effect of this class of drugs. For patients with active stomatitis, frequent coughing may lead to increased pain and irritation (Thompson, 1995). In patients with severe stomatitis and no contraindications to other agents, a change of therapy may be warranted.

Decongestants

Decongestants are sympathomimetic agents, and include phenylpropanolamine and pseudoephedrine. Their mechanism of action is vasoconstriction, with shrinking of the upper respiratory mucous membrane and decreased secretion production. The water component of secretions is reduced to a greater extent than the mucin component, causing the secretions that are present to be relatively thickened (Thompson, 1995). Although practitioners are unlikely to prescribe decongestants for their patients with xerostomia or mucositis, they are present in a multitude of combination over-the-counter products.

Psychotropic Agents

Tricyclic antidepressants have long been recognized to have significant anticholinergic properties, leading to drying of the mucosa of the upper respiratory tract. Although anticholinergic effects are less prominent with serotonin selective reuptake inhibitors, dry mouth is one of the leading side effects reported by patients. Dryness of the vocal tract mucosa is almost always observed in patients using antipsychotics of the phenothiazine class, but again, the negative impact of this side effect on the patient's oral environment must be balanced against his or her need for the medication (Thompson, 1995).

CONCLUSIONS

In conclusion, pharmacological agents play a central role in the treatment of cancers. Pharmacological agents are one of the most effective tools used in the treatment and cure of many different types of cancers. In addition, medications assist in providing relief and palliation from the unpleasant symptoms that often accompany disease progression and aggressive chemotherapy treatment regimens. More careful selection of chemotherapy agents (treatment design) can reduce the intensity of mucosal damage. Greater attention toward avoiding substances that could increase or magnify a patient's discomfort can also lead to a more tolerable and comfortable treatment experience for patients.

REFERENCES

Ahmann, F. R., Garewal, H., & Greenburg, B. (1986). Phase II trial of high-dose continuous infusion 5-fluorouracil with allopurinol modulation in colon cancer. *Oncology, 43,* 83.

Allison, R. R., Vongtama, V., Vaughan, J., & Shin, K. H. (1995). Symptomatic acute mucositis can be minimized or prophylaxed by the combination of sucralfate and fluconazole. *Cancer Investigation, 13,* 16–22.

Atkinson, K., Biggs, J. C., Downs, K., et al. (1991). GM-CSF after allogeneic bone marrow transplantation: Accelerated recovery of neutrophils, monocytes, and lymphocytes. *Australian and New Zealand Journal of Medicine, 21,* 686–696.

Barker, G., Loftus, L., Cuddy, P., & Barker, B. (1991). The effects of sucralfate suspension and diphenhydramine syrup plus kaolin-pectin on radiotherapy-induced mucositis. *Oral Surgery, Oral Medicine, and Oral Pathology, 71,* 288–293.

Barrett, A. P. (1984). Evaluation of nystatin in prevention and elimination of oropharyngeal *Candida* in immunosuppressed patients. *Oral Surgery, 58,* 148.

Berger, A., Henderson, M., Nadoolman, W., et al. (1995). Oral capsaicin provides temporary relief for oral mucositis pain secondary to chemotherapy/radiation therapy. *Journal of Pain and Symptom Management, 10,* 243–248.

Berger, A., & Kilroy, T. (1997). Oral complications. In V. T. De Vita (Ed.), *Cancer: Principles and practice of oncology* (5th ed.). Philadelphia: Lippincott-Raven.

Bianco, J. A., Appelbaum, F. R., Nemunaitis, J., et al. (1991). Phase I–II trial of pentoxifylline for the prevention of transplant-related toxicities following bone marrow transplantation. *Blood, 78,* 1205–1211.

Bronchud, M. H., Howell, A., Crowther, D., et al. (1989). The use of granulocyte colony-stimulating factor to increase the intensity of treatment with doxorubicin in patients with advanced breast and ovarian cancer. *British Journal of Cancer, 60,* 121–125.

Carl, W., & Emrich, L. S. (1991). Management of oral mucositis during local radiation and systemic chemotherapy: A study of 98 patients. *Journal of Prosthetic Dentistry, 66,* 361.

Childers, N. K., Stinnett, E. A., Wheeler, P., et al. (1993). Oral complications in children with cancer. *Oral Surgery, Oral Medicine, and Oral Pathology, 75,* 41–47.

Clark, P. I., & Slevin, M. L. (1985). Allopurinol mouthwashes and 5-fluorouracil induced oral toxicity. *European Journal of Surgical Oncology, 11,* 267.

Degregorio, M. W., Lee, W. M., & Ries, C. A. (1982). *Candida* infections in patients with acute leukemia: ineffectiveness of nystatin prophylaxis and relationship between oropharyngeal and systemic candidiasis. *Cancer, 50,* 2780.

DiPiro, J. T., Talbert, R. L., Yee, G. C., et al. (1997). *Pharmacotherapy: A pathophysiologic approach* (3rd ed.). Norwalk, CT: Appleton & Lange.

Dodd, M. J., Larson, P. J., Dibble, S. L., et al. (1996). Randomized clinical trial of chlorhexidine versus placebo for prevention of oral mucositis in patients receiving chemotherapy. *Oncology Nurses' Forum, 23,* 921–927.

Dorr, W., Jacubek, A., & Kummermehr, J. (1995). Effects of stimulated repopulation on oral mucositis during conventional radiotherapy. *Radiotherapy in Oncology, 37,* 100.

Duenas-Gonzalez, A., Sobrevilla-Calvo, P., Frias-Mendivil, M., et al. (1996). Misoprostol prophylaxis for high-dose chemotherapy-induced mucositis: A randomized double-blind study. *Bone Marrow Transplant, 17,* 809–812.

Epstein, J. B., & Stevenson-Moore, P. (1986). Benzydamine hydrochloride in prevention and management of pain in oral mucositis associated with radiation therapy. *Oral Surgery, Oral Medicine, and Oral Pathology, 62,* 145.

Epstein, J. B., Stevenson-Moore, P., Jackson, S., Mohamed, J. H., & Spinelli, J. J. (1989). Prevention of oral mucositis in radiation therapy: A controlled study with benzydamine hydrochloride rinse. *International Journal of Radiation Oncology, Biology, Physics, 16,* 1571–1575.

Epstein, J. B., Stevenson-Moore, P., & Scully, C. (1992). Management of xerostomia. *Journal of the Canadian Dental Association, 58,* 140.

Epstein, J. B., Vickers, L., Spinelli, J., & Reece, D. (1992). Efficacy of chlorhexidine and nystatin rinses in prevention of oral complications in leukemia and bone marrow transplantation. *Oral Surgery, Oral Medicine, and Oral Pathology, 73,* 682–689.

Epstein, J. B. & Wong, F. L. (1994). The efficacy of sucralfate suspension in the prevention of oral mucositis due to radiation therapy. *International Journal of Radiation Oncology, Biology, Physics, 28,* 693.

Feber, T. (1996). Management of mucositis in oral irradiation. *Clinical Oncology Review, Colleges of Radiology, 8*, 106.

Ferraro, J. M. & Mattern, J. G. (1984). Sucralfate suspension for stomatitis. *Drug Intelligence in Clinical Pharmacology, 18*, 153.

Ferretti, G. A., Largent, B. M., Ash, R. C., et al. (1987). Chlorhexidine for prophylaxis against oral infections and associated complications in patients receiving bone marrow transplants. *Journal of the American Dental Association, 114*, 461–467.

Fidler, P., Loprinzi, C. L., O'Fallon, J. R., et al. (1996). Prospective evaluation of a chamomile mouthwash for prevention of 5-FU induced oral mucositis. *Cancer, 77*, 522–525.

Finley, R. S. (1991). *Concepts in oncology therapeutics: A self instructional course.* Bethesda, MD: American Society of Hospital Pharmacists.

Foote, R. L., Loprinzi, C. L., Frank, A. R., et al. (1994). Randomized trial of a chlorhexidine mouthwash for alleviation of radiation-induced mucositis. *Journal of Clinical Oncology, 12*, 2630–2633.

Fox, P. C., Atkinson, J. C., Macynski, A. A., et al. (1991). Pilocarpine treatment of salivary gland hypofunction and dry mouth (xerostomia). *Archives of Internal Medicine, 151*, 1149–1152.

Franzen, L., Henriksson, R., Littbrand, B., & Zackrisson, B. (1995). Effects of sucralfate on mucositis during and following radiotherapy of malignancies in the head and neck region. A double-blind, placebo-controlled study. *Acta Oncologica, 34*, 219–223.

Futran, N. D., Trotti, A., & Gwede, C. (1997). Pentoxifylline in the treatment of radiation-related soft tissue injury: Preliminary observations. *Laryngoscope, 107*, 391.

Gabrilove, J. L., Jakubowski, A., Scher, H., et al. (1988). Effect of granulocyte colony-stimulating factor on neutropenia and associated morbidity due to chemotherapy for transitional-cell carcinoma of the urothelium. *New England Journal of Medicine, 318*, 1414–1422.

Garewal, H. S., & Meyskens, F. (1992). Retinoids and carcinoids in the prevention of oral cancer: A critical appraisal. *Cancer Epidemiology Biomarkers and Prevention, 1*, 155.

Greenspan, D., & Daniels, T. E. (1987). Effectiveness of pilocarpine in postradiation xerostomia. *Cancer, 59*, 1123.

Hamlet, S., Faull, J., Klein, B., et al. (1997). Mastication and swallowing in patients with postirradiation xerostomia. *International Journal of Radiation Oncology, Biology, Physics, 37*, 789–796.

Holmes, S. (1991). The oral complications of specific anticancer therapy. *International Journal of Nursing Studies, 28*, 343.

Howell, S. B., Wung, W. E., Taetle, R., Hussain, F., & Romine, J. S. (1981). Modulation of 5-fluorouracil toxicity by allopurinol in man. *Cancer, 48*, 1281–1289.

Ilveskoski, I., Saarinen, U. M., Wiklund, T., et al. (1996). Ototoxicity in children with malignant brain tumors treated with the "8 in 1" chemotherapy protocol. *Medical and Pediatric Oncology, 27*, 26–31.

Jebb, S. A., Osborne, R. J., Maughan, T. S., et al. (1994). 5-Fluorouracil and folinic acid-induced mucositis: No effect of oral glutamine supplementation. *British Journal of Cancer, 70*, 732–735.

Johnson, J. T., Ferretti, G. A., Nethery, W. J., et al. (1993). Oral pilocarpine for post-irradiation xerostomia in patients with head and neck cancer. *New England Journal of Medicine, 329*, 390–395.

Kannan, V., Bapsy, P. P., Anantha, N., et al. (1997). Efficacy and safety of granulocyte macrophage-colony stimulating factor (GM-CSF) on the frequency and severity of radiation mucositis in patients with head and neck carcinoma. *International Journal of Radiation Oncology, Biology, Physics, 37*, 1005–1010.

Kim, J. H., Chu, F. C., Lakshmi, V., & Houde, R. (1986). Benzydamine HCl, a new agent for the treatment of radiation mucositis of the oropharynx. *American Journal of Clinical Oncology, 9*, 132–134.

Kuhrer, I., Kuzmits, R., Linkesch, W., & Ludwig, H. (1986). Topical PGE_2 enhances healing of chemotherapy-associated mucosal lesions. *Lancet, 1*, 623.

Labar, B., Mrsic, M., Pavleric, A., et al. (1993). Prostaglandin E_2 for prophylaxis of oral mucositis following BMT. *Bone Marrow Transplant, 11*, 379–382.

Langslet, A., Olsen, I., Lie, S. O., & Lokken, P. (1974). Chlorhexidine treatment of oral candidiasis in seriously diseased children. *Acta Paediatrica Scandinavia, 63*, 809–811.

Lever, S. A., Dupuis, L. L., Chan, H. S. (1987). Comparative evaluation of benzydamine oral rinse in children with antineoplastic-induced stomatitis. *Drug Intelligence and Clinical Pharmacy, 21*, 359.

Lieschke, G. J., Ramenghi, U., O'Connor, M. P., et al. (1992). Studies of oral neutrophil levels in patients receiving G-CSF after autologous marrow transplantation. *British Journal of Haematology, 82*, 589–595.

Loprinzi, C. L., Dose, A. M., Burnham, N. L., et al. (1990). A controlled evaluation of an allopurinol mouthwash as prophylaxis against 5-fluorouracil-induced stomatitis. *Cancer, 65*, 1879–1882.

Loprinzi, C. L., Ghosh, C., Camoriano, J., et al. (1997). Phase III controlled evaluation of sucralfate to alleviate stomatitis in patients receiving fluorouracil-based chemotherapy. *American Journal of Clinical Oncology, 15*, 1235–1238.

Maciejewski, B., Zajusz, A., Pilecki, B., et al. (1992). Acute mucositis in the stimulated oral mucosa of patients during radiotherapy for head and neck cancer. *Radiotherapy and Oncology, 22*, 7–11.

Mahood, D. J., Dose, A. M., Loprinzi, C. L., et al. (1991). Inhibition of fluorouracil-induced stomatitis by oral cryotherapy. *Journal of Clinical Oncology, 9*, 449–452.

Makkonen, T. A., Bostrom, P., & Vilja, P. (1994). Sucralfate mouth washing in the prevention of radiation-induced mucositis: A placebo-controlled, double-blind, randomized study. *International Journal of Oncology, Biology, Physics, 30*, 177–182.

Martin, F. G. (1988). Drugs and vocal function. *Journal of Voice, 2*, 338.

Matejka, M., Nell, A., Kment, G., et al. (1990). Local benefits of prostaglandin E$_2$ in radiochemotherapy-induced oral mucositis. *British Journal of Oral and Maxillofacial Surgery, 28*, 89–91.

McGaw, W. T., & Belch, A. (1985). Oral complications of acute leukemia: Prophylactic impact of a chlorhexidine mouth rinse regimen. *Oral Surgery, Oral Medicine, and Oral Pathology, 60*, 275.

Meredith, R., Salter, M., Kim, R., et al. (1997). Sucralfate for radiation mucositis: Results of a double-blind randomized trial. *International Journal of Radiation Oncology, Biology, and Physics, 37*, 275–279.

Mills, E. E. (1988). The modifying effect of beta-carotene on radiation and chemotherapy induced oral mucositis. *British Journal of Cancer, 57*, 416.

National Institutes of Health. (1989). Oral complications of cancer therapies: Diagnosis, prevention, and treatment. *Connecticut Medicine, 53*, 595–601.

Osaki, T., Ueta, E., Yoneda, K., Hirota, J., & Yamamoto, T. (1994). Prophylaxis of oral mucositis associated with chemoradiotherapy for oral carcinoma by Azelastine hydrochloride (Azelastine) with other antioxidants. *Head and Neck, 16*, 331–339.

Oshitani, T., Okada, K., Kushima, T., et al. (1990). Clinical evaluation of sodium alginate on oral mucositis associated with radiotherapy. *Journal of the Japanese Society of Cancer Therapists, 25*, 1129–1137.

Pettengell, R., Gurney, H., Radford, J. A., et al. (1992). Granulocyte colony-stimulating factor to prevent dose-limiting neutropenia in non-Hodgkin's lymphoma: A randomized controlled trial. *Blood, 80*, 1430–1436.

Pfeiffer, P., Madsen, E. L., Hansen, O., & May, O. (1990). Effect of prophylactic sucralfate suspension on stomatitis induced by cancer chemotherapy. *Acta Oncologica, 29*, 171–173.

Pillsbury, H. C., Webster, W. P., & Rosenman, J. (1986). Prostaglandin inhibitor and radiotherapy in advanced head and neck cancers. *Archives of Otolaryngology and Head and Neck Surgery, 112*, 552.

Porta, C., Moroni, M., & Nastasi, G. (1994). Allopurinol mouthwashes in the treatment of 5-fluorouracil-induced stomatitis. *American Journal of Clinical Oncology, 17*, 246.

Porteder, H., Rausch, E., Kment, G., et al. (1988). Local prostaglandin E$_2$ in patients with oral malignancies undergoing chemo- and radiotherapy. *Journal of Cranio-Maxillo-Facial Surgery, 16*, 371–374.

Pourreau-Schneider, N., Soudry, M., Franquin, J. C., et al. (1992). Soft-laser therapy for iatrogenic mucositis in cancer patients receiving high-dose fluorouracil: A preliminary report. *Journal of the National Cancer Institute, 84*, 358–359.

Rocke, L. K., Loprinzi, C. L., Lee, J. K., et al. (1993). A randomized clinical trial of two different durations of oral cryotherapy for prevention of 5-fluorouracil-related stomatitis. *Cancer, 72*, 2234–2238.

Rothwell, B. R., & Spektor, W. S. (1990). Palliation of radiation-related mucositis. *Special Care in Dentistry, 10*, 21–25.

Rutkauskas, J. S. & Davis, J. W. (1993). Effects of chlorhexidine during immunosuppressive chemotherapy. A preliminary report. *Oral Surgery, Oral Medicine, and Oral Pathology, 76*, 441–448.

Samaranayake, L. P., Robertson, A. G., MacFarlane, T. W., et al. (1988). The effect of chlorhexidine and benzydamine mouthwashes on mucositis induced by therapeutic irradiation. *Clinical Radiology, 39*, 291–294.

Seiter, K., Kemeny, N., Martin, D., et al. (1993). Uridine allows dose escalation of 5-fluorouracil when given with N-phosphonacetyl-L-aspartate, methotrexate, and leucovorin. *Cancer, 71*, 1875–1881.

Sharon, A., Berdicevsky, I., Ben-Aryeh, H., & Gutman, D. (1977). The effect of chlorhexidine mouth rinses on oral *Candida* in a group of leukemic patients. *Oral Surgery, Oral Medicine, and Oral Pathology, 44*, 201–205.

Shenep, J. L., Kalwinsky, D. K., Hutson, P. R., et al. (1988). Efficacy of oral sucralfate suspension in prevention and treatment of chemotherapy-induced mucositis. *Journal of Pediatrics, 113*, 758–763.

Skubitz, K. M. & Anderson, P. M. (1996). Oral glutamine to prevent chemotherapy induced stomatitis: A pilot study. *Journal of Laboratory and Clinical Medicine, 127*, 223.

Solomon, M. A. (1986). Oral sucralfate suspension for mucositis. *New England Journal of Medicine, 315*, 459.

Sonis, S. T., Clairmont, F., Lockhart, P., & Connolly, S. F. (1985). Benzydamine HCl in the management of chemotherapy induced mucositis. 1. Pilot study. *Journal of Oral Medicine, 40*, 67–71.

Spijkervet, F. K., van Saene, H. K., Panders, A. K., et al. (1989). Effect of chlorhexidine rinsing on the oropharyngeal ecology in patients with head and neck cancer who have irradiation mucositis. *Oral Surgery, Oral Medicine, and Oral Pathology, 67*, 154–161.

Spijkervet, F. K., van Saene, H. K., Panders, A. K., et al. (1991). Effect of selective elimination of the oral flora on mucositis in irradiated head and neck cancer patients. *Journal of Surgical Oncology, 46,* 167–173.

Symonds, R. P., McIlroy, P., Khorrami, J., et al. (1996). The reduction of radiation mucositis by selective decontamination antibiotic pastilles: A placebo-controlled double-blind trial. *British Journal of Cancer, 74,* 312–317.

Thompson, A. R. (1995). Pharmacologic agents with effects on voice. *American Journal of Otolaryngology, 16,* 12.

Tsavaris, N., Caragiauris, P., & Kosmidis, P. (1988). Reduction of oral toxicity of 5-fluorouracil by allopurinol mouthwashes. *European Journal of Surgical Oncology, 4,* 89.

van Groeningen, C. J., Peters, G. J., Leyva, A., Laurensse, E., & Pinedo, H. M. (1989). Reversal of 5-fluorouracil-induced myelosuppression by prolonged administration of high-dose uridine. *Journal of the National Cancer Institute, 81,* 157–162.

van Zaanen, H. C., van-der-Lelie, H., Timmer, J. G., Furst, P., & Sauerwein, H. P. (1994). Parenteral glutamine dipeptide supplementation does not ameliorate chemotherapy-induced toxicity. *Cancer, 74,* 2879–2884.

Verdi, C. J. (1993). Cancer therapy and oral mucositis: An appraisal of drug prophylaxis. *Drug Safety, 9,* 185.

Wadleigh, R. G., Redman, R. S., Graham, M. L., et al. (1992). Vitamin E in the treatment of chemotherapy-induced mucositis. *American Journal of Medicine, 92,* 481–484.

Wahlin, Y. B. (1989). Effects of chlorhexidine mouthrinses on oral health in patients with acute leukemia. *Oral Surgery, Oral Medicine, and Oral Pathology, 68,* 279.

Weisdorf, D. J., Bostrom, B., Raether, D., et al. (1989). Oropharyngeal mucositis complicating bone marrow transplantation: Prognostic factors and the effect of chlorhexidine rinse. *Bone Marrow Transplantation, 4,* 89–95.

Weiss, G. R., Green, S., Hannigan, E. V., et al. (1990). A phase II trial of cisplatin and 5-fluorouracil with allopurinol for recurrent or metastatic carcinoma of the uterine cervix: A Southwest Oncology Group trial. *Gynecologic Oncology, 37,* 354–358.

Williams, C., Whitehouse, J. M., Lister, T. A., & Wrigley, P. F. (1977). Oral anticandidal prophylaxis in patients undergoing chemotherapy for acute leukemia. *Medical and Pediatric Oncology, 3,* 275–280.

Zimmerman, R. P., Mark, R. J., Tran, L. M., & Juillard, G. F. (1997). Concomitant pilocarpine during head and neck irradiation is associated with decreased posttreatment xerostomia. *International Journal of Radiation Oncology, Biology, Physics, 37,* 571–575

15

Psychological Care of Cancer Patients with Swallowing and Communication Disorders

Paul B. Jacobsen, Ph.D., and Michael A. Weitzner, M.D.

In the oncology setting, communication and swallowing disorders are most commonly observed among patients with cancers of the head and neck region (e.g., oral cavity, larynx, pharynx). In addition to possible impairments in communication and swallowing, many patients with head and neck cancer experience the loss of normal facial appearance as well as loss of sight, taste, or smell. Although the diagnosis of any form of cancer is likely to give rise to psychological distress, these features of head and neck cancer pose special problems for psychosocial adaptation.

Further compounding the risk of psychosocial problems is the fact that head and neck cancer most often occurs in individuals with histories of tobacco use and excessive alcohol use. As a result, patients with this disease are likely to have multiple psychological and psychiatric symptoms and to require considerable psychosocial care. This chapter outlines the range of psychosocial problems that clinicians working with this patient population are likely to encounter. Recommendations for the psychosocial care of head and neck

cancer patients during the period of active cancer treatment as well as during the period of rehabilitation are also provided.

IMPACT OF DISEASE AND TREATMENT ON PSYCHOSOCIAL FUNCTIONING

The potential sources of psychological distress for patients with head and neck cancer are many. They include pain as well as fears of disease recurrence and disease progression. In addition to these factors, which are common across disease sites, there are additional sources of distress for patients with disease in the head and neck region. Because of the nature of this disease and its treatment, patients may also experience psychological distress due to changes in their facial appearance, their ability to eat, and their ability to perceive or to communicate. These structural and functional alterations are among the most potent and common sources of psychological distress in this patient population. In general, head and neck cancer patients who experience greater disfigurement and dysfunction experience more problems with loss of self-esteem, social isolation, and psychological distress (Breitbart & Holland, 1988). Thus, the degree of physical disfigurement and the severity of communication and swallowing problems are essential factors to consider in assessing the potential for psychosocial problems.

The severity of structural and functional alterations can be assessed using either clinician rating measures or patient self-report instruments. The Dysfunction/ Disfigurement Scale (Dropkin, Malgady, Scott, Oberst, & Strong, 1983) is an example of a clinician rating measure. This scale provides explicit criteria for rating the severity of physical disfigurement as well as the severity of functional impairment due to sensory loss, communication problems, and eating problems. The Performance Status Scale for Head and Neck Cancer (PSS; List, Ritter-Sterr, & Lansky, 1990) is another example of a clinician-rated measure. This instrument yields ratings of the normalcy of diet, understandability of speech, and difficulties in eating.

A thorough evaluation of dysfunction and disfigurement should not be limited to clinician ratings alone. Patients' self-perceptions may be even more valuable in understanding individual reactions to diagnosis and treatment of head and neck cancer. In recent years, a number of self-report instruments have been developed to assess the quality-of-life of cancer patients. At least two quality-of-life measures also incorporate disease-specific modules for head and neck cancer. These are the Functional Assessment of Cancer Therapy (Cella et al., 1993; List et al., 1996) and the European Organization for Research and Treatment of Cancer Quality of Life Questionnaire (Aaronson et al., 1993; Bjordal & Kaasa, 1992). Another quality-of-life measure, the University of Washington Quality of Life Questionnaire, is designed specifically for use with head and neck cancer patients. This brief (9-item) scale, which includes items assessing disfigurement, eating, and speech, may be particularly useful for routine clinical use.

The preoperative period provides a good opportunity to assess and address any psychosocial problems. A thorough preoperative psychosocial assessment includes evaluation of premorbid personality, coping skills, family supports, financial and vocational problems, and alcohol and substance abuse histories. A major purpose of the psychosocial assessment is to identify those patients who would benefit from a psychiatric consultation, particularly those with a history of alcohol or other substance abuse as well as those with past psychiatric problems. The psychiatrist is an important member of the treatment team in that he or she can provide an overall assessment of emotional distress and evaluate alcohol-related disorders such as malnutrition and cognitive impairment. Careful assessment of cognition is important in the determination of whether a patient adequately comprehends the nature of the planned procedure. Competency to give consent may be a major question, as well as the ability to cooperate in self-care.

The surgeon and the nurse can play an important role in preparing the patient psychologically for surgery. Through preoperative counseling, they can prepare the patient for what to expect in the postoperative period, particularly with details of the procedure to be performed and the surgical defects that can be expected. The preoperative counseling should also include the radiation oncologist and medical oncologist if those treatment modalities are to be used. Other health care professionals who have essential roles in the preoperative period include the dentist and the speech-language pathologist. The opportunity for the dentist to meet with the patient preoperatively goes a long way toward providing continuity of service because the dental prosthesis needed in the postoperative period will require frequent adjustments. Likewise, a preoperative meeting with the speech-language pathologist can help allay any fears the patient may have about postoperative speech and swallowing.

The postoperative period is a critical time for beginning rehabilitation. The major rehabilitative concerns of this period include eating, speaking, and body image. Optimally, attention to these concerns should begin in the hospital right after surgery, with a particular emphasis on patients' concerns regarding their facial appearance. Patients who refuse to look at their face following surgery are likely to have a poor adjustment and to be less able to cooperate in their rehabilitation (Gamba et al., 1992). Research suggests that the 5th postoperative day is the critical point in recovery relative to acceptance of the defect, participation in self-care, and resocialization (Dropkin et al., 1983). Delay in undertaking self-care beyond 5 days is predictive of both poorer coping and poorer rehabilitative outcome.

Early socialization can be encouraged through attendance at in-hospital support group meetings of patients and families. These support groups are appropriate venues for psychosocial issues to be addressed as well. An altered body image can lead to anxiety and depression because the face carries both physical and emotional significance (Bronheim, Strain, & Biller, 1991). Fear and insecurity regarding disfigurement can lead to further social isolation, thus perpetuating both anxiety and depression (Strauss, 1989). This establishes a vicious cycle, because anxiety and depression can also contribute to distorted perceptions of body image. These distortions can be confronted in a support group through reality testing (Bronheim et al., 1991). Anxiety and depression are not limited to issues of body image. Concerns regarding eating and speech can also generate anxiety and depression. For example, ongoing problems with the ability to eat can have profound effects on lifestyle and family interactions (Schmitz, 1990). Some of the problems encountered by this patient population are increased time for eating, untidy food consumption, special food preparation needs, special nutritional management, and oral inconsistency (List et al., 1990). Support groups are instrumental in addressing these impor-

tant issues. The value of these support groups continues after discharge, aiding both patient and family to feel more confident in managing psychosocial problems that may arise at home.

TOBACCO AND ALCOHOL USE

As stated previously, head and neck cancer is most likely to occur in individuals with histories of tobacco use and excessive alcohol use. These features can seriously complicate the clinical management of patients with head and neck disease. Patients who are hospitalized for treatment of head and neck disease may experience symptoms of acute nicotine withdrawal (e.g., anxiety, depressed mood, irritability, restlessness) once tobacco use is restricted. These symptoms can usually be relieved by initiating transdermal nicotine replacement therapy (i.e., use of nicotine patch) on admission. Of even greater concern is the possibility of acute alcohol withdrawal in patients who abruptly discontinue excessive alcohol use on hospital admission. Patients are most at risk for alcohol withdrawal within the first 24 hr after their last drink. However, patients remain at risk for an alcohol withdrawal delirium (delirium tremens) until approximately 10 days following their last drink. Symptoms of alcohol withdrawal are predominantly autonomic in nature and include tachycardia, elevated diastolic blood pressure, diaphoresis, tremulousness, and elevated temperature. An alcohol withdrawal delirium will also be characterized by a waxing and waning mental status affecting all areas of a patient's psychological functioning (i.e., cognition, perception, affect, and behavior).

It is critical to provide proper medical management during alcohol withdrawal, using pharmacological detoxification with a cross-tolerant drug (Miller, 1993). The benzodiazepines, particularly lorazepam, are considered the preferred agents for management of alcohol withdrawal in the hospitalized cancer patient because of their safety and efficacy (Breitbart &

Holland, 1988; Miller, 1993). Other medications have been used in the treatment of alcohol withdrawal, including beta-blockers, clonidine, anticonvulsants, and neuroleptic agents. However, these alternative agents are currently considered adjuvants (Miller, 1993). Perhaps the most widely used adjunctive medication administered with a benzodiazepine in this population is haloperidol. The addition of haloperidol in a medically ill patient who is experiencing alcohol withdrawal or alcohol withdrawal delirium makes it possible to use less lorazepam. Lower dosages of lorazepam cause less sedation and allow the patient to be extubated faster.

Many head and neck patients who use tobacco and alcohol just prior to diagnosis are at risk for resuming use of these substances once discharged from the hospital. Along these lines, one survey found that 35% of head and neck cancer patients continued to use tobacco following surgical treatment (Ostroff et al., 1995). Continued use of tobacco and alcohol can pose a variety of problems. First and foremost, continued use of tobacco and alcohol by patients with head and neck disease is associated with an increased risk for development of a second cancer (Day et al., 1994). Second, continued tobacco and alcohol use can exacerbate disease-related or treatment-related problems with nutrition and respiration. The association between excessive alcohol use and malnutrition is of particular concern in this patient population. Third, continued use of tobacco and alcohol is likely to complicate rehabilitation efforts. Patients who continue to use these substances against medical advice are likely to have difficulties adhering to other treatment recommendations. Moreover, to the extent that patients continue to use alcohol excessively, they are likely to manifest social and cognitive deficits that will interfere with rehabilitative efforts to improve nutrition and restore communication.

For patients who continue to use tobacco, smoking cessation counseling should be considered a part of their cancer treatment. Gritz et al. (1993) have demonstrated how physicians and dentists can be trained to deliver a smoking cessation intervention to head and neck cancer patients during routine follow-up visits. The intervention consists of repeated advice to quit smoking, a specified quit date, tailored written materials, and booster advice sessions following cessation of tobacco use. These techniques, combined with use of transdermal nicotine replacement therapy (now available without prescription), can be very effective in promoting smoking cessation following diagnosis of head and neck cancer.

It is well recognized that heavy alcohol users usually have a myriad of psychosocial problems relating to different areas of functioning including marital, family, and social relationships; work performance; and finances (Breitbart & Holland, 1988). Discontinuation of alcohol consumption is an important and laudable goal, but is rarely achieved due to impaired decision-making, low motivation, and cognitive impairment due to dementia. Physical health in this population may be further compromised by several alcohol-related medical problems (e.g., cardiomyopathy, liver dysfunction, malnutrition, pancreatitis, and portal hypertension; Breitbart & Holland, 1988). Therefore, the immediate goal for these patients is abstinence during the preperioperative and immediate postoperative periods. Further abstinence following discharge from the hospital may be addressed in the outpatient clinic. At that time, referral to community resources for alcohol rehabilitation treatment (e.g., Alcoholics Anonymous) should be made routinely. Newer approaches to problem drinking, directed at enhancing motivation for change, may also be quite useful in this population (Miller & Rollnick, 1991).

ANXIETY AND DEPRESSION

A period of acute emotional crisis is part of a normal response to the diagnosis of a life-threatening illness such as cancer. In most instances, acute emotional turmoil subsides within a few weeks following diagnosis as patients accommodate and adapt to changes in their lives. Emotional reactions that persist beyond a few weeks or interfere with the optimal delivery of medical care are causes for concern. In such instances, treatment providers should consider obtaining a psychiatric consultation because patients are likely to require psychopharmacological management and/or ongoing psychotherapy.

Symptoms of anxiety (see Table 15–1) are common among cancer patients and reflect, in part, realistic concerns about cancer and its treatment. Among head and neck patients, symptoms of anxiety can be particularly severe or chronic for several reasons. First, many patients with head and neck disease use alcohol and/or nicotine to "self-medicate" underlying problems with anxiety. Once deprived of these substances, the patient experiences a reemergence of anxiety symptoms that can

be exacerbated by the concurrent experience of a withdrawal syndrome. A second factor contributing to anxiety is the enormous psychological investment most individuals have in the head and neck area. Treatments that may result in functional or structural changes can be particularly threatening to patients because social interaction and emotional expression depend to a great extent on facial expressiveness and verbal interaction (Breitbart & Holland, 1988). Consequently, many patients report intense preoperative anxiety as they prepare to undergo procedures that may result in disfiguring facial alterations or loss of communicative abilities.

Initial treatment of anxiety depends on whether there is a premorbid anxiety disorder in addition to anxiety related to cancer diagnosis and treatment. Any premorbid anxiety disorder, such as panic disorder, generalized anxiety disorder, or pho-

TABLE 15–1. Signs and Symptoms of Anxiety

Symptom Type	Symptom
Cognitive	Excessive worry
	Feelings of unreality
	Feeling detached from oneself
	Fears of losing control or going crazy
	Intrusive thoughts or images of distressing events
	Recurrent dreams of distressing events
	Difficulty concentrating
Behavioral	Avoidance of feared objects or situations
	Difficulty falling or staying asleep
	Irritability or outbursts of anger
	Restlessness
Physiological	Palpitations
	Sweating
	Trembling or shaking
	Shortness of breath
	Chest pain or discomfort
	Nausea or abdominal distress
	Feeling dizzy, lightheaded, or faint
	Numbness or tingling sensations
	Chills or hot flushes
	Exaggerated startle response
	Muscle tension
	Fatigue

Source: *Diagnostic and Statistical Manual of Mental Disorders* (4th ed.), by the American Psychiatric Association, 1994, Washington, DC: Author.

bic disorder, must be stabilized before one can use psychological treatments for the current anxiety component. Benzodiazepines play an integral role in the treatment of these premorbid conditions. Panic disorder and generalized anxiety disorder may be treated with intermediate-acting benzodiazepines, such as clonazepam, which provide more consistent coverage than shorter-acting ones, such as alprazolam. The selective serotonin reuptake inhibitors (e.g., paroxetine, sertraline) are also of potential use in the treatment of panic disorder and generalized anxiety disorder in this population group. These may be used with or in lieu of benzodiazepines, although patients usually do not derive a clinical benefit from these antidepressants for a minimum of 2–4 weeks. Fluoxetine, however, is to be avoided in these patients because of its significant drug-drug interactions and long half-life. Although medications may be of benefit for panic and generalized anxiety disorders, they are not as efficacious for phobic disorders. Certainly, anxiolytic medications may have some benefit, but other psychological treatments are indicated and are often preferred to medications. The first is relaxation training, in which patients learn to relax through instruction in deep breathing and progressive muscle relaxation exercises. Patients mastering this technique often feel that they regain some degree of mental and physical control over their situation. Desensitization provides another means for patients to overcome their anxiety, through gradual exposure to fearful or anxiety-provoking thoughts, images, and environmental stimuli. Cognitive restructuring is another commonly used technique, in which patients are taught to "check out" their cognitions to see whether they are realistic or not. This technique helps patients gain insight into their thought patterns and teaches them how to rework their thoughts so that they reduce rather than exacerbate symptoms of anxiety.

Symptoms of depression (see Table 15–2) are also common among cancer patients. The frequency of depressive symptoms can be explained, in part, by the fact that some symptoms attributable to depression in physically healthy individuals (e.g., fatigue, loss of appetite) can be present in cancer patients as a consequence of the disease and its treatment. In general, the presence of cognitive symptoms of depression (e.g., dysphoric mood, suicidal ideation, feelings of worthlessness) is considered a more reliable indicator of a depressive disorder in physically ill individuals.

Surveys suggest that rates of depression are particularly high among patients with head and neck cancer. Among the general oncology population, it is estimated that 25% of patients experience clinically significant depressive symptoms (Bukberg, Penman, & Holland, 1984). Among patients with head and neck cancer, the prevalence is reported to be as high as 40% (Baile, Gibertini, Scott, & Endicott, 1992; Morton, Davies, Baker, Baker, & Stell, 1984). In a pattern that is consistent with these differences, at least one study has found that patients with head and neck cancer are twice as likely to commit suicide as patients with other forms of cancer (Faberow, Ganzler, Cutter, & Reynolds, 1971). The high rates of depression and suicidality among head and neck patients have been attributed to several factors. One factor often cited is preexisting psychopathology (Baile et al., 1992; Breitbart & Holland, 1988). Given the relation between excessive alcohol use and head and neck disease, it is likely that many patients have emotional problems that predate the diagnosis of cancer. A second factor is the severe psychosocial challenge posed by changes in facial appearance and/or loss of communicative abilities. Finally, there may be an interaction between these two factors that contributes to the high rates of depression.

When severe psychosocial challenges occur to individuals who are vulnerable to emotional problems and have limited coping resources, depression is a likely outcome. As stated previously, many individuals with head and neck cancer have a history of difficulty dealing with life stres-

TABLE 15–2. Signs and Symptoms of Depression

Symptom Type	Symptom
Cognitive	Feelings of sadness and emptiness Loss of interest or pleasure in usual activities Feelings of worthlessness Excessive or inappropriate guilt Indecisiveness Ruminative thinking Low self-esteem Feelings of hopelessness Difficulty concentrating Recurrent thoughts of death Suicidal ideation
Behavioral	Tearfulness Psychomotor agitation or retardation Suicide attempt
Physiological	Significant weight loss or weight gain Decrease or increase in appetite Insomnia or hypersomnia Fatigue or loss of energy

Source: Diagnostic and Statistical Manual of Mental Disorders (4th ed.), by the American Psychiatric Association, 1994, Washington, DC: Author.

sors. The presence of a communication disorder, an eating disorder, facial disfigurement, or poorly controlled pain may lead some individuals predisposed to emotional problems to become depressed and suicidal.

The clinician should be aware of the signs and symptoms of depression that are outlined in Table 15–2. As might be expected, diagnosing depression can be problematic in patients who are already having difficulty with sleep, speech, swallowing, and appetite. Other signs to look for specifically with head and neck cancer patients include excessive neediness, anger, withdrawn behavior, little eye contact, feeling hopeless and helpless, excessive pain, and unwillingness to cooperate with the medical regimen (Bronheim et al., 1991). The more subtle, nonverbal cues expressed in both gestures and expressions further indicate the mood of the patient. Factors related to increased risk of suicide are prior suicide attempts, presence of a plan and a means to carry it out, persistent thoughts of suicide, having a family member who has committed sui-

cide, substance abuse currently or in the past, and perpetual feelings of hopelessness and despair (Lucente, Strain, & Wyatt, 1987). Additional risk factors, particularly relevant to head and neck cancer, include increased age, low social support, delirium, advanced disease, and disfigurement (Depression Guideline Panel, 1993). It is important to assess a depressed patient's suicide potential because it may not be freely volunteered. Patients generally feel relieved to have the issue raised; it makes them feel safer and cared about.

Treatments available for major depression are multimodal in nature. The first issue in treatment is to determine the necessity for antidepressant medication. Certainly, if a major depression includes symptoms of social withdrawal and isolation, ruminative thinking, emotional liability, and, particularly, suicidal ideation, treatment with an antidepressant is indicated. Treatment with the selective serotonin reuptake inhibitors (e.g., paroxetine, sertraline) is often the best choice, given the rather innocuous side effect profile. Treatment with tricyclic antidepressants is problematic given the side effect profile, particularly the dry mouth, which adds to the xerostomia already experienced by patients as a result of surgery and/or radiation treatment. Fluoxetine is not indicated in this group due to its long half-life and drug-drug interactions. Venlafaxine is a good alternative to the selective serotonin reuptake inhibitors, although orthostatic hypotension is a potential problem in this malnourished population. All in all, antidepressants have proved to be effective with head and neck cancer patients (Bronheirn et al., 1991). Supportive psychotherapy and cognitive therapy are also effective in mobilizing patients and helping them to develop healthy coping strategies. Support from both the family and the medical treatment team is therapeutic as well (Breitbart & Holland, 1988; Shapiro & Kornfeld, 1987).

CONCLUSIONS

Among cancer patients with communication and swallowing disorders, individuals with head and neck disease pose the greatest challenge in terms of psychosocial care. In addition to swallowing and communication problems, these patients frequently experience chronic pain and the loss of normal facial appearance.

Compounding the risk for psychosocial problems is the fact that head and neck cancer most often occurs in individuals with histories of tobacco use and excessive alcohol use. Not surprisingly, many patients with head and neck disease require considerable psychosocial care. The recommended forms of care depend on the nature and severity of the patient's problems. Almost all patients are likely to benefit from attendance in support groups that seek to decrease social isolation and promote rehabilitation. Patients who are functioning poorly are likely to have symptoms of anxiety and depression that require more intensive treatment.

REFERENCES

Aaronson, N. K., Ahmedzai, S., Bergman, B., Bullinger, M., Cull, A., & Duez, N. J. (1993). The European Organization for Research and Treatment of Cancer QLQ-C30: A quality of life instrument for use in international clinical trials in oncology. *Journal of the National Cancer Institute, 85,* 365–376.

Baile, W. F., Gibertini, M., Scott, L., & Endicott, J. (1992). Depression and tumor stage in cancer of the head and neck. *Psycho-Oncology, 1,* 15–24.

Bjordal, K., & Kaasa, S. (1992). Psychometric validation of the EORTC Core Quality of Life Questionnaire, 30-item version and a diagnosis-specific module for head and neck cancer patients. *Acta Oncologica, 31,* 311–321.

Breitbart, W., & Holland, J. C. (1988). Psychosocial aspects of head and neck cancer. *Seminars in Oncology, 15,* 61–69.

Bronheim, H., Strain, J. J., & Biller, H. F. (1991). Psychiatric aspects of head and neck surgery: Part II: Body image and psychiatric intervention. *General Hospital Psychiatry, 13,* 225–232.

Bukberg, J., Penman, D., & Holland, J. (1984). Depression in hospitalized cancer patients. *Psychosomatic Medicine, 46,* 199–212.

Cella, D. F., Tulsky, D. S., Gray, G., Sarafian, B., Linn, E., & Bonomi, A. (1993). The Functional Assessment of Cancer Therapy Scale: Development and validation of the general measure. *Journal of Clinical Oncology, 11,* 570–579.

Day, G. L., Blot, W. J., Shore, R. E., McLaughlin, D. F., Austin, D. F., & Greenberg, R. S. (1994). Second cancers following oral and pharyngeal cancers: Role of tobacco and alcohol. *Journal of the National Cancer Institute, 86,* 131–137.

Depression Guideline Panel (1993). *Depression in primary care: Volume 1. Detection and diagnosis. Clinical practice guideline, number 5.* (AHCPR Publication No. 93-0550). Rockville, MD: U.S. Department of Health and Human Services, Public Health Service, Agency for Health Care Policy and Research.

Dropkin, M. J., Malgady, R. G., Scott, D. W., Oberst, M. T., & Strong, E. W. (1983). Scaling of disfigurement and dysfunction in postoperative head and neck patients. *Head and Neck Surgery, 8,* 559–570.

Faberow, N. L., Ganzler, S., Cutter, N., & Reynolds, D. (1971). An eight year survey of hospital suicides. *Life-Threatening Behavior, 1,* 184–210.

Gamba, A., Romano, M., Grosso, I. M., Tamburini, M., Cantu, G., Molinari, R., & Ventafridda,V. (1992). Psychosocial adjustment of patients surgically treated for head and neck cancer. *Head and Neck, 14,* 218–223.

Gritz, E. R., Carr, C. R., Rapkin, D., Abemayor, E., Chang, L. C., & Wong, W. K. (1993). Predictors of long-term smoking cessation in head and neck cancer patients. *Cancer Epidemiology, Biomarkers, and Prevention, 2,* 261–270.

Hassan, S. J., & Weymuller, E. A. (1993). Assessment of quality of life in head and neck cancer patients. *Head and Neck, 15,* 485–496.

List, M. A., D'Antonio, L. L., Cella, D. F., Siston, A., Mumby, P., & Haraf, D. (1996). The Performance Status Scale for Head and Neck Cancer and the Functional Assessment of Cancer Therapy-Head and Neck Scale. *Cancer, 77,* 2294–2301.

List, M. A., Ritter-Sterr, C., & Lansky, S. B. (1990). A performance status scale for head and neck cancer patients. *Cancer, 66,* 564–569.

Lucente, F. E., Strain, J. J., & Wyatt, D. A. (1987). Psychological problems of the patient with head and neck cancer. In S. E. Thawley & W. R. Panje (Eds.), *Comprehensive management of head and neck tumors* (pp. 69-78). Philadelphia: W. B. Saunders.

Miller, L. J. (1993). Pharmacologic treatment of acute alcohol withdrawal. *Cancer Bulletin, 45,* 465–466.

Miller, W. R., & Rollnick, S. (1991). *Motivational interviewing: Preparing people to change addictive behavior.* New York: Guilford Press.

Morton, R. P., Davies, A. D., Baker J., Baker, G. A., & Stell, P. M. (1984). Quality of life in treated head and neck cancer patients. *Clinical Otorhinolaryngology, 9,* 181–185.

Ostroff, J. S., Jacobsen, P. B., Moadel, A. B., Spiro, R., Shah, J. P., & Strong, E. W. (1995). Prevalence and predictors of continued tobacco use after treatment of patients with head and neck cancer. *Cancer, 75,* 569–576.

Schmitz, J. (1990). Dysphagia. In D. J. Gines (Ed.), *Nutrition management in rehabilitation* (pp. 141–157). Rockville, MD: Aspen.

Shapiro, P. A., & Kornfeld, D. S. (1987). Psychiatric aspects of head and neck cancer surgery. *Psychiatric Clinics of North America, 10,* 87–100.

Strauss, R. P. (1989). Psychosocial responses to oral and maxillofacial surgery for head and neck cancer. *Journal of Oral and Maxillofacial Surgery, 47,* 343–348.

16

Care for the Child With Early Onset of Cancer

Margie Wells-Friedman, M.S., CCC-SLP

According to the National Cancer Institute (NCI, 1996, p. 1), "cancer in children is rare." The majority of childhood cancers are central nervous system cancers, with 11,300 new pediatric cases diagnosed annually (Reichley, 1994). The most frequently occurring types of childhood cancers include leukemia, neuroblastoma, brain tumor, Hodgkin's disease or other lymphoma, osteosarcoma, Wilms' tumor, Ewing's sarcoma, rhabdomyosarcoma, and retinoblastoma (American Cancer Society [ACS], 1992).

Although cancer is the primary cause of death from disease among children between the ages of 1 and 15 years, the rate of death has dropped approximately 60% over the last 40 years (ACS, 1992). Of the leukemias, acute lymphocytic leukemia (ALL) has an outcome cure rate of about 70%. Acute myelogenous leukemia (AML), a less frequently occurring and more resistant form, has a cure rate of only approximately 40% (Odom, 1995).

It is widely asserted that treatment should be conducted "at a major medical center with experience in treating children" (NCI, 1996, p. 1). This is best accomplished through the cooperative care of a qualified team of pediatric specialists including, but not limited to, hematologists/oncologists, physicians, radiologists and radiation therapists, nurses, pathologists, physiatrists, rehabilitation therapists (speech-language pathologists, occupational therapists, and physical therapists), audiologists, nutritionists/dietitians, child life therapists, teachers, social workers, chaplains, and psychiatrists. These individuals work together to treat the cancer itself and the consequences of cancer treatment.

Children with cancer are caught up in the process of growth and development, which continues throughout the period of their treatment and beyond. The families are profoundly influenced by the disease and its treatment and side effects (NCI, 1988b). Medical and rehabilitation specialists must take it upon themselves to become aware of the many types of treatment and of the consequences of the disease on the developing child and family. There is a need to understand the roles of other team members and to link them to the overall plan of care for each child requiring rehabilitation. The ultimate goal of the plan of care is to achieve the best quality of life and outcome possible for each child and his or her family.

The speech-language pathologist's role on the rehabilitation team for a child with cancer varies depending on the diagnosis, stage, and sequelae of the disease and its treatment. The role will involve assessment

257

and intervention/rehabilitation of communication disorders, dysphagia, and eating disorders. Intervention may occur in the acute, periodic acute, outpatient, and reintegrated stages of recovery. This chapter attempts to define the role of the speech-language pathologist in relation to pediatric hematology/oncology under the general guidelines of the stages of recovery, specific pediatric considerations, and common diagnoses. The more frequently occurring cancer types and the wide variety of their sequelae are discussed with illustrative examples where possible. A single chapter cannot provide detailed information relative to the specific evaluation and treatment of speech-language and swallowing deficits in pediatrics. Therefore, references are made to more inclusive literature and readings on these topics.

CONSIDERATIONS RELATED TO CANCER TREATMENT IN PEDIATRICS

Audiology

As with all pediatric patients, children in treatment for cancer should receive an audiological evaluation to rule out hearing loss prior to speech-language treatment and, often, prior to cancer treatment. Given the use of ototoxic drugs during some chemotherapies, it is essential that periodic audiological evaluation and follow-up be completed. The primary ototoxins implicated in recent research have been cisplatin and carboplatin (Fausti, Schechter, Rappaport, Frey, & Mass, 1982; Helson, Okonkwo, Anton, & Cvitkovic, 1978; Komune & Snow, 1981; Simpson, Schwan, & Rintelmann, 1992). Schell et al. (1989) found that hearing loss in their sample of children and young adults "was directly related to the cumulative dose of cisplatin" (p. 754). They also noted that patients receiving radiation treatment followed by cisplatin had a high probability of acquiring a significant hearing loss. Further, the use of serial audiograms was recommended for patients whose cumulative dose of

cisplatin exceeded 360 mg/m^2 as well as for "irradiated patients, very young children (who must be conditioned to respond to conventional audiometry), patients receiving cisplatin with other known or suspected ototoxins, and patients receiving cisplatin in combination with new investigational agents" (p. 759). Although pediatric cancer centers throughout the country have established protocols for audiological evaluations, it is essential that the speech-language pathologist monitor hearing status and alert physicians to any changes and to the need for further evaluation throughout the cancer patient's treatment process.

Nutrition

The side effects of chemotherapy that may influence feeding, swallowing, and nutrition in pediatrics include, but may not be limited to, nausea and vomiting, mouth sores and ulcers (oral mucositis), altered taste, constipation, lethargy, tiredness, and lack of coordination (NCI, 1994). Should neurological impairment occur as a result of brain tumor, neurosurgery, chemoradiation therapy, or other treatments or complications, impairment can occur in the swallowing process itself, resulting in impaired nutritional intake. Children are particularly prone to developing food refusals as well as malnutrition, which can result in immune suppression and infections (Van Eys, 1984). As members of dysphagia or feeding teams at pediatric cancer centers, speech-language pathologists must work closely with physicians and nutritionists in providing preventive and interventive care for children receiving chemotherapy.

Aspects of feeding and nutritional support may include parent counseling and education to assist the family and patient in coping with the diet and behavioral changes required to maintain adequate nutrition and hydration (Dunn Klein & Delaney, 1994; van Eys, 1984). The primary interventionists at this level will most often be the nurse and nutritionist, who educate patient and family as well as monitor for outcome. Occasional direct mealtime intervention by a speech-language pathologist may be required for patients and families to develop functional behavioral plans to improve intake, decrease food refusals, and alter diets. For instance, a child may experience oral mucositis, as in approximately 39% of those treated with high-dose methotrexate (Rask, Albertoni, Schroder, & Peterson, 1996), and may require a soft, moist, bland, or blenderized diet to maintain oral intake (Dunn Klein & Delaney, 1994). The family that experiences difficulty coping with a child during such changes may require the assistance of a speech-language pathologist experienced in treating food refusals and behavior management. Should a child require supplemental feeding via nasogastric tubing or other means, direct treatment may assist the family in continuing with some minimal level of oral intake. Several excellent resources to providing such therapy include Chatoor, Dickson, Schaefer, and Egan (1986); Dunn Klein and Delaney (1994); NCI (1988a, 1988b, 1990, 1994, 1996); and Satter (1992).

Dysphagia

Feeding and swallowing disorders are associated with a wide variety of etiologies and systems within the body and require a team approach to effectively manage the patient's care. The team evaluation and treatment of pediatric dysphagia is especially valuable in pediatric cancer treatment with the many drugs, drug interactions, treatments, and their effects. This medical complexity necessitates the involvement of a group of health care professionals with varying expertise (Arvedson & Brodsky, 1993). According to Logemann (1983) the speech-language pathologist, or the "swallowing therapist" on the dysphagia team, is essential to team success. The speech-language pathologist evaluates the swallowing and feeding of the child with both bedside and radiographic methods, provides direct treatment to the child, educates the family, and communicates all aspects of the dysphagia treatment plan to the other

team members. In cancer treatment the successful plan of care will take into account specific nutritional needs, medical aspects of the diagnosis, drug interactions and side effects, as well as family involvement.

Many of the patients undergoing posterior fossa brain tumor (PFBT) resection will experience cranial nerve paralysis leading to dysphagia. Levine (1988) lists the nerves most at risk during such surgeries as cranial nerves V, VII, IX, X, and XII. This may lead to problems with chewing, decreased intraoral or pharyngeal sensation with subsequent loss or reduction in protective gag/cough reflexes, asymmetries, poor lip seal/function, delayed swallow reflex, nasopharyngeal or gastroesophageal reflux, and aspiration (Arvedson & Brodsky, 1993; Groher, 1992; Logemann, 1983). Treatments with drugs such as methotrexate and vincristine as well as chemoradiation therapy can have deleterious effects on neurological function, resulting in swallowing disorders, especially in children (Allen, 1978).

Components of Pediatric Dysphagia Evaluation

A dysphagia evaluation including an oral pharyngeal motility study (OPMS) or modified barium swallow (MBS) is a complex evaluation usually completed by a speech-language pathologist in association with a radiologist. Often there is a formal team, or, on a case-by-case basis, an informal team may be developed (Wolf & Glass, 1992). Members involved in the evaluation process may include speech-language pathologist, physiatrist, occupational therapist, primary and consulting physicians, radiologist, dietitian/nutritionist, and family. Much detailed literature exists on the methods to be employed in a dysphagia evaluation (Arvedson & Brodsky, 1993; Groher, 1992; Kramer & Eicher, 1993; Logemann, 1983; Palmer, Kuhlemeier, Tippett, & Lynch, 1993; Wolf & Glass, 1992).

The evaluation typically begins with obtaining detailed medical histories and impressions from the treating physicians as well as parental report of the history of the child's problem in detail. This should include detailed information relative to type of cancer, treatment plan, phase of treatment, medications, side effects, eating and swallowing abilities prior to diagnosis, and current feeding or swallowing symptoms. This is followed by a standard pediatric bedside/chairside feeding evaluation during which the therapist assesses the child's tone, movement, head control, and seating. The oral mechanism is evaluated for symmetry, structure, motor abilities, and protective reflexes. Also included are the timing and sound characteristics of the pharyngeal swallow via cervical ausculatation, self-feeding, parent-child interaction, and voice. The speech-language pathologist and the physician are concerned with clinical signs of aspiration, respiratory changes, secretion management, signs or symptoms of gastroesophageal reflux, and behavioral influences.

If an OPMS or MBS has been requested or is indicated following the bedside/chairside feeding evaluation, the child and parent are taken to the radiology department. The child is seated in a similar position to that used at home and/or at school. The parent feeds the child during the radiographic procedure if the therapist believes that it will help the child remain cooperative and calm and if it will better replicate the typical feeding methods. The child is fed various thicknesses, textures, and bolus sizes as each swallow is evaluated for oral motor, pharyngeal motility, and control as well as the presence of aspiration. Therapeutic techniques are attempted during the OPMS to evaluate their effectiveness in improving the swallow and to maintain the patient's ability to eat at least some portion of the diet orally. This procedure is captured on videotape for review, analysis, and baseline measurement.

On completion of the evaluation, a post-diagnostic conference is held to view the videotaped swallowing examination with the parent. At that time the therapist may review the preliminary results, provide suggestions, demonstrate therapeutic methods, provide written information, and make therapy recommendations to the parent. Re-

sults are made available to the referring physician, nurses are informed, and a report is placed in the medical record immediately following the evaluation in most cases. Referrals for further evaluation or consultation with such services as gastroenterology, otolaryngology, and pulmonology may result, depending on the joint findings of the primary physician and the speech-language pathologist.

The following case presentation serves as an illustration of the complexity of dysphagia evaluation and treatment with a pediatric patient experiencing treatment for cancer. It demonstrates also the many interrelated aspects of cancer treatment and the consequences for deglutition.

Case Presentation

A male, aged 1 year 2 months, presented to the emergency room with exacerbation of chronic sinusitis and otitis media treated with intravenous antibiotics delivered at home. Two weeks later he was observed to have difficulty walking and right eye deviation inward and was taken to the emergency room. A computed tomography scan of the brain revealed a large brain tumor in the cerebellar hemisphere totally filling the fourth ventricle along with significant hydrocephalus. Posterior fossa craniotomy with excision of the anaplastic ependymoma, insertion of intraventricular catheter and insertion of a ventriculoperitoneal shunt and Mediport were the surgical procedures conducted during the acute phase.

Two days after the PFBT excision, a bedside feeding evaluation by the speech-language pathologist revealed severe dysphagia with decreased frequency of swallowing; right-sided facial paresis; hoarse, wet voice; noisy, wet cervical auscultation during the limited swallows; intermittent nonnutritive sucking; and no swallow to taste stimulation. Recommendations were for OPMS, daily dysphagia treatment, and thickening of formula presentations.

Treatment consisted of parent and staff training to decrease the irritability and/or hypersensitivity by providing maximal positional support and decreasing environmen-

tal stimulation present during feeding attempts. A gradual increase in presentations of nonnutritive sucking on a pacifier to increase soft palate movement and tongue and cheek function, taste presentations of thickened formula and baby food, and finally, slow, gentle bottle presentations of thickened formula were also components of treatment. Formula was thickened to increase acceptance of liquids by slowing the flow and to lessen the chance of aspiration. Therapy goals emphasized increasing vocalizations for improving vocal fold closure. Over the next 16 days the child improved rapidly to wean from the nasogastric tube and began taking total oral nutrition with increased frequency of swallowing, clear cervical auscultation, and no clinical signs of aspiration. Chemotherapy was in progress including cyclophosphamide, vincristine, and cisplatin. He was subsequently diagnosed with a severe-profound sensorineural hearing loss in the right ear with a probable etiology of eighth nerve damage during tumor excision. The child's hearing status was periodically reevaluated during the course of his treatment.

Prior to or during the second course of chemotherapy, the patient developed persistent episodes of choking on liquids. An OPMS or MBS revealed severe pharyngeal dysphagia with delayed initiation of swallow, pooling in the valleculae and pyriform sinuses, and excessive residue after the swallow. With thicker textures the patient emitted gag/cough/vomit cycles with nasopharyngeal reflux, gastroesophageal reflux, and several episodes of minimal aspiration. A hoarse vocal quality was noted which was later diagnosed by the otolaryngologist as bilateral vocal fold paralysis in the paramedian position. A gastrostomy tube was subsequently placed and developmental and oral motor therapies were initiated.

A follow-up OPMS several months later was conducted at the mother's request, as she had been giving the patient his bolus gastrostomy feeds as well as "tastes of baby food and sips of iced tea" (against medical advice) with no obvious signs of aspiration. Results indicated ongoing moderate-severe dysphagia with functional swallows for pudding consistency only, and continuing problems with velopharyngeal closure and pharyngeal motility. The recommendation to the physician was to consider continuing gastrostomy feeding as the primary source of nutrition with supplemental oral feedings of pudding-level consistencies allowing dry swallows to clear each bolus. Parent training at the conclusion of the evaluation included review and explanation of the OPMS videotape, as well as discussion and demonstration of precautions and treatments such as thickening procedures and consistencies, as the family resided far from the hospital site. Dysphagia therapy was recommended, with referral to sites closer to the family locale.

SPECIFIC DIAGNOSES

Leukemia

As the most frequently occurring cancer among children, leukemia presents a daunting prospect to the developing child. Various aspects of the treatment can potentially influence normal development, such as the many visits to clinics, frequent and lengthy hospitalizations, chemotherapy, and chemoradiation therapy (Haupt et al., 1994). One study of long-term survivors of standard-risk ALL suggested "minimal intellectual toxicity" of methotrexate and 18-Gy chemoradiation therapy, with increased risk for those patients receiving more aggressive treatments (Mulhern, Ochs, & Fairclough, 1992, p. 480). Neuropsychological outcome is of importance to the speech-language pathologist, as it so closely relates to language functioning in general.

Children with cancer who receive chemoradiation therapy may suffer structural changes in the brain such as calcifications, which can result in difficulties with information processing, memory, and attention deficits 1 to 3 years later. These consequences vary widely and seem related to age at treatment, dosage, size and location of the radiation field, and so forth (Copeland, 1992). Combination treatments including chemotherapy with chemoradiation therapy can result in deficits in areas such as visual processing speed, visual-motor integration, sequencing, and short-term memory (Cousens, Water, Said, & Stevens, 1988). Murdoch, Boon, and Ozanne (1994) found a wide variation of language outcomes, and specific impairments in the areas of receptive semantics and syntax; expressive semantics, syntax, and vocabulary; and listening, reading, and written language and syntax have been reported to occur following central nervous system prophylaxis for ALL. They also suggested "a tendency for the proportion of children treated for ALL exhibiting a language impairment to increase with the time post-treatment" (p. 121). Haupt et al. (1994) further indicated that IQ reductions can be observed 3 years posttreatment and the greatest reduction may be measured 5 years posttreatment for ALL survivors. Given these late effects of treatment, referrals for appropriate management must be made by informed parents, educators, and health care professionals involved with such patients. Typically, treatment for these late effects will not occur during the acute phase of the recovery in the pediatric cancer center. Consequently, speech-language pathologists treating patients in all types of settings (e.g., outpatient clinics, school systems, and private clinics) must be made aware of the potential for the above-described problems to occur.

Brain Tumor

Brain tumors are the third most common type of cancer in children, with posterior fossa tumors (infratentorial) constituting two thirds of the pediatric tumors (NCI, 1996). Medulloblastoma, cerebellar astrocytoma, ependymoma, and brainstem glioma, as well as the associated treatments, are well described in other areas of this text. From a pediatric standpoint, prediagnosis and postdiagnosis abilities and skill levels related to cognitive and language domains are primary considerations of the speech-language pathologist. Outcomes may include decreased capacities in the areas of global intellectual skill, per-

ception, attention, memory, and executive function as well as in receptive and expressive language abilities (Hudson & Murdoch, 1992a, 1992b, 1992c; Hudson, Murdoch, & Ozanne, 1989; Mulhern, 1996). These deficits may occur only in the acute stages of the disorder/recovery, may surface later in treatment, or may become chronic and long-term.

Long-term language impairment can be a consequence of postsurgical radiation-therapy for brain tumor (Hudson et al., 1989) or a result of a combination of influences such as central nervous system prophylaxis, age at diagnosis, type of tumor, presence and severity of hydrocephalus, and duration of pretreatment symptoms (Murdoch & Hudson-Tennent, 1994a). Reportedly mild and sometimes transient language impairments may occur also in patients undergoing PFBT resection (Hudson & Murdoch, 1992a). The sensory, motor, and cognitive impairments listed above will impede a child's ability to achieve and learn academically (Mulhern, 1996). In addition, these learning difficulties may have a delayed emergence, making it essential that speech-language pathologists be aware of their presence and the need for early intervention. This can be accomplished through family education, yearly follow-up, neuropsychological and speech-language evaluation, and periodic review of the changing needs of the child.

Various levels of academic support are available to the child returning to school. Mulhern (1996) has identified five different levels that may be available for children upon their return to school. These levels are outlined in Table 16–1. Mutism and dysarthria as postsurgical complications of PFBT excision, with or without chemoradiation therapy, have been reported since at least the early 1980s (Al-Jarallah, Cook, Gascon, Kanaan, & Sugueira, 1994; Dailey, McKhann, & Bergerm, 1995; Kingma, Mooij, Metzemaekers, & Leeuw, 1994; Pollack, Polinko, Albright, Towbin, & Fritz, 1995; Rekate, Grubb, Aram, Hahn, & Ratcheson, 1985). The following terms have been used in the literature concerning PFBT: pseudobulbar palsy, cerebellar mutism, transient

TABLE 16–1. Levels of Academic Support for Children in Schools

Level	Description
1	Fully mainstreamed
2	Mainstreamed with resource room assistance from learning disabilities teachers and therapists
3	Part-time placement in exceptional education classes with some mainstreaming
4	Self-contained fulltime exceptional education class (i.e., specific learning disability or traumatic brain injury)
5	Homebound education (e.g., for acute or chronically ill patients)

mutism, oral pharyngeal apraxia, posterior fossa mutism, transient cerebellar mutism, and mutism and subsequent dysarthria.

Descriptions of the disorder have varied and range from brief anecdotal observations (Rekate et al., 1985) to more detailed analyses (Murdoch & Hudson-Tennent, 1994a, 1994b). The characteristics that have been included in various descriptions of children with PFBT appear in Table 16–2.

The reported incidence of postsurgical mutism following posterior fossa brain tumor resection varies in the literature. Van Calenbergh, Van De Laar, Plets, Goffin, and Casaer (1995) suggest it may be as low as 7.9%, whereas Van Dongen, Castman-Berrevoets, and Van Mourik (1994) suggest a rate as high as 30%. In the more comprehensive reviews the rates are generally considered to be lower than 10% of the total number of PFBT resection cases. Therefore, a speech-language pathologist working with a pediatric population should be aware of the possible symptoms and treatments as well as the expected recovery. Evaluation and treatment techniques for motor speech disorders are well represented in the literature (Caruso, 1995; Murdoch & Hudson-Tennent, 1994b).

The following case presentation serves as an illustration of the many possible side effects of brain tumor and its treatment via PFBT resection and chemoradiation therapy. In addition, it describes the type and extent of speech-language and dysphagia treatment required.

Case Presentation

A female, aged 5 years 2 months, experienced a 2 to 3-week history of irritability, *headaches, hallucinations, and difficulty with balance (ataxia) prior to hospital admission. A computed tomography scan revealed hydrocephalus and a PFBT predominantly involving the fourth ventricle. Preoperative teaching was conducted by the child life therapist and neurosurgeon. Initial surgery was for placement of a unilateral occipital ventriculoperitoneal shunt followed by craniotomy 8 days later for tumor excision. The postoperative period was eventful for one-time use of the word Mom followed by several weeks of "mutism," emotional lability, severe ataxia, severe dysarthria, feeding difficulties, and urinary retention.*

The patient was evaluated during the acute phase of the initial hospitalization by occupational therapy, physical therapy, and speech-language pathology. In addition, the child life therapist provided intervention as necessary for preprocedure teaching, sibling intervention, and parent education to support the child's overall psychosocial well-being. The speech-language pathologist completed communication and bedside feeding evaluations 10 days after craniotomy. These evaluations resulted in the following abbreviated list of symptoms:

1. *Initial inability to voice on command (mute), able to exhale on command, using voice to moan and groan primarily.*
2. *100% reliability of yes/no response, smiling, and head nods to orientation, memory, and general knowledge questions.*
3. *Severe flaccid dysarthria with*
   ■ *Left facial weakness, low tone, asymmetries*
   ■ *Right tongue weakness, low tone, asymmetries*

TABLE 16–2. Characteristics of Children with Posterior Fossa Brain Tumors

Characteristic	Reference
Complete mutism in a conscious state	(Van Calenbergh et al., 1995)
Immediate or delayed onset of mutism	(Al-Jarallah et al., 1994; Kingma et al., 1994; Van Calenbergh et al., 1995)
Variable duration of mute stage: from 17 days to 6 months	(Hudson et al., 1989)
May have emotional lability	(Pollack et al.,1995)
May affect deglutition/swallowing	(Dailey et al., 1995; Pollack et al., 1995)
May affect other volitional movements such as eye opening, voiding	(Pollack et al., 1995)

- *Velopharyngeal weakness, depressed gag response, hypernasality*
- *Decreased respiratory support for speech and motor acts*
- *Decreased loudness control, monotonous*
- *Decreased pitch control, limited range, monotonous, pitch breaks*

4. *Moderate oral stage dysphagia (pureed diet, thickened liquids, 3 weeks of nasogastric tube supplementation)*

Speech-language pathology treatment in the acute phase encompassed several areas, including parent counseling, education, and training; improvement of oral control for speech and feeding; provision of temporary augmentative communication method; as well as improvement of control of exhalation and voicing for speech production. Initial treatment was 1–2 times daily progressing to once daily prior to discharge to home, 4 days after initial speech-language pathology consult. Acute phase activities included the following:

1. *Oral motor exercises to increase volitional control of the mechanism through massage, physical assistance to complete oral motor commands, and later alternating movements of the articulators.*
2. *Parent education regarding dysarthria and its expected progression, feeding and swallowing, safety concerns relating to decreased communication skills,*

nonverbal communication methods, and emotional lability.

3. *Voicing control exercises to increase volitional control for speech through laryngeal jiggling to stimulate cough and tickling to stimulate laugh. These and any other spontaneous voicing events were called to the patient's attention, and attempts were made at repeating the voicing with reinforcement following.*
4. *Breath support to provide volitional control of exhalation for speech via exercises to increase abdominal/diaphragmatic breathing, prolong exhalation for blowing bubbles and feathers, and later combining breath control with voice control.*

Treatment continued in the periodic acute and outpatient phases with occupational therapy, physical therapy, and speech-language pathology provided in the home setting for approximately 2 full years. Further language testing revealed difficulties with both recent and remote recall of auditorily presented material. Clinical treatments by the speech-language pathologist consisted of 40 hour-long sessions over an 8-month period. Treatment activities included continuation and expansion of the early phase oral motor exercises interspersed with functional feeding and articulation activities; memory-enhancing exercises to teach strategies; abdominal breathing exercises extending the length and control of exhalation for blowing and speech; and vocal exercises to improve pitch control, stress and intonation, and loudness control. The patient improved from the levels described in the acute phase to producing intelligible, slightly slowed speech in phrases and sentences of approximately eight syllables in length. She had a slight nasal quality notable to the trained ear, pitch breaks, and a limited singing voice. Memory for verbal material improved to immediate and delayed recall of strings of up to 5 words and three-step related oral commands. Memory for facts from simple short stories and story retelling was also improved. She went on to attend prekindergarten for several weeks accompanied by her mother for half days initially. She attended regular education in kindergarten with mobility problems related to balance and ataxia, as well as problems with dysarthria and socialization.

A second surgery was performed 5 years after the first for a recurrence. This was followed by chemoradiation therapy. Neuropsychological testing was conducted before and after chemoradiation therapy. Academic difficulties became apparent again in the fourth grade, with overall slow speed of writing and reading comprehension, and ongoing problems with physical education and socialization. In the fifth grade at 6 years after initial surgery she was transferred to a special education private school where she received physical therapy, occupational therapy, speech-language pathology treatments, and small class instruction. Neuropsychological testing and program updates are conducted yearly to assist the family in providing for this child.

CONCLUSIONS

Children with cancer are at risk for communication, swallowing, and feeding disorders, as well as cognitive or learning disorders, at many points during and following their treatment. Younger children, and those receiving chemoradiation therapy, high-dose chemotherapy, or neurosurgical removal of brain tumors appear to be at particularly high risk. The speech-language pathologist has an active role to play in the diagnosis and treatment of these varied disorders throughout the many phases of cancer treatment and beyond. This can be accomplished through evaluation and periodic reevaluation; supporting other professional disciplines; providing direct therapy to patients; educating family members, staff, and teachers; and functioning as a child advocate.

REFERENCES

Al-Jarallah, A., Cook, J. D., Gascon, G., Kanaan, I., & Sugueira, E. (1994). Transient mutism following posterior fossa surgery in children. *Journal of Surgical Oncology, 55*, 126–131.

Allen, J. C. (1978). The effects of cancer therapy on the nervous system. *Journal Pediatrica, 93*, 903–909.

American Cancer Society. (1992). *Facts on childhood cancer* (Rev. ed.) [Brochure]. ACS Publication No. 2081.

Arvedson, J. C., & Brodsky, L. (1993) *Pediatric swallowing and feeding.* San Diego, CA: Singular Publishing Group.

Caruso, A. J. (Ed.). (1995). Motor speech disorders in children. *Seminars in Speech and Language, 16.*

Chatoor, I., Dickson, L., Schaefer, S., & Egan, J. (1986). A developmental classification of feeding disorders associated with failure to thrive: Diagnosis and treatment. In D. Drotar (Ed.), *New directions in failure to thrive: Implications for research and practice.* New York: Plenum Press.

Copeland, D. R. (1992). Neuropsychological and psychosocial effects of childhood leukemia and its treatment. *CA: A Cancer Journal for Clinicians, 42*, 283–295.

Cousens, P., Waters S., Said J., & Stevens, M. (1988). Cognitive effects of central nervous system prophylactic treatment of cancer in children. *Journal of Clinical and Experimental Neuropsychology, 10*, 495–538.

Dailey, A. T., McKhann, G. M., II, & Bergerm, M. S. (1995). The pathophysiology of oral pharyngeal apraxia and mutism following posterior fossa tumor resection in children. *Journal of Neurosurgery, 83*, 467–475.

Dunn Klein, M., & Delaney, T. A. (1994). Nutrition and feeding for the child with cancer. In *Feeding and nutrition for the child with special needs* (pp. 353–358). Tucson, AZ: Therapy Skill Builders.

Fausti, S. A., Schechter, M. A., Rappaport, B. Z., Frey, R. H., & Mass, R. E. (1982). Early detection of cisplatin ototoxicity. *Cancer, 53*, 224–231.

Groher, M. (Ed.). (1992). *Dysphagia: Diagnosis and management*. Stoneham, MA: Butterworth-Heinemann, Reed.

Haupt, R., Fears, T. R., Robison, L. L., Mills, J. L., Nicholson, H. S., Zeltzer, L. K., Meadows, A. T., & Byrne, J. B. (1994). Educational attainment in long-term survivors of childhood acute lymphoblastic leukemia. *JAMA, 272*, 1429–1432.

Helson, L., Okonkwo, E., Anton, L., & Cvitkovic, E. (1978). Cis-platinum ototoxicity. *Clinical Toxicology, 13*, 469–478.

Hudson, L. J., & Murdoch, B. E. (1992a). Chronic language deficits in children treated for posterior fossa tumour. *Aphasiology, 6*, 136–150.

Hudson, L. J., & Murdoch, B. E. (1992b). Language recovery following surgery and CNS prophylaxis for the treatment of childhood medulloblastoma: prospective study of three cases. *Aphasiology, 6*, 17–28.

Hudson, L. J., & Murdoch, B. E. (1992c). Spontaneously generated narratives of children treated for posterior fossa tumour. *Aphasiology, 6*, 549–566.

Hudson, L. J., Murdoch, B. E., & Ozanne, A. E. (1989). Posterior fossa tumours in childhood: Associated speech and language disorders post-surgery. *Aphasiology, 3*, 1–18.

Kingma, A., Mooij, J. J. A., Metzemaekers, M. D. M., & Leeuw, J. A. (1994). Transient mutism and speech disorders after posterior fossa surgery in children with brain tumours. *Acta Neurochirurgica, 131*, 74–79.

Komune, A., & Snow, J. B. (1981). Potentiating effects of cisplatin and ethracrynic acid in ototoxicity. *Archives of Otolaryngology, 107*, 594–596.

Kramer, S. S., & Eicher, P. M. (1993). The evaluation of pediatric feeding abnormalities. *Dysphagia, 8*, 215–224.

Levine, T. L. (1988). Swallowing disorders following skull base surgery. *Otolaryngologic Clinics of North America, 21*, 751–759.

Logemann, J. (1983). *Evaluation and treatment of swallowing disorders*. Austin, TX: Pro-Ed.

Mulhern, R. K. (1996, November). *Evaluation and intervention for learning-impaired children with cancer*. Paper presented at the 20th Annual Seminar: Advances in Pediatric Hematology/Oncology of the Florida Association of Pediatric Tumor Programs, Tampa, FL.

Mulhern, R. K., Ochs, J., & Fairclough, D. (1992). Deterioration of intellect among children surviving leukemia: IQ test changes modify estimates of treatment toxicity. *Journal of Consulting and Clinical Psychology, 60*, 477–480.

Murdoch, B. E., Boon, D. L., & Ozanne, A. E. (1994). Variability of language outcomes in children treated for acute lymphoblastic leukemia: An examination of 23 cases. *Journal of Medical Speech-Language Pathology 2*, 113–123.

Murdoch, B. E., & Hudson-Tennent, L. J. (1994a). Differential language outcomes in children following treatment for posterior fossa tumours. *Aphasiology, 8*, 507–534.

Murdoch, B. E., & Hudson-Tennent, L. J. (1994b). Speech disorders in children treated for posterior fossa tumours: Ataxic and developmental features. *European Journal of Disorders of Communication, 29*, 379–397.

National Cancer Institute. (1988a). *Diet and nutrition—A resource for parents of children with cancer*. NIH Publication No. 88–2038.

National Cancer Institute. (1988b). *Young people with cancer: A handbook for parents* (Rev. ed.) NIH Publication No. 92–2378.

National Cancer Institute. (1990). *Eating hints: Recipes and tips for better nutrition during cancer treatment*. NIH Publication No. 912079.

National Cancer Institute. (1994). *Managing your child's eating problems during cancer treatment*. NIH Publication No. 94–2038.

National Cancer Institute. (1996). *PDQ information for health care professionals: Childhood acute lymphocytic leukemia* [On-line]. Available: CancerNet.

Odom, L. (1995). *Acute leukemia of childhood and adolescence* [On-line]. Available: OncoLink, Pediatric Leukemias, University of Pennsylvania.

Palmer, J. B., Kuhlemeier, K. V., Tippett, D. C., & Lynch, C. (1993). A protocol for the videofluorographic swallowing study. *Dysphagia, 8*, 209–214.

Pollack, I. F., Polinko, P., Albright, A. L., Towbin, R., & Fitz, C. (1995). Mutism and pseudobulbar symptoms after resection of posterior fossa tumors in children: Incidence and pathophysiology. *Neurosurgery, 37*, 885–893.

Rask, C., Albertioni, F., Schroder, H., & Peterson, C. (1996). Oral musocitis in children with acute lymphoblastic leukemia after high-dose methotrexate treatment without delayed elimination of methotrexate: Relation to pharmacokinetic parameters of methotrexate. *Pediatric Hematology and Oncology, 13*, 359–367.

Reichley, M. L. (1994, June 27). Rehab role vital in pediatric oncology. *Advance for Speech-Language Pathologists and Audiologists, 4,* 21.

Rekate, H. L., Grubb, R. L., Aram, D. M., Hahn, J. F., & Ratcheson, R. A. (1985). Muteness of cerebellar origin. *Archives of Neurology, 42,* 697–698.

Satter, E. (1992). The feeding relationship. *Zero to Three, 12,* 1–9.

Schell, M. J., McHaney, V. A., Green, A. A., Kun, L. E., Hayes, F. A., Horowitz, M., & Meyer, W. H. (1989). Hearing loss in children and young adults receiving cisplatin with or without prior cranial irradiation. *Journal of Clinical Oncology, 7,* 754–760.

Simpson, T. H., Schwan, S. A., & Rintelmann, W. F. (1992). Audiometric test criteria in the detection of cisplatin ototoxicity. *Journal of the American Academy of Audiology, 3,* 176–185.

Van Calenbergh, F., Van De Laar, A., Plets, C., Goffin, J., & Casaer, P. (1995). Transient cerebellar mutism after posterior fossa surgery in children. *Neurosurgery, 37,* 894–898.

Van Dongen, H. R., Catsman-Berrevoets, C. E., & Van Mourik, M. (1994). The syndrome of cerebellar mutism and subsequent dysarthria. *Neurology, 44,* 2040–2046.

Van Eys, J. (1984). The concept of rehabilitation in pediatric oncology. In A. E. Gunn (Ed.), *Cancer rehabilitation* (pp. 195–218). New York: Raven Press.

Wolf, L., & Glass, R. (1992). *Feeding and swallowing disorders in infancy: Assessment and management.* Tucson, AZ: Communication Skill Builders.

17

Hearing Management

Annelle V. Hodges, Ph.D., and Brenda L. Lonsbury-Martin, Ph.D.

Communication skills, while of primary importance to all humans, become even more crucial during serious illness. Such abilities are necessary so that the patient can maintain an open dialogue with health care providers that ensures therapeutic compliance. In addition, communication skills are critical so that the patient preserves satisfactory interactions with significant family members and friends at the time of a grave affliction. The initial stage of the communication process involves the ear's capability to process sound stimuli. Without the ability to hear, conversational interchange becomes extremely difficult, especially for patients who are mentally and/or physically compromised because of the severity of their disease.

It is notable that many of the treatments for oncologic diseases, particularly the chemotherapeutic ones, have the potential to cause hearing impairment due to their innate ototoxicity. Additionally, radiation therapy involving the head and neck and, specifically, the temporal bone region also has the capability of directly harming the peripheral hearing apparatus. Finally, even treatments that appear not to purposely target the ear, such as the filtered-air therapies used for some immunologically compromised patients, can potentially cause

hearing loss due to the damaging effects that the noisy laminar airflow units can have directly on the cochlea's hair-cell receptor cells.

The principal approach toward avoiding or alleviating treatment-related hearing problems in severely ill patients is to evaluate the baseline status of their hearing capability and to serially assess the effects of the treatment on hearing at regular intervals during the therapeutic period. Due to some of the delayed effects of ototoxic compounds as well as radiation therapy, an argument can also be made for evaluating hearing capability regularly for up to 1 year following the completion of treatment. A detailed knowledge about the encroachment of illness-related therapy on the communication skills of the patient should affect the patient's treatment. That is, information that the patient's hearing is deteriorating should alert the primary health care provider so that the patient and family can be reminded about the potential adverse consequences of the treatment, and, perhaps, the informed consent agreement should be renewed. However, most importantly, if at all possible the treatment plan should be modified so that less ototoxic agents are used or a less toxic dosing regimen is instituted. Clearly, the choice between hearing impairment and death makes such risky treatments understandable. However, a discerning awareness of the consequent levels of exposure to damaging treatments is necessary to reduce risk, limit any actual loss, and facilitate management of the patient whose hearing is adversely affected.

The following discussion reviews the essential components of the standard diagnostic audiological test battery as a mechanism for assessing pretreatment, intratreatment, and posttreatment hearing abilities. In addition, some special-purpose tests aimed at sensitively detecting the onset stages of treatment-related hearing loss are also discussed. Finally, detailed information about the application of these tests in patients who are being treated for oncologic diseases is presented.

DIAGNOSTIC AUDIOLOGICAL TEST BATTERY

The routine diagnostic audiological assessment protocol consists of the pure-tone audiogram to examine hearing sensitivity, speech audiometry to assess the reception and discrimination of speech sounds at both threshold and suprathreshold levels, and aural-acoustic immittance testing, which evaluates the functional status of the outer and middle ear's sound-transmission apparatus. The conventional air-conduction pure-tone audiogram tests the frequency range extending from 0.25–8 kHz. This examination is typically performed in octave steps (i.e., 0.25, 0.5, 1, 2, 4, and 8 kHz), but testing at the semioctave frequencies of 3 and 6 kHz is commonly included as well. Hearing thresholds are considered to be normal by convention when they are ≤ 20 dB HL. It is not uncommon for a mean or pure-tone average hearing level to be reported for the frequencies that most prominently contribute to speech understanding (e.g., 1, 2, and 3 kHz).

In cases where impaired hearing is noted, it is standard practice to use bone-conduction testing to determine hearing thresholds in the absence of the outer and middle ear sound-transmission system. In this manner, a bone vibrator that is typically placed on the mastoid process of the temporal bone is used to test frequencies from about 0.25-6 kHz. Any identified difference between the air- and bone-conducted thresholds is designated as an air-bone gap, and such discrepancies are attributed to a dysfunctional middle ear sound-transmission system. Under normal-hearing conditions, the thresholds for bone-conducted signals are essentially equivalent to the air-conducted ones.

The speech reception or recognition threshold (SRT) is the hearing threshold for speech sounds. The SRT is defined as the lowest hearing level at which a patient correctly recognizes standardized, usually recorded, speech stimuli 50% of the time. The SRT is most commonly determined for speech stimuli in the form of spondaic words, i.e., bisyllabic words with equal stress on both syllables. The hearing level outcome of the SRT test should be in accordance with the pure-tone audiometric hearing levels. In addition, as part of the speech audiometry diagnostic battery, speech-discrimination ability is established by testing the intelligibility of suprathreshold, phonetically balanced, monosyllabic words. Typically, normal-hearing individuals exhibit speech-discrimination scores that are better than about 90%. Once pure-tone thresholds have deteriorated, both tests show appreciable changes in that the SRT becomes elevated and the speech-discrimination score decreases.

Finally, as part of the immittance-audiometry battery of tests, both tympanometry and acoustic-reflex testing are performed. Tympanometry, which establishes the static compliance and pressure of the middle ear, is usually performed using a low-frequency probe tone around 200–230 Hz. Static compliance is considered to be normal at values >2 acoustic mmhos, whereas middle ear pressures between about −100 and +100 daPa are assumed to be normal. As part of this examination of middle ear function, thresholds for the middle ear's acoustic reflex are also determined for eliciting stimuli applied both ipsilaterally (probe tone and eliciting tones are applied to the same test ear) and contralaterally (probe tone is applied to the ipsilateral test ear, whereas the eliciting stimulus is in the contralateral ear). Typically, ipsilateral thresholds are established for eliciting tones at 1 and 2 kHz, whereas contralateral thresholds are obtained for 0.5-, 1-, 2-, and 4-kHz tones. Acoustic-reflex thresholds are considered normal, if they are ≤100 dB HL.

The determination of hearing thresholds and speech recognition ability are behavioral tests in that the audiologist depends on the patient to signal that a tone or word is heard. Such tests are considered to be subjective in that the examiner must depend on the patient's cooperation in fully complying with the accompanying instruction set. In contrast, the immittance-related tests are objective in that the patient simply sits quietly while the middle-ear evaluation is performed by the examiner.

SPECIAL-PURPOSE AUDIOLOGICAL TESTING

Special audiological tests include high-frequency audiometry, auditory brainstem responses (ABRs), and evoked otoacoustic emissions (OAEs). High-frequency audiometry or determining the threshold levels for the perception of pure tones that are higher in frequency than the highest test frequency examined by the conventional audiogram at 8 kHz is, again, a behavioral test in which the patient must contribute a high degree of compliance to ensure that a valid test is achieved. In contrast, both the ABR and OAE tests are objectively based, and, because they are automatically performed, they require only minimal compliance from the patient. That is, the only obligation that the patient has is to follow the instructions to remain as physically quiescent and as acoustically quiet as possible. OAEs differ from the ABR in that they represent an acoustic, rather than an electrically based, response measure. Thus, rather than being susceptible to the interfering properties of poor electrical environments (e.g., 60-Hz "hum"), OAEs are more vulner-

able to the ambient noise levels of test surroundings that include sounds made by both test personnel and nearby medical support equipment, as well as the patient (e.g., coughing, snoring, respiratory rales). Details of these three special-purpose audiometric tests are described below.

High-Frequency Audiometry

Testing of the extended frequency range usually includes the frequencies from 9–20 kHz. Whereas the lower extent of this range is typically tested at approximately 1-kHz intervals (e.g., at 9, 10, 11.2, and 12.5 kHz), the frequencies higher than about 12 kHz are examined in 2-kHz intervals (e.g., 14, 16, 18, and 20 kHz). The testing of higher frequencies, which is an option that is common to many of the commercially available audiometers, requires a special set of headphones and calibration procedures that are distinct from those needed to achieve a valid examination of the lower frequencies that make up the conventional assessment range. Normative data are not available for the high frequency audiometric test range. However, it is commonly assumed that thresholds >80 dB HL represent abnormal sensitivity.

Auditory Brainstem Responses

ABRs are obtained using electrophysiological recording techniques that are based on stimulus-locked averaging. Thus, to effect a differential-recording montage, a set of surface electrodes, which act as the active and reference sites, is attached, typically to the vertex of the scalp and to either the mastoid or earlobe ipsilateral to the ear receiving the stimuli, respectively. In addition, a common or ground electrode is affixed, usually to the forehead or neck. With this configuration, a series of electrical potentials consisting of five to seven sequential waveforms that occur within 10 ms of the onset of a brief stimulus (e.g., click) is recorded.

The ABR represents the activity of the initial auditory neural pathway coursing from the output of the cochlea to the upper brainstem region. Although the source of each ABR wave is not exactly known, it is well accepted that the structures that contribute to the formation of these potentials include the auditory portion of the eighth cranial nerve; the lower brainstem auditory relay nuclei, consisting of the cochlear nucleus and the nuclei of the superior olivary complex; and the midbrainstem region consisting of the lateral lemniscus. It is clear that, although the ABR can measure electrical activity from the auditory pathway that is specific to each ear by application of monaural stimuli, each record represents the contributions of the neurons and connecting fiber tracts (e.g., trapezoid body) that course between ipsilateral and contralateral structures as part of the primary ascending auditory pathway. Although it is possible to limit the electrophysiological examination to the cochlea itself by using a procedure referred to as electrocochleography (ECoG), this procedure is not frequently used as a special-purpose audiometric test. The major reasons that the ECoG is not commonly used to evaluate the condition of the initial stage of the auditory nervous system is that lengthy protocols are required to assess the minuscule electrical responses of the cochlea, and only a few relatively expensive instruments are in the marketplace.

Otoacoustic Emissions

Evoked OAEs are sounds made by the cochlea during its normal processing of incoming acoustic signals (Kemp, 1978). The OAEs represent a relatively new response measure that is unique in that it primarily assesses the operation of the cochlea's outer hair cell (OHC) system (Brownell, 1990), that is, the auditory receptor that makes the principal contribution to the ear's ability to sensitively detect sounds. This feature of OAEs to specifically test OHC function contributes a major benefit toward the evaluation of the peripheral auditory system, because it is precisely this class of receptor cell that is most vulnerable to diseases and external agents that cause the majority of hearing problems. In particular, the OHCs are especially vulnerable to ototoxins and to excessive noises in that both these external agents initially damage or destroy these sensory cells. Moreover, because OHCs are primarily responsible for the fine threshold of hearing and sharp frequency tuning manifested by normal ears, they are sensitive to the early stages of hearing loss, which initially affect these threshold-related attributes. Additionally, because OAEs are acoustic rather than electrical signals, they can be recorded in a straightforward manner. Thus, they are noninvasively measured by merely placing an acoustic probe containing a miniaturized microphone assembly securely in the outer ear canal.

The evoked OAEs that are used most commonly in clinical settings include the transient evoked and the distortion-product OAEs. The transient evoked OAEs (TEOAEs) are recorded by methods that are similar to the ABR in that a series of brief acoustic stimuli, such as clicks, are presented to each ear separately, and a response is determined through a time-locked averaging of the resulting signals emitted by the ear (Glattke & Robinette, 1997; Kemp, 1978; Kemp, Ryan, & Bray, 1990). Because of the acoustic features of the click used by the commercially available instrumentation, TEOAEs best test the frequency region extending from about 500 Hz to 4 kHz for adult ears, and from about 1-6 kHz for the ears of infants and children. The distortion-product OAEs (DPOAEs) represent a slightly more complex test of the OHC system, because they are elicited by two pure tones, related in frequency, that are applied simultaneously to the test ear (Kemp, 1979; Kimberley, Brown, & Allen, 1997; Lonsbury-Martin, Martin, & Whitehead, 1997). Because of the tonal nature of the eliciting stimuli, DPOAEs provide precise information that is more frequency related than do TEOAEs. The commercial instrumentation available to test DPOAEs typically assesses the frequency region from 0.5–8 kHz, with some instruments extending the upper-frequency test range to about 10 kHz. This type of analysis is usually referred to as a DP-gram, and it essentially describes the frequency pattern of remaining OHCs that are functioning reasonably normally.

There is no question that evoked OAEs make an ideal test for monitoring patient ears for a potential ototoxic drug reaction due to their special ability to specify the status of OHC function and the knowledge that the OHC system represents the primary target of such agents. However, there are several important limitations to OAE measures. First, more than 50% of the population over about 65 years has a hearing loss (Wax & DiPietro, 1991), which typically involves frequencies >4 kHz. Unfortunately, it is this age group that exhibits the more serious diseases that require treatment with ototoxic drugs such as cisplatinum (CP) and the aminoglycoside antibiotics. Because OAEs are reduced or absent as hearing levels decline to about 35-55 dB HL, many of the older patients who would benefit from OAE monitoring have no measurable emissions for the frequencies maximally affected by ototoxins (Lonsbury-Martin, Cutler, & Martin, 1991; Stover & Norton, 1993). Second, to ensure a valid measure of OAEs, it is absolutely essential that the middle ear system operate normally due to the critical role of its conduction apparatus in transmitting both the evoking stimulus from the ear canal to the cochlea, and the emission from the cochlea to the ear canal (Owens, McCoy, Lonsbury-Martin, & Martin, 1992; Margolis & Trine, 1997). Fortunately, a fairly small percentage of elderly patients have incapacitating middle ear problems, but if they exist, it is impossible to test OHC function adequately using OAEs.

It is also important to note that, although OAE, ABR, and immittance measures do not require a sound-treated testing environment, the traditional audiological test battery as well as high frequency testing are routinely administered within the confines of a conventional double-walled test chamber situated in the audiology clinic. Because, during treatment, therapy often sickens patients, they frequently are incapable of traveling between diagnostic areas that usually are distributed over great distances within a medical center. Thus, abbreviated "screening" versions of the audiological examination are available, and can be per- formed within the treatment area. Consequently, in order to document baseline function reasonably accurately, it is advantageous to administer screening versions of the audiogram, ABR, and evoked OAEs in the oncologic clinic setting, rather than in the standard audiological sound-treated environment.

HEARING LOSS IN ONCOLOGIC DISEASE

In most cases, other than primary tumors of the outer and middle ear, acoustic neuromas, or some skull-base glomus tumors that affect the blood supply to the inner ear, the underlying carcinoma itself is unlikely to affect the hearing of the patient. However, nasopharyngeal tumors, for example, can sometimes invade the middle ear space and adversely influence the sound-conduction pathway in a direct manner. Most commonly, though, the adverse influence of malignancies on hearing comes from the injurious effects that the treatment modalities can have on the hearing apparatus itself. Such treatment effects frequently include ototoxicity caused by drug agents that are generally included in chemotherapeutic treatments, and/or irradiation damage produced by radiation therapy to structures critical to the hearing process.

After surgery, the current treatment for curing or palliating advanced cancer relies mainly on chemotherapy based on platinum compounds, of which the most widely used is CP or cis-diamminedichloroplatinum II. CP can be administered alone, but, typically, it is given in combination with other pharmacological agents. The most active regimens combine CP with 5-fluorouracil, or with vincristine and methotrexate (Planting, de Mulder, de Graeff, & Verweij, 1997). The ototoxicity of CP is well known (Cersosimo, 1989), as is the influence of the dose, schedule, and mode of administration (Vermorken, Kapteyn, Hart, & Pinedo, 1983) on the amount of drug-induced hearing loss. It is also clear that definitions of ototoxicity and the methods of auditory testing also influence the incidence of CP toxicity reported in the literature (Wake, Takeno, Ibrahim, & Harrison, 1994). However, it is indisputable that the ear is most affected by single, high-dose injections, and that the cumulative ototoxic effects of repeated low-dose treatments have also been noted. There is also a considerable interpatient variability in the ototoxic effect, evidenced by observations in the literature that report the incidence of CP ototoxicity when administered intravenously to range from 11–100% (Brock, Bellman, Yeomans, Pinkerteon, & Pritchard, 1991; Cohen, Zweidler, Goldwein, Malloy, & Packer, 1990; Corden, Strauss, & Killmond, 1991; Reddel et al., 1982; Schweitzer, 1993). Some of the susceptibility factors alleged to predispose an individual toward developing ototoxicity are age (i.e., very young and very old), the existence of a previous hearing loss, and a poor general medical condition (van der Hulst, Sahola, Hazanka, & Rajashekar, 1988; Weatherly, Owens, Catlin, & Mahoney, 1991). Clearly, patient selection also influences dramatically the reported incidence of CP ototoxicity in a given study.

The ototoxic action of CP is limited to the neurosensory epithelium of the cochlea, and does not involve either the central auditory pathway or the vestibular portion of the inner ear (Myers, Blakely, & Schwan, 1993). Examination of the ultrastructure of the temporal bones from patients treated with CP indicate that the primary site of its ototoxicity initially is the OHCs of the basal turn of the cochlea (Strauss et al., 1983; Wright & Schaefer, 1982). The damage then progresses apically and to the inner hair cells. Where the OHC damage is most extensive in the basal turn, changes in spiral ganglion cells (Strauss et al., 1983) and in the myelinated fibers (Wright & Schaefer, 1982) have also been reported, although it is unclear if these changes resulted from the acute ototoxic effects or from degenerative changes caused by the drug-induced destruction of the corresponding receptor cells. Although the fundamental mechanism of CP ototoxicity remains unknown, there is evidence that the drug blocks the mechanoelectrical transduction processes of the OHCs, and that this blockage even-

tually leads to cytoxicity within affected OHCs. In particular, it was inferred from the experiments of McAlpine and Johnstone (1990), who used iontophoretic methods to infuse CP into the scala media of an animal model, that CP blocked the transduction channels, which results in a reduction in hair cell receptor current and subsequent hearing loss. This imbalance of the OHC's ionic environment affects the cell's metabolic-enzyme system, which eventually results in fatal morphological damage to the receptor.

The symptoms and audiological findings in patients with ototoxicity induced by CP are most consistent with a cochlear process, which is most pronounced in the basal turn. The resulting hearing loss is commonly characterized in adults by a mild to moderate impairment of up to 40 dB that initially affects the high frequencies (i.e., frequencies >4 kHz) and that usually is bilateral, symmetrical, and permanent. However, additional treatment courses, higher dose levels, or protracted dosing schedules can eventually produce a hearing loss that extends down to affect the major speech frequencies that include those greater than 1–2 kHz. The concomitant use of diuretics such as furosemide or aminoglycosides (e.g., gentamicin) with CP exacerbates the hearing loss (Reddel, et al., 1982).

There are reports in the literature of partial recovery of hearing following completion of CP therapy (Skinner, Pearson, Amineddine, Mathias, & Craft, 1990). However, it is more common for the hearing loss to progress further within days of the termination of treatment (Sie & Norton, 1997). Indeed, the CP-induced hearing loss may begin shortly after the initiation of treatment (Yung & Dorman, 1986), or may initially appear several days after treatment. Along with the reported hearing loss problems, other common symptoms reportedly associated with CP ototoxicity include tinnitus, loudness recruitment, and otalgia (Reddel et al., 1982).

Another common treatment for cancer is postoperative focal radiation therapy to prevent local regional recurrence after resection of a malignant tumor. Despite refinements in therapies based on ionizing radiation, tumors in areas such as the parotid gland, nasopharynx, tonsil, tongue, palate, and hypopharynx expose the temporal bone, because of the standard strategy of encompassing the tumor volume with an adequate surrounding margin. Thus, a portion of the outer ear, the middle and inner ear, and adjacent brainstem are often unavoidably exposed to a significant radiation dose. Similar to the factors that increase a patient's risk for developing ototoxicity, the dose fraction and total dosage of radiation are directly related to the resulting hearing loss. Thus, daily fractions of 2–2.5 Gy and total doses of 50 Gy have been shown to cause permanent changes to inner ear as well as auditory nerve and brainstem structures (Anteunis et al., 1994).

The hearing impairment reported as a radiation sequela, which can be delayed for months or years after exposure, is often initially a mixed or conductive hearing loss due to a concomitant radiation-induced secretory otitis media. The development of middle ear disease is caused by the basic reaction of the mucosal membrane of the middle ear to irradiation, which includes an inflammation of the endothelium of blood vessels leading to vasodilation and destruction of the vascular lumen as well as desquamation (Varghese, Sahola, Hazanka, & Rajashekar, 1996). The latter effect causes the mucosa to become edematous, which subsequently leads to the formation and collection of fluid within the middle ear cavity, thus resulting in radiation otitis media with conductive hearing loss. On otoscopic examination, evidence for a secretory otitis media and erythema of the tympanic membrane are typically noted.

It also is not uncommon for a sensorineural hearing loss to develop that is more severe at the higher frequencies. In fact, recently, Grau and Overgaard (1996) found that such sensorineural hearing losses develop in about one third of patients following the application of curative radiation doses, usually within 0.5–1 year after radiation. This impairment is likely due to radiation-induced atrophic changes to the

structures of the organ of Corti, including the basilar membrane, spiral ligament, and stria vascularis, as well as to the destruction of the hair cells (Schuknect & Karmody, 1965). If the absorption of radiation is sufficient to involve the bony structures of the peripheral ear, the death of osteocytes and alterations in new bone formation appear to significantly delay the onset of hearing loss. In addition, radiation-induced retrocochlear changes such as the emergence of abnormal ABRs have also been demonstrated, particularly in patients treated for nasopharyngeal carcinoma (Lau, Wei, Sham, Choy, & Hui, 1992).

In recent years, radiation therapy and CP-based chemotherapy have been increasingly combined for the treatment of advanced malignancies following surgery (Grau & Overgaard, 1996). Unfortunately, there is evidence that the combination of ionizing radiation with CP chemotherapy can result in enhanced ototoxic effects. For example, Schell et al. (1990) prospectively tested a reasonably large group of patients who received either CP, cranial irradiation, or both. These investigators found that there was a significantly greater potentiation of ototoxicity when the two types of therapy were used together. There is also evidence that, if radiation therapy is used in conjunction with CP chemotherapy, the hearing loss associated with CP administration may be progressive beyond the termination of the drug treatment (Sweetow & Will, 1993). Moreover, prior radiation therapy to the temporal bone region may also increase a patient's risk for developing an ototoxic reaction to chemotherapy. In fact, there is evidence of a synergistic effect here, too, in that if a patient has received irradiation prior to chemotherapy, there may be augmented ototoxicity (Sweetow & Will, 1993; Walker, Pillow, Waters, & Keir, 1989).

Although the combination chemotherapy regimens in association with radiation therapy are the most popular treatments for advanced head and neck malignancies, there has been an increased interest in therapies based on the single-agent CP given at high, frequent doses, along with high doses of radiation. For example, one new recommended chemoradiation protocol incorporates high-dose intra-arterial CP therapy together with high-dose external beam radiation of about 70 Gy (Madasu, Ruckenstein, Leake, Steere, & Robbins, 1997) in order to provide a high concentration of the treatment to the site of the tumor. It is not surprising, however, that the use of such a focused and high-exposure level treatment regimen results in over half of the patients exhibiting ototoxicity, with frequencies >2 kHz maximally affected.

Applications of the Audiological Test Battery to Oncologic Disease

There is no doubt that the side effects of drug therapy should be controlled to minimize the number of patients who become ototoxic patients. This consensus is largely based on the realization that, due to the increased efficacy of treatments for cancer that are limiting the growth and spread of tumors, life expectancy is increasing. Thus, cancer patients are achieving a longer life span, and it is imperative that they also receive a better quality of life. It is also clear that proper counseling about loudness recruitment and/or tinnitus effects would significantly alleviate the patient's apprehension concerning imminent hearing difficulties. It is highly recommended, then, that careful monitoring of those exposed to ototoxic treatments should be performed so that fewer patients are left with a hearing loss.

The American Speech-Language-Hearing Association (1994) has published standardized clinical guidelines for monitoring ototoxic effects. The primary strategy recommended for identifying hearing loss related to the administration of potentially ototoxic compounds is the use of behavioral audiometry in the form of serial audiograms. For use as an ototoxicity monitor, audiometric testing depends on intrasubject comparison methods so that each patient serves as his or her own control and the criterion for identifying a critical effect is computed relative to baseline measures. Thus, to document the ototoxic

effects of drug therapy, it is necessary to perform quantitative observations of auditory function systematically during treatment. The typical protocol for monitoring pure-tone sensitivity involves obtaining a baseline audiogram before treatment begins, and then performing serial retests before each administration of the ototoxic agent.

The usual audiometric approach is to identify ototoxicity by testing with the conventional pure-tone audiogram extending from 0.25–8 kHz. Some studies, though, have focused on identifying changes only for frequencies from 1–4 kHz, based on the notion that these frequencies, which are predominately represented in the vowel sounds, are the most critical for verbal communication (e.g., Blakley, Gupta, Myers, & Schwan, 1994). However, it is important to stress that the higher frequencies from 4–8 kHz, which are represented in some of the consonant sounds (e.g., *f*) as well as the voiceless fricatives (e.g., *th*), are also critical for speech audibility. Most importantly, though, once a hearing loss is detected within the conventional frequency-test range, it is clearly too late to prevent an ototoxic reaction that has the potential of affecting speech understanding, because the hair cells tuned to the frequencies associated with drug-induced elevations in threshold have already been irreparably damaged and/or destroyed. Thus, it is widely recognized that screening over the conventional test range cannot detect the early changes of cochleotoxic effects.

The rationale for evaluating hearing above the conventional test range is based on the knowledge that hearing loss as a result of CP treatment has been shown to typically begin in the highest frequency region corresponding to the basal end of the cochlea. A number of investigators have evaluated hearing above 8 kHz in patients treated with ototoxic compounds, and they have found that it is these higher-frequency thresholds that are usually affected first, with hearing loss progressing to the lower frequencies throughout the course of treatment (Fausti, Schechter,

Rappaport, Frey, & Mass, 1984; Kopelman, Budnick, Sessions, Kramer, & Wong, 1988; Dreschler, Van der Hulst, Tange, & Urbanus, 1989). Thus, because the high-frequency thresholds are affected first, identification of the initial hearing loss at these frequencies provides the earliest possible warning before the loss includes frequencies crucial for verbal communication. It is important to note that, although the usefulness of high frequency audiometry in monitoring for ototoxicity was reported over a decade ago, it is still not commonly used in the serial evaluation of the effects of ototoxic treatment regimens on hearing.

There is no doubt that behavioral audiometry is the gold standard for identifying ototoxicity-induced hearing loss. However, there are reasons for using a less subjective test in documenting such changes in hearing status. For example, at times critically ill patients simply cannot adequately comply with subjective testing paradigms. In these instances, objective testing is needed.

A number of clinical studies have shown that the ABR is an efficient way of demonstrating or monitoring ototoxicity (Guerit, Mahieu, Houben-Giurgea, & Herbay, 1981; Hotz, Kaufmann, & Allum, 1990). In general, the most common observation is an increased latency in Waves I and V, with a resulting increase in the Wave I–V interlatency interval (Hotz et al., 1990). This outcome is expected in conditions in which the cochlea is the target structure for ototoxins, because Wave I is thought to assess the output of the cochlea at the level of the cochlear nerve. Thus, it would be most sensitive to any treatment-induced changes in cochlear function.

Early experimental work in both animals and humans showed that the simple, non-invasive technique of OAE testing was extremely sensitive to cochlear condition (Avan, Bonfils, Loth, Narcy, & Trotoux, 1990; Harris & Probst, 1991; Lonsbury-Martin, Martin, & Balkany, 1994; Martin, Franklin, Harris, Ohlms, & Lonsbury-Martin, 1990). Because the OAEs reflect the functional status of OHCs, with known

OHC damage, OAEs are greatly reduced or even absent. Thus, the evoked OAEs have properties that are ideal for ototoxicity-monitoring programs in which the primary goal is to identify the initial signs of an ototoxic-drug reaction of the ear. Because OHCs are the primary target of ototoxic compounds, it is not surprising that a number of case studies have appeared in the literature that document the aftereffects of CP treatment on both TEOAEs and DPOAEs (e.g., Ozturan, Jerger, Lew, & Lynch, 1996).

For example, in Figure 17–1, the results of CP treatment in a 26-year-old female patient with a neuroblastoma are shown by comparing pretreatment versus posttreatment measures. Comparison of the pretreatment (solid circles) and posttreatment (open circles) audiograms shown in Figure 17–1A for the patient's right ear indicate that, following the initial bolus injection, the ototoxic agent produced a mild hearing loss of about 30–40 dB for frequencies above 4 kHz, and appeared to elevate thresholds above control levels for all test tones above 2 kHz. Similarly, the DP-grams illustrated in Figure 17–1B reflect a drug-induced reduction from baseline measures for frequencies greater than about 3 kHz. However, as might be expected based on the frequency-specific elevation in hearing thresholds, the spectral configuration of the corresponding TEOAEs (pretreatment: Figure 17–1C; posttreatment: Figure 17–1D) showed little difference in emission levels over the approximately 1- to 4-kHz range tested with the standard click stimuli. These results demonstrate that OAEs (in this case, particularly DPOAEs) can act as objective indicators of a developing, frequency-specific ototoxicity.

The plots of Figure 17–2 show in another patient the satisfactory ability of OAEs to track the frequency pattern of a resulting CP-induced hearing loss. This 8-year-old female patient was also diagnosed with a neuroblastoma. In these plots, the hearing and emission results are compared for the right ear between the baseline record (solid circles) and those obtained after the

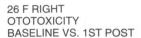

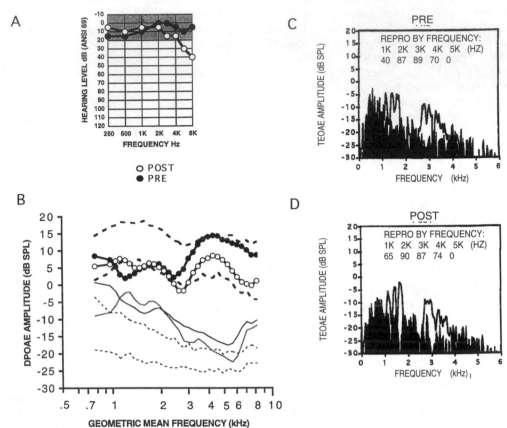

Figure 17–1. Hearing and evoked-emission test results for the right ear of a 26-year-old female patient with a neuroblastoma obtained before (solid circles) and after treatment (open circles) with a bolus injection of CP. In **A**, the conventional behavioral audiogram shows that before drug injection hearing was normal. The stippling indicates the region considered clinically normal. After treatment, note the hearing levels for 6 and 8 kHz were elevated to 30–40 dB HL. The DP-gram plot of **B** shows the DPOAE levels for this ear before and following CP administration as a function of the geometric-mean frequency of the primary tones ($f_2/f_1 = 1.21$; $L_1 = L_2 = 75$ dB SPL). The top pair of bold dashed lines around 3–15 dB SPL shows the ± 1 standard deviation (SD) boundaries of the mean DPOAE levels measured with these stimulus parameters from 94 ears of normal-hearing adults, to indicate the expected DPOAE amplitudes for normal ears. The lower pair of light dashed lines show the ± 1 SD limits of the corresponding noise-floor levels. It is clear that the pretreatment DPOAE levels (solid circles) were essentially within the normal range from 0.8–8 kHz. Following CP (open circles), the DPOAE levels for frequencies ≥ 5 kHz were reduced below normal limits, which was consistent with the elevated hearing thresholds for 6–8 kHz depicted in the behavioral audiogram. The lower solid lines indicate the average noise floor for this patient associated with the pretreatment and posttreatment records. The spectrum of the pretreatment TEOAE responses evoked by click stimuli of approximately 80 dB $_{peak}$SPL, measured using the ILO88 device, is shown in **C**. TEOAE components (open area) were present above the background noise (filled area) between approximately 1–4 kHz during the baseline period, as expected for a normal adult ear. The percentage values ("REPRO BY FREQUENCY") given at the top right of each TEOAE panel are measures of the reproducibility of the TEOAE response, determined by cross-correlation of the two independently averaged TEOAE waveforms. In general, a reproducibility value >50% indicates the presence of a genuine TEOAE response. The posttreatment TEOAE spectrum shown in **D** is essentially identical to the baseline record of **C**. Note that in the other examples of patient test results presented in the following figures, the format of the plots illustrating the results of behavioral hearing, DPOAE, and TEOAE tests are the same as in this figure.

278

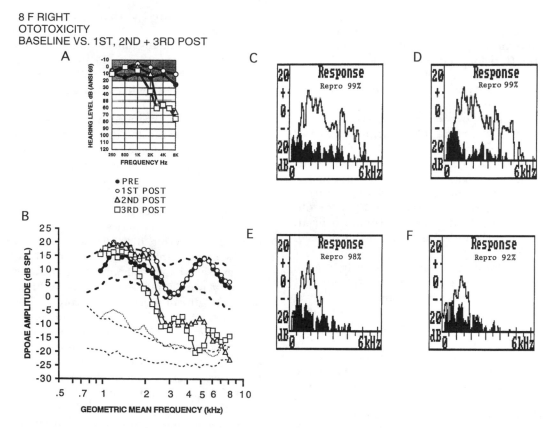

Figure 17–2. Hearing and evoked-emission test results for the right ear pretreatment (filled circles) and post-treatments #1 (open circles), #2 (open triangles), and #3 (open squares) with a bolus injection of CP for an 8-year old female with a neuroblastoma. Note that for the results of behavioral-audiogram testing shown in **A**, there was a slight improvement in the pattern of normal hearing following dose #1. However, doses #2 and #3 elevated hearing thresholds to 55–75 dB HL for frequencies >2 kHz. The DP-grams of **B** indicate emission levels within normal limits for the pretreatment and posttreatment #1 records. However, doses #2 and #3 reduced DPOAE levels to essentially noise-floor levels for frequencies greater than about 2 kHz. Similar findings are shown in **C–F** for TEOAEs in that the baseline (**C**) and posttreatment #1 records (**D**) were almost identical, whereas the TEOAEs recorded following doses #2 and #3 (**E** and **F**, respectively) show that this emission was immeasurable for frequencies greater than about 2 kHz.

first (open circles), second (open triangles), and third (open squares) CP-infusion sessions. It is clear from the data depicted in Figure 17–2A that, after the initial drug treatment in the form of a bolus injection, a notable improvement in hearing occurred. Similarly, although the post-treatment #1 TEOAE spectrum in Figure 17–2D appeared similar to the baseline record of Figure 17–2C in its frequency extent, level, and repeatability (i.e., "Repro" factors of 99%), DPOAEs for frequencies from 0.8–3 kHz also improved. In contrast,

a few weeks later, the second treatment produced a high-frequency hearing loss of about 60 dB for frequencies above 2 kHz. This considerable hearing loss was clearly reflected in both the corresponding DPOAE and TEOAE recordings (Figures 17–2B and 17–2E, respectively), which showed reduced OHC activity for frequencies greater than about 2–3 kHz. Moreover, after the third CP treatment, hearing levels declined even further (Figure 17–2A), with frequencies above 1 kHz being maximally affected. Similarly, the corresponding DP-gram (Figure 17–2B) and TEOAE spectrum (Figure 17–2F) again indicated that the ototoxic drug essentially abolished OHC function for frequencies above 1.5 kHz. The CP infusions affected the related measures of this patient's contralateral left ear in a manner that was identical to that described above for the right ear.

The patient example presented in Figure 17–3 underscores how evoked OAEs can contribute additional information about ototoxic damage that assists the audiologist in developing a valid intervention strategy. In this case, the 59-year-old female with advanced epithelial ovarian cancer had undergone several schedules of chemotherapy that included CP. It is clear from the clinical audiograms in Figure 17–3A for the left (solid circles) and right (open circles) ears that the ototoxic drug had produced a permanent, bilateral hearing loss for frequencies above 3–4 kHz. However, considering the configuration of the hearing loss, which maximally affected the high frequencies of the conventional hearing range, the patient unexpectedly complained about having difficulties with distorted hearing and in conversing with others, particularly in the presence of background noise. In fact, she had come to the otology/audiology clinic specifically to request a hearing aid that she anticipated would improve her communication skills. Understandably, the attending audiologist was reluctant to prescribe this rehabilitative approach to her problem until her OAE records were reviewed. It is clear from the DP-grams shown in Figure 17–3B that, surprisingly, the DPOAE levels for this patient were abnormally low, across the entire frequency-test range. Similarly, rather than displaying the approximately 10-dB levels typically exhibited by adults, on average, the TEOAEs illustrated in Figures 17–3C and 17–3D, for the right and left ears, respectively, also reflected abnormally low levels of emission activity. Together, these OAE findings implied that the patient would probably benefit from a hearing-aid effected amplification of sound for frequencies less than about 4 kHz. Indeed, the patient

was fully satisfied with her corrective amplification.

Several systematic clinical studies reported in the literature have documented the efficacy of evoked OAEs to detect ototoxicity due to treatment with aminoglycoside antibiotics. The configuration of the resulting hearing loss produced by these agents is essentially identical to the pattern caused by CP: an initial impairment in high-frequency hearing that progressively involves the mid to lower frequencies as treatment continues. For example, Hotz, Harris, and Probst (1994) used TEOAEs to monitor amikacin therapy in a series of nine patients, who were receiving high doses because of life-threatening infections. These investigators discovered a partially reversible decrease in the overall TEOAE level after, at least, 16 days of treatment. Because the reproducibility index, which is automatically calculated by the commercial device used to test TEOAEs (the ILO88, Otodynamics Ltd), exhibited greater sensitivity to the deterioration of emissions at the higher frequencies around 4 kHz than did the amplitude measure, the authors recommended its usefulness as a monitor of the ototoxic effects of, at least, aminoglycoside treatment.

In a more recent study, Mulheran and Degg (1997) examined DPOAEs in a group of 15 young patients with cystic fibrosis, who had been treated regularly with the ototoxic antibiotic gentamicin for recurrent respiratory infections. These investigators showed that DPOAEs were reduced in the majority of the patients, especially around 4 kHz, in the presence of normal hearing. They concluded that OAEs are sensitive to the earliest reductions in OHC activity caused by an ototoxic drug, although the effects of the cystic fibrosis condition, itself, on cochlear function were not ruled out.

Zorowka, Schmift, and Gutjahr (1993) were first to report the serial use of evoked OAEs in combination with pure-tone audiometry to monitor auditory changes in a small population of eight child and young-adult patients receiving CP therapy as an antitumor treatment. In this study,

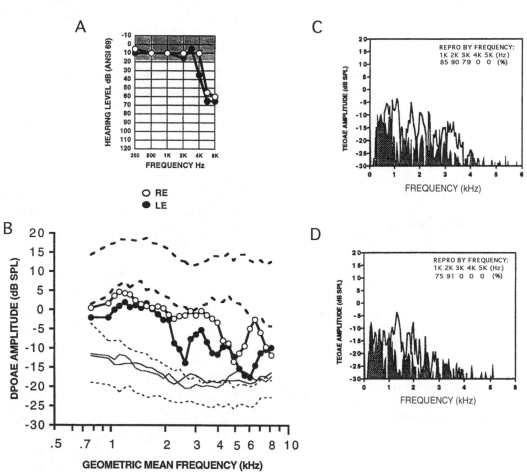

Figure 17–3. Hearing and evoked-emission test results for the left (filled circles) and right (open circles) ears of a 59-year-old female who received CP as part of her antitumor therapy for ovarian cancer. Note in **A** the bilateral high-frequency hearing loss associated with ototoxicity. The DP-grams of **B** indicate that DPOAE levels were abnormally low across the entire test range, with the left ear exhibiting lower levels than the right ear. The TEOAE plots for the left (**C**) and right (**D**) ears also reflected this asymmetry in that the frequency extent for the left ear extended only to approximately 3 kHz, whereas the right ear exhibited responses up to approximately 4 kHz.

click-based TEOAE testing was performed immediately before and after various numbers of drug doses. Zorowka et al. (1993) reported a reduction in the peak levels of TEOAEs following treatment in all patients. Their detailed Fourier analysis of the TEOAE waveforms typically showed amplitude reductions over the whole spec-

trum of frequencies tested (i.e., 0.6–6 kHz). In about one half of the patients, the audiometric hearing impairment correlated well with the absence of corresponding TEOAE frequencies, particularly for those frequencies where a permanent hearing loss of more than 30–35 dB HL occurred. In several patients, however, TEOAEs for frequencies around 4 kHz were absent posttreatment, in the absence of any related changes in the pure-tone audiogram. Like the findings reported above for the Mulheran and Degg (1997) study, these latter results, again, suggest that OAEs may be a more sensitive detector than conventional audiometry of initial cochlear dysfunction due to ototoxic agents.

Our own laboratory has performed a pilot study aimed at documenting the utility of evoked OAE testing in a series of 33 oncologic patients with a variety of advanced pulmonary and head and neck tumors, who were undergoing treatment with a regimen of antineoplastic pharmacological agents that included CP. One goal of the study was to evaluate the effectiveness of TEOAEs compared to DPOAEs in detecting drug-induced changes in hearing ability. A further aim was to determine if OAEs could detect reduced cochlear function within the conventionally tested hearing range before a clinical hearing loss was evident. The study population included several patients who were commencing a second or even a third course of chemotherapy, as well as some who had previously undergone radiation therapy to the affected anatomic region. The experimental protocol was designed to encourage excellent patient follow-up by testing on the day that patients returned to the hospital for their next round of chemotherapy. Thus, each record was acquired approximately 3 weeks after the previous drug treatment, immediately prior to the next infusion of CP.

Overall, the OAEs, particularly the higher frequency DPOAEs between 4–8 kHz, detected drug-induced OHC dysfunction in 92% of the patients, whereas hearing thresholds for the standard and/or high-frequency pure tones were elevated by CP exposure in 82% of the patients. Thus, in some patients, the OAEs were more sensitive than measures of behavioral hearing to the earliest ototoxic changes in OHC function. It is interesting to note, though, in many of the patients who had exhibited baseline thresholds that were testable by high-frequency audiometry, CP-induced increases in hearing thresholds were measurable along with reductions in the lower frequency OAEs.

Figures 17–4 and 17–5 illustrate the behavioral and OAE findings for the right and left ears, respectively, of a 59-year-old female patient with a non-small cell lung carcinoma and metastasis, who received two relatively high-dose (100 mg/m²) CP treatments, in combination with the cytotoxic agents vincristine and 5-fluorouracil. The initial baseline audiogram (solid circles) illustrated in Figure 17–4A for the right ear showed a mild hearing loss of about 10–20 dB for frequencies above 3 kHz that was likely due to presbycusis. The mild loss was reflected in the pretreatment high-frequency audiogram of Figure 17–4B, which was measurable only to 10 kHz with thresholds ≤ 80 dB HL. However, the pretreatment DP-gram of Figure 17–4C showed that, even though the DPOAE levels for frequencies above 2 kHz were closer to the –1 standard deviation limit than were those for frequencies below 2 kHz, they still were clearly within normal limits. Similarly, the corresponding baseline TEOAE record of Figure 17–4D showed click-evoked emission activity that extended up to about 5 kHz, in the presence of several odd "notched" regions, in which TEOAEs were either very low-level (approximately 1.5–2 kHz), or absent (approximately 3.5–4 kHz). Following the first dose of CP (open circles), hearing thresholds became more elevated for test frequencies above 3 kHz, DPOAEs were reduced from their control levels for frequencies greater than about 2.5 kHz, and the peak of TEOAE activity (Figure 17–4E) observed between 4–5 kHz was diminished. The open triangles of Figures 17–4A–C indicate that, after the second CP treatment, hearing thresholds essentially stabilized at levels >35 dB HL, for frequencies above 3 kHz, whereas DPOAE levels continued to decrease for frequencies greater than about 3 kHz, and became immeasurable, at noise-floor levels, for frequencies greater than about 5.5 kHz. The TEOAE spectrum of Figure 17–4F also indicates that the peaks

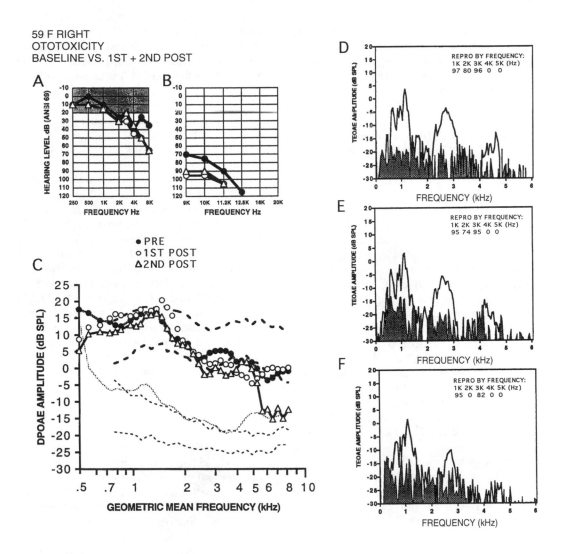

Figure 17–4. Hearing and evoked-emission test results for the right ear of a 59-year-old female with a non-small cell lung carcinoma receiving high-dose CP (100 mg/m²) in combination with 5-fluorouracil and vincristine. Plots of both conventional (**A**) and high-frequency (**B**) behavioral audiometry, obtained before (solid circles) and after #1 (open circles) and #2 (open triangles) treatments show that before treatment hearing was normal up to approximately 2 kHz, above which a mild hearing loss, likely associated with presbycusis, was observed over the higher frequency range. Three weeks following the initial treatment (open circles), hearing thresholds in the conventional range above 3 kHz were elevated to 35 dB HL or greater, whereas the testable high-frequency thresholds were shifted about 20–25 dB. After the second treatment (open triangles), there was little change in behavioral hearing. In **C**, the DP-gram shows that before treatment (solid circles) DPOAE levels were essentially within normal limits for this ear, with a tendency toward being at low-normal levels for frequencies >2 kHz. Following the first drug treatment (open circles), DPOAE levels decreased from their baseline amplitudes, especially for frequencies from about 2–5 kHz. However, after treatment #2 (open triangles), DPOAEs were below their baseline levels for frequencies greater than about 2.5 kHz, and even fell to noise-floor levels for frequencies >5 kHz. The TEOAE plots at the right show little change between the baseline (**D**) and first-treatment (**E**) records. However, the TEOAE plot in **F** shows lower levels for emissions greater than about 1.5 kHz following treatment #2. In fact, the low-level TEOAEs around 2 kHz essentially disappeared as indicated by the 0 value for the corresponding reproducibility index.

of TEOAE activity around 2–3 and 4–5 kHz were also considerably reduced by the second dose of CP. Interestingly, the TEOAEs around 2 kHz, which were very low-level during the pretreatment recording period and after dose #1, effectively disappeared, as indicated by the related 2-kHz reproducibility index, which fell from 74% after CP dose #1 in Figure 17–4D to 0% after dose #2 in Figure 17–4F.

Figure 17–5 shows complementary plots for the opposite left ear of the patient illustrated in Figure 17–4. The patterns of the CP-induced loss in hearing and cochlear function were generally similar between the two ears. However, a comparison between the effects of doses #1 and #2 supports the notion that some ototoxic ears are capable of showing improved performance following a recovery period. It is clear from the open triangles of Figures 17–5A–C that, after dose #2, hearing thresholds and DPOAE amplitudes actually recovered to near-baseline performance levels for frequencies between about 2–4 kHz. Additionally, comparing the corresponding records of Figures 17–5E and 17–5F for the TEOAEs, a notable improvement in emission activity for frequencies between 2–4 kHz was also apparent. Thus, the findings for this patient illustrate the possibility that ototoxins can differentially affect the right and left ears of the same individual, and that some improvement in peripheral ear function is feasible, at times, following chemotherapy.

A final informative example from this CP-serial monitoring study is illustrated in Figure 17–6, which shows, for a 43-year-old female patient with an adenocarcinoma of the left lung, the possibility of using OAEs for detecting the early signs of an ototoxic-induced change in cochlear function. The records of Figure 17–6 compare the baseline measures to responses obtained after the initial infusion of a low dose (50 mg/m^2) of CP along with the cytotoxin vincristine. It is clear from the pretreatment responses (solid circles) that the patient's hearing (Figures 17–6A and 17–6B) and DPOAEs (Figure 17–6C) were essentially within normal limits. Similarly,

the control TEOAEs in Figure 17–6D showed a relatively normal adult frequency pattern for emissions from about 1–4 kHz. However, following the initial chemotherapeutic dose, although hearing (open circles) over the conventional test range was minimally affected, there was a clear elevation in the thresholds of the sensitive high-frequency pure tones at 9–12.5 kHz of about 5–10 dB. Similarly, the DPOAEs of Figure 17–6C were reduced from baseline levels for frequencies above 2 kHz, and, in fact, decreased to noise floor levels for the highest test stimuli around 7–8 kHz. Moreover, the posttreatment TEOAEs of Figure 17–6E showed some reduction in activity around 3-4 kHz, as indicated by the reproducibility scores decreasing from about 83% and 87%, respectively, to 0%. Together, the evoked OAE results indicate that emissions can provide early evidence of ototoxic-induced decrements in the function of the peripheral ear in the absence of notable changes in hearing ability.

CONCLUSIONS

Hearing loss caused by treatment with ototoxic drugs and procedures is irreversible, so prevention is critical. The practice of audiological monitoring, however, during CP treatment and following the cessation of CP dosing, with or without an accompanying radiation treatment, unfortunately is not universally accepted or followed. There is no question that patients with cancer are achieving a longer life span due to improvements in their treatment. Although in many cases hearing loss is not considered relevant in the face of life-threatening disease, it is vital that these patients be monitored for such communication deficiencies, because every possible action should be taken to ensure that the prolonged life now possible has both richness and quality as well as quantity (Mencher, Novotny, Mencher, & Gulliver, 1995). Moreover, a preexisting hearing loss, which many of the older patients have, places them at a greater risk than the normal-hearing patient, because any addi-

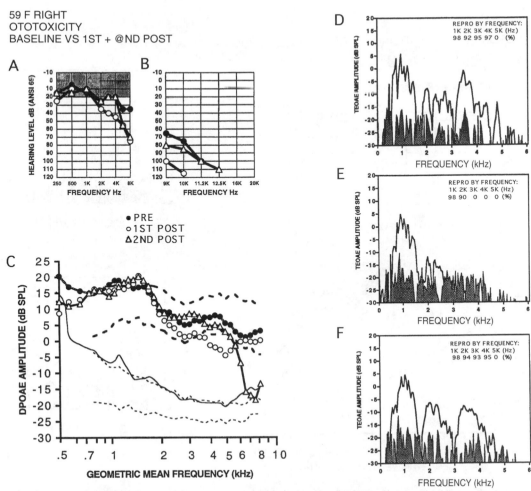

Figure 17–5. Hearing and evoked-emission test results for the left ear of the 59-year-old female patient of Figure 17–4. Plots of the results for conventional (**A**) and high-frequency (**B**) audiometry are displayed for the pre- (solid circles) and posttreatments #1 (open circles) and #2 (open triangles). Before treatment, hearing was normal up to about 4 kHz, above which a mild hearing loss was observed over the conventional test range, with high-frequency hearing being reasonably measurable only at 9 and 10 kHz. Three weeks following the initial treatment (open circles), hearing thresholds ≥1 kHz were elevated to 35 dB HL or greater, with the high frequencies becoming essentially immeasurable. After the second treatment (open triangles), behavioral hearing improved for frequencies from 2–4 kHz, and for 9 and 10 kHz. The DP-gram in **C** shows that before treatment (solid circles) DPOAE levels were essentially within normal limits for this ear. However, following the first drug treatment (open circles), DPOAE levels decreased from their control values for frequencies >2 kHz. Similar to the improvements observed for behavioral hearing, the posttreatment #2 DP-gram (open triangles) showed baselinelike levels for DPOAEs up to about 4 kHz, and then amplitudes that were further reduced for the higher frequencies. In fact, for frequencies >6 kHz, DPOAEs were essentially at noise-floor levels. The TEOAE plots at the right show considerable reductions for frequencies >2 kHz between the baseline (**D**) and first-treatment (**E**) records. However, after treatment #2 (**F**), TEOAEs returned almost to normal levels.

tional loss can immediately affect their speech-communication ability, and, thus, adversely affect their quality of life. It is widely recognized that the far-reaching and emotional effects of hearing loss are often underestimated in practice. However,

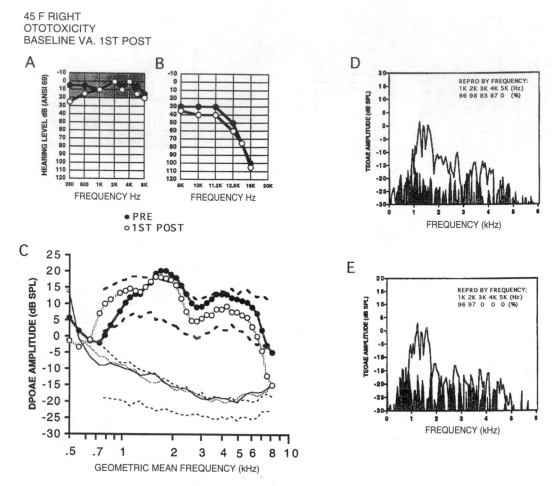

45 F RIGHT
OTOTOXICITY
BASELINE VA. 1ST POST

● PRE
○ 1ST POST

Figure 17–6. Hearing and evoked-emission test results for the right ear of a 43-year-old female with an adenocarcinoma of the left lung who received a combination chemotherapy infusion of low-dose CP (60 mg/m²) and vincristine. **A**: Pretreatment behavioral hearing (filled circles) showing normal thresholds over the conventional test range, and 50 dB HL or better thresholds for frequencies from 9–12.5 kHz. However, following CP therapy (open circles), whereas conventional hearing remained essentially normal, the high-frequency thresholds were elevated by about 10 dB. **B**: Pretreatment DP-gram (solid circles) showing DPOAE levels within normal limits compared to posttreatment DPOAEs (open circles), which were reduced for frequencies greater than about 2 kHz, and even dropped to noise-floor levels for the very highest test frequencies. Note the slight improvement in the low-frequency DPOAEs from approximately 0.7–1 kHz. **C**: Pretreatment TEOAE spectrum showing a frequency distribution from about 1–4 kHz that represents a relatively normal adult pattern. **D**: Posttreatment TEOAE spectrum showing essentially the same frequency distribution as displayed in **C**, but with lower emission levels for frequencies from 3–4 kHz as evidenced by the 0 values for these reproducibility indices.

the risk of serious hearing problems for these patients is even more likely in the future, because the newer, aggressive strategies incorporate high-dose CP, which has been shown to cause profound deafness (Buhrer, Weinel, Sauter, Reiter, & Riehm, 1990).

Audiological monitoring is crucial to the early identification of cochlear damage and the resulting hearing impairment. The benefits of early identification of change in hearing include the option to change the chemotherapeutic protocol to prevent further damage, or to allow for early rehabilitative measures if further damage is unavoidable. There is no doubt that the earlier a hearing loss is identified, the sooner an appropriate amplification device can be used to minimize the adverse effects of high-frequency hearing loss on communication abilities.

A highly recommended monitoring protocol is to assess cochlear function before, during, and at the completion of drug treatment whenever possible (Shulman, 1979). It is an ethical necessity that all patients undergo audiological testing before applying potentially ototoxic therapeutic modalities, and they should also be adequately informed about the potential sequelae of such treatment. Because significant changes in auditory ability have been reported for frequencies above 8 kHz, the inclusion of high-frequency audiometry in the monitoring of potential ototoxic patients is also advisable. From our knowledge of the well-described progression of ototoxicity from such known pharmacological agents as CP from high to low frequencies, identifying a drug-induced hearing loss before it affects the frequency range associated with the majority of speech sounds would alert care providers to the onset of a communication disorder. Similarly, if radiation therapy to the head and neck region is part of the treatment plan, hearing audiometry performed for both the conventional and high-frequency ranges, immittance testing, and OAE and ABR audiometry should be performed to document the baseline condition of the auditory pathway that extends from the outer ear to the higher brainstem region.

Finally, given the cost-conscious concerns of present-day medicine, it is likely that new tests will be developed that will make it possible to monitor even the most critically ill patients as well as fiscally practical to track the hearing of all patients receiving potentially ototoxic treatments. For example, the relatively newly proposed strategy of targeting a limited number of the highest measurable test frequencies that can be obtained within a reasonably brief period offers a method of testing that could be tolerated by a greater number of patients as well as being cost-effective (Fausti et al., 1994). Moreover, for patients who cannot provide the active cooperation and attention that behavioral hearing threshold measures require, evoked OAE testing provides a practical alternative. Certainly, economical OAE-testing equipment is available in the marketplace (Decker, 1997), and sensitive detection strategies (e.g., Sutton, Lonsbury-Martin, Martin, & Whitehead, 1994) and methods of predicting the corresponding hearing level (e.g., Gorga, Stover, Neely, & Montoya, 1996) are at hand. There is no question that the tools are available to prevent a communicatively handicapping hearing loss due to cancer treatment.

REFERENCES

American Speech-Language-Hearing Association. (1994). Guidelines for the audiologic management of individuals receiving cochleotoxic drug therapy. *ASHA, 36* (Suppl. 12), 11–19.

Anteunis, L. J. C., Wanders, S. L., Hendriks, J. J. T., Langendijk, J. A., Manni, J. J., & de Jong, J. M. A. (1994). A prospective longitudinal study on radiation-induced hearing loss. *American Journal of Surgery, 168*, 408–411.

Avan, P., Bonfils, P., Loth, D., Narcy, P., & Trotoux, J. (1991). Quantitative assessment of human cochlear function by evoked otoacoustic emissions. *Hearing Research, 52*, 99–112.

Balkany, T. J., Telischi, F. F., Lonsbury-Martin, B. L., & Martin, G. K. (1994). Otoacoustic emissions in clinical practice. *American Journal of Surgery, 15* (Suppl. 1), 29–38.

Blakley, B. W., Gupta, A. K., Myers, S. T., & Schwan, S. (1994). Risk factors for ototoxicity due to cisplatin. *Archives of Otolaryngology—Head and Neck Surgery, 120*, 541–546.

Brock, P. R., Bellman, S. C., Yeomans, E. C., Pinkerton, C. R., & Pritchard, J. (1991). Cisplatin ototoxicity in children: A practical grading system. *Medical and Pediatric Oncology, 19*, 295–300.

Brownell, W. E. (1990). Outer hair cell electromotility and otoacoustic emissions. *Ear and Hearing, 11*, 82–92.

Brownell, W. E., Bader, C. R., Bertrand, D., & Ribaupierre, Y. (1985). Evoked mechanical responses of isolated outer hair cells. *Science, 227*, 194–196.

Buhrer, C., Weinel, P., Sauter, S., Reiter, A., & Riehm, H. (1990). Acute deafness in a 4-year-old girl after a single infusion of cis-platinum. *Pediatric Hematology and Oncology, 7*, 145–148.

Cersosimo, R. J. (1989). Cisplatin neurotoxicity. *Cancer Treatment Reviews, 16*, 195–211.

Cohen, B. H., Zweidler, P., Goldwein, J. W., Molloy, J., & Packer, R. J. (1990). Ototoxic effect of cisplatin in children with brain tumors. *Pediatric Neurosurgery, 16*, 292–296.

Corden, B. J., Strauss, L. C., & Killmond, T. (1991). Cisplatin, ara-C and etoposide (PAE) in the treatment of recurrent childhood brain tumor. *Journal of Neuro-Oncology, 11*, 57–63.

Decker, T. N. (1997). General recording considerations and clinical instrument options. In M. S. Robinette & T. J. Glattke (Eds.), *Otoacoustic emissions: Clinical applications* (pp. 307–332). New York: Thieme.

Dreschler, W. A., van der Hulst, R. J. A. M., Tange, R. A., & Urbanus, N. A. M. (1989). Role of high-frequency audiometry in the early detection of ototoxicity. *Audiology, 28*, 211–220.

Fausti, S. A., Schechter, M. A., Rappaport, B. Z., Frey, R. H., & Mass, R. E. (1984). Early detection of cisplatin ototoxicity: Selected case reports. *Cancer, 53*, 224–231.

Fausti, S. A., Larson, V. D., Noffsinger, D., Wilson, R. H., Phillips, D. S., & Fowler, C. G. (1994). High-frequency audiometric monitoring strategies for early detection of ototoxicity. *Ear and Hearing, 15*, 232–239.

Glattke, T. J., & Robinette, M. S. (1997). Transient evoked otoacoustic emissions. In M. S. Robinette & T. J. Glattke (Eds.), *Otoacoustic emissions: Clinical applications* (pp. 63–82). New York: Thieme.

Gorga, M. P., Stover, L., Neely, S. T., & Montoya, D. (1996). The use of cumulative distributions to determine critical values and levels of confidence for clinical distortion product otoacoustic emission measurements. *Journal of the Acoustical Society of Amerca, 100*, 968–977.

Grau, C., & Overgaard, J. (1996). Postirradiation sensorineural hearing loss: A common but ignored late radiation complication. *International Journal of Radiation Oncology, Biology, Physics, 36*, 515–517.

Guerit, J.-M., Mahieu, P., Houben-Giurgea, S., Herbay, S. (1981). The influence of ototoxic drugs on brainstem auditory potentials in man. *Archives of Otorhinolaryngology, 233*, 189–199.

Harris, F. P., & Probst, R. (1991). Reporting click-evoked and distortion-product otoacoustic emission results with respect to the pure-tone audiogram. *Ear and Hearing, 12*, 399–405.

Hotz, M. A., Kaufmann, G., & Allum, J. H. J. (1990). Shifts in brainstem response latencies following plasma-level controlled aminoglycoside therapy. *European Archives of Oto-Rhino-Laryngology, 247*, 202–205.

Hotz, M. A., Harris, F. P., & Probst, R. (1994). Otoacoustic emissions: An approach for monitoring aminoglycoside-induced ototoxicity. *Laryngoscope, 14*, 1130–1134.

Kemp, D. T. (1978). Stimulated acoustic emissions from within the human auditory system. *Journal of the Acoustical Society of America, 64*, 1386–1391.

Kemp, D. T. (1979). Evidence of mechanical nonlinearity and frequency selective wave amplification in the cochlea. *Archives of Oto-Rhino-Laryngology, 224*, 37–45.

Kemp, D. T., Ryan, S., Bray, P. (1990). A guide to the effective use of otoacoustic emissions. *Ear and Hearing, 11*, 93–105.

Kimberley, B.P., Brown, D.K., & Allen, J. B. (1997). Distortion product otoacoustic emissions and sensorineural hearing loss. In M. S. Robinette & T. J. Glattke (Eds.), *Otoacoustic emissions: Clinical applications* (pp. 181–204). New York: Thieme.

Kopelman, J., Budnick, A. S., Sessions, R. B., Kramer, M. B., & Wong, G. Y. (1988). Ototoxicity of high-dose cisplatin by bolus administration in patients with advanced cancers and normal hearing. *Laryngoscope, 98*, 858–864.

Lau, S. K., Wei, W. I., Sham, J. S. T., Choy, D. T. K., & Hui, Y. (1992). Early changes of auditory brain stem evoked response after radiotherapy for nasopharyngeal carcinoma—A prospective study. *Journal of Laryngology and Otology, 106*, 887–892.

Lonsbury-Martin, B. L., Cutler, W. M., Martin, G. K. (1991). Evidence for the influence of aging on distortion-product otoacoustic emissions in humans. *Journal of the Acoustical Society of America, 89*, 1749–1759.

Lonsbury-Martin, B. L., Martin, G. K., Balkany, T. (1994). Clinical applications of otoacoustic emissions. In F. E. Lucente (Ed.), *Highlights of the instructional courses—1994* (pp. 343–355). Alexandria, VA: American Academy of Otolaryngology—Head & Neck Surgery.

Lonsbury-Martin, B. L., Martin, G. K., & Whitehead, M. L. (1997). Distortion product otoacoustic emissions. In M. S. Robinette & T. J. Glattke (Eds.), *Otoacoustic emissions: Clinical applications* (pp. 83–109). New York: Thieme.

Madasu, R., Ruckenstein, M. J., Leake, F., Steere, E., & Robbins, K. T. (1997). Ototoxic effects of supradose cisplatin with sodium thiosulfate neutralization in patients with head and neck cancer. *Archives of Otolaryngology—Head and Neck Surgery, 123*, 978–981.

Margolis, R. H., & Trine, M. B. (1997). Influence of middle-ear disease on otoacoustic emissions. In M. S. Robinette & T. J. Glattke (Eds.), *Otoacoustic emissions: Clinical applications* (pp.130–150). New York: Thieme.

Martin, G. K., Franklin, D. J., Harris, F. P., Ohlms, L. A., & Lonsbury-Martin, B. L. (1990). Distortion-product emissions in humans: III. Influence of hearing pathology. *Annals of Otology, Rhinology, and Laryngology.* Supplement, 236, 29–44.

McAlpine, A., & Johnstone, B. M. (1990). The ototoxic mechanism of cisplatin. *Hearing Research, 47,* 191–204.

Mencher, G. T., Novotny, G., Mencher, L., & Gulliver, M. (1995). Ototoxicity and irradiation: Additional etiologies of hearing loss in adults. *Journal of the American Academy of Audiology, 6,* 351–357.

Myers, S. F., Blakley, B. W., & Schwan, S. (1993). Is *cis*-platinum vestibulotoxic? *Otolaryngology—Head and Neck Surgery, 108,* 322–328.

Mulheran, M., & Degg, C. (1997). Comparison of distortion product OAE generation between a patient group requiring frequent gentamicin therapy and control subjects. *British Journal of Audiology, 31,* 5–9.

Owens, J. J., McCoy, M. J., Lonsbury-Martin, B. L., & Martin, G. K. (1992). Influence of otitis media on evoked otoacoustic emissions in children. *Seminars in Hearing, 13,* 53–66.

Ozturan, O., Jerger, J., Lew, H., & Lynch, G. R. (1996). Monitoring of cisplatin ototoxicity by distortion-product otoacoustic emissions. *Auris, Nasus, Larynx, 23,* 147–151.

Planting, A. S. T., de Mulder, P. H. M., de Graeff, A., & Verweij, J. (1997). Phase II study of weekly high-dose cisplatin for six cycles in patients with locally advanced squamous cell carcinoma of the head and neck. *European Journal of Cancer, 33,* 1–65.

Reddel, R. R., Kefford, R. F., Grant, J. M., Coates, A. S., Fox, R. M., & Tattersall, M. H. (1982). Ototoxicity in patients receiving cis-platin: Importance of dose and method of administration. *Cancer Treatment Reports, 66,* 19–23.

Schell, M. J., McHaney, V. A., Green, A. A., Kun, L. E., Hayes, F. A., Horowitz, M., & Meyer, W. H. (1990). Hearing loss in children and young adults receiving cisplatin with or without prior cranial irradiation. *Journal of Clinical Oncology, 7,* 754–760.

Schuknect, H. F., & Karmody, C. S. (1965). Radionecrosis of the temporal bone. *Laryngoscope, 76,* 1416–1428.

Schweitzer, V. G. (1993). Ototoxicity of chemotherapeutic agents. *Otolaryngologic Clinics of North America, 26,* 759–789.

Shulman, J. B. (1979). Ototoxicity. In V. Goodhill (Ed.), *Ear: Diseases, deafness, and dizziness* (pp. 691–704). Hagerstown, MD: Harper & Row.

Sie, C. Y., & Norton, S. J. (1997). Changes in otoacoustic emissions and auditory brain stem response after cis-platinum exposure in gerbils.

Otolaryngology—Head and Neck Surgery, 116, 585–592.

Skinner, R., Pearson, A. D. J., Amineddine, H. A., Mathias, D. B., & Craft, A. W. (1990). Ototoxicity of cisplatinum in children and adolescents. *British Journal of Cancer, 61,* 779–787.

Stover, L., & Norton, S. J. (1993). The effects of aging on otoacoustic emissions. *Journal of the Acoustical Society of America, 94,* 2670–2681.

Strauss, M., Towfighi, J., Lord, S., Lipton, A., Harvey, H. A., & Brown, B. (1983). Cis-platinum ototoxicity: Clinical experience and temporal bone histopathology. *Laryngoscope, 93,* 1554–1559.

Sutton, L. A., Lonsbury-Martin, B. L., Martin, G. K., & Whitehead, M. L. (1994). Sensitivity of distortion-product otoacoustic emissions in humans to tonal over-exposure: Time course of recovery and effects of lowering L_2. *Hearing Research, 75,* 161–174.

Sweetow, R. W., & Will, T. I. (1993). Progression of hearing loss following the completion of chemotherapy and radiation therapy: Case report. *Journal of the American Academy of Audiology, 4,* 360–363.

van der Hulst, R. J. A. M., Dreschler, W. A., & Urbanus, N. A. M. (1988). High frequency audiometry in monitoring for ototoxicity. *Archives of Oto-Rhino-Laryngology, 97,* 133–137.

Varghese, G., Sahola, J. S., Hazanka, P., & Rajashekar, B. (1996). Hearing anomalies following radiation therapy for head and neck cancers. *Indian Journal of Experimental Biology, 34,* 878–879.

Vermorken, J. B., Kapteyn, T. S., Hart, A. A. N., & Pinedo, H. M. (1983). Ototoxicity of cis-diamminedichloroplatinum II. Influence of dose, schedule and mode of administration. *European Journal of Cancer and Clinical Oncology, 19,* 53–58.

Wake, M., Takeno, S., Ibrahim, D., & Harrison, R. (1994). Selective inner hair cell ototoxicity induced by carboplatin. *Laryngoscope, 104,* 488–493.

Walker, D. A., Pillow, J., Waters, K. D., & Keir, E. (1989). Enhanced cisplatinum ototoxicity in children with brain tumours who have received simultaneous or prior cranial irradiation. *Medical and Pediatric Oncology, 17,* 48–51.

Wax, T., & DiPietro, L. (1991). Managing hearing loss in later life. National Information Center on Deafness (NICD). Washington, DC: Gallaudet University.

Weatherly, R. A., Owens, J. J., Catlin, F. I., & Mahoney, D. H. (1991). Cis-platinum ototoxicity in children. *Laryngoscope, 101,* 917–924.

Whitehead, M. L., Stagner, B. B., Lonsbury-Martin, B. L., & Martin, G. K. (1994). Measurement of otoacoustic emissions for hearing assessment. In O. Ozdamar (Ed.), *Hearing and speech* (pp. 210–226). IEEE Engineering in Medicine and Biology.

Wright, C. G., & Schaefer, S. D. (1982). Inner ear histopathology in patients treated with cisplatin. *Laryngoscope, 92,* 1408–1413.

Yung, M. W., & Dorman, E. B. (1986). Electrocochleography during intravenous infusion of cisplatin. *Archives of Otolaryngology—Head and Neck Surgery, 112,* 823–826.

Zorowka, P. G., Schmitt, H. J., & Gutjahr, P. (1993). Evoked otoacoustic emissions and pure tone threshold audiometry in patients receiving cisplatinum therapy. *International Journal of Pediatric Otorhinolaryngology, 25,* 73–80.

18

Rehabilitation of Speech and Voice Deficits Following Cancer Treatments

Donna S. Lundy, M.A., CCC-SLP, and Roy R. Casiano, M.D.

Communication may be affected directly by the treatment of cancer involving the structures of the head and neck or indirectly from the complications or side effects of adjuvant treatment for carcinoma elsewhere in the body. The primary goal of speech rehabilitation in cancer patients is to optimize the potential for communication in the least amount of time. Toward this end, treatment considerations need to focus on the ability to achieve complete tumor removal while minimizing the amount of cosmetic or functional deficit. Treatment decisions also need to consider realistic goals that are consistent with the patient's medical and speech prognosis. In some cases, palliation may be the best treatment option. A patient's status may change over time due to recurrent disease, complications, side effects of treatment, aging, or the development of other medical conditions, and rehabilitation efforts must also conform to these changing demands.

Changes in the ability to produce intelligible speech are common after ablative surgery and reconstruction of the oral structures. In addition, complications from reconstruction may adversely affect articulation, voice, and resonance. Trismus, or limited oral aperture, may decrease the size of the resonating oral cavity and thus diminish vocal quality. If severe, trismus may also compromise articulation. Xerostomia (dry mouth) is a common side effect of radiation treatment secondary to inadequate salivation. Dryness may interfere with swallowing function by preventing a dry bolus from being cohesively manipulated. The excursion of solid foods through the pharynx and esophagus may be affected also. Xerostomia may also affect the resonance of sound through a dry vocal tract.

This chapter focuses on the major components of speech production that are most frequently affected by treatment of head and neck cancer: articulation, resonance, and voice. Each section presents the types of deficits seen and methods of treatment. Surgical, prosthetic, and speech rehabilitation options are discussed.

ARTICULATION

Adequate control of the lips, tongue, and palate is vital for the production of intelligible speech. Any impairment in the range of motion, strength, and/or flexibility of these dynamic articulators may affect the ability to make the precise individual speech movements and coarticulations needed in connected speech. The resulting articulatory impairments typically cluster along placement, manner, and/or voicing parameters as opposed to misarticulation of an individual or isolated phoneme. These impairments may develop following direct surgical manipulation, scarring, or an interruption in neuromuscular integrity.

Any compromise in the neuromuscular integrity along the course of the nerve roots can result in a dysarthria. Dysarthrias may develop also due to compression of nerves from primary or metastatic brain lesions. Occasionally, the effects may be temporary when nerves are stretched during surgery (neuropraxia), from the side-effects of radiation therapy, or from compression by the primary tumor itself. In other cases, resection of the nerve may be necessary and result in deinervation.

Treatment: Speech Therapy

Management of articulatory deficits that may develop following head and neck cancer treatment typically follows three paradigms. Initial efforts frequently need to be aimed at improving strength and control of the musculature. Second, traditional articulation therapy may be needed to work on specific difficulties with manner, placement, and/or voicing parameters of the disordered sounds. Third, compensatory strategies may need to be taught when the potential for adequate production is not realistic. Preliminary data indicate that patients who initiate therapy within the first 3 months posttreatment benefit the most (Logemann, Pauloski, Rademaker, & Colangelo, 1997).

Oral Facilitative Exercises

Oral facilitative exercises, or "oral aerobics," are commonly prescribed exercises designed to increase strength, range of motion, and flexibility of the oral articulators. These same exercises may also improve swallowing function, as adequate control of the oral musculature is necessary to prepare and propel a bolus from the oral cavity to the oropharynx to initiate swallowing. However, generalization between these practiced exercises and improvements in speech and/or swallowing has not been fully researched. Furthermore, although it is generally accepted that adequate strength and range of motion of the dynamic articulators are vital for intelligible speech, critical values have not been established. In a study of 102 patients who received range of motion exercises following surgical treatment for oral and oropharyngeal cancer, significant differences in global measures of swallowing and improvement in speech intelligibility were found at 3 months posttreatment (Logemann et al., 1997).

The development of strength in specific muscle groups and overall conditioning have been extensively studied by exercise physiologists. In general, muscular strength and endurance can be improved through three basic types of exercises: isometric, isotonic, and isokinetic (Saxon & Schneider, 1995). Also, it is important to consider specificity of function. The applicability of these factors to the speech musculature is unknown at this time. Thus, although the following theories apply to the skeletal muscles and overall conditioning, only selective applications may be relevant to the oral articulators.

Isometric, or static, training involves resistance without movement (Fox, Kirby, & Fox, 1987). An example of an isometric exercise to increase tongue strength would be to squeeze the dorsum of the tongue against the palate as hard as possible. Clark (1973) has found that maximal isometric contractions of 6-s duration repeated 5–10 times daily produce the best results. Atha (1982) has studied the effects of isometric exercises and found that they should be performed at maximal effort, last long enough to involve all muscle fibers, and be repeated several times daily.

Isometric exercises can also be used to develop increased range of motion. For example, tongue elevation can be practiced by forcing the tongue tip against the upper alveolar ridge.

Isotonic, or dynamic, exercises use the principles of resistance with added motion. This requires both a concentric or shortening contraction of the muscle and an eccentric or lengthening contraction. The advantage of this type of exercise is that it strengthens the targeted muscle through a range of motion as opposed to a static point. An example of an isotonic exercise to increase tongue control might be to rapidly produce with force the phoneme *cha*.

Isokinetic exercises combine resistance techniques at a constant speed of repetition. The target muscle shortens against an accommodating resistance that matches the force produced by the muscle throughout the full range of motion (Heyward, 1991). An example of this type of exercise applied to improving tongue motion and strength might be to forcefully move the tongue laterally while applying a resisting pressure from the back of a metal spoon at a constant rate of repetition (Figure 18–1).

In addition to strength and range of motion, rapidity and flexibility exercises may be performed to improve the ability to quickly move from one articulatory position to another as accurately as possible. Rapid productions of consonant-vowel syllables may assist not only production of the targeted sound but also the ability to make the rapid adjustments needed for coarticulation.

Directed Articulation Therapy

Directed articulation therapy is frequently indicated to improve production of specific phonemes and phoneme groups. Patients who have undergone anterior or lateral tongue resections may have difficulty with sounds requiring tongue elevation, tip plosion, and/or tongue protrusion. The ability to generate adequate oral air pressure for production of fricatives and plosives may

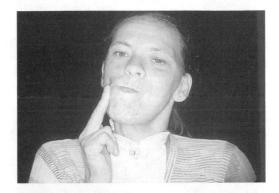
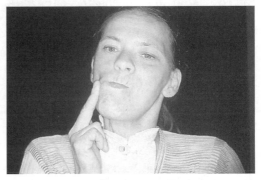

Figure 18–1. Patient performing tongue isokinetic exercises with the application of resistant pressure against the cheek (**A**) and tongue depressor (**B**).

also be compromised in patients who have undergone base of tongue resections, as the remaining tongue tissue may not be able to produce adequate and controlled forceful movements. Patients with lip incompetence following lip resections or neural compromise to that area may experience difficulties with bilabial sounds and developing adequate lip plosion. Traditional articulation therapy may improve the production of these groups of sounds.

Compensatory Techniques

Compensatory techniques may need to be considered when the patient does not have the potential for correct placement of a targeted sound or group of sounds. For example, patients who have undergone extended tonsilar/palatal resections with base of tongue involvement may be unable to produce velar consonants even after directed articulation therapy. They may, however, be able to substitute a coughlike sound for the targeted /k/ sound, which facilitates adequate intelligibility. It is interesting to note that compensatory patterns differ between patients who have undergone total glossectomy versus those that have had a partial glossectomy. Partial glossectomees have been found to make use of the residual tongue stump in adaptive movements approximating the normal movement, whereas total glossectomees use true compensatory strategies (Imai & Michi, 1992; Skelly, 1973). The primary purpose of the compensatory strategy is to improve the intelligibility of speech in the most inconspicuous manner possible. Some compensatory strategies are developed unconsciously by the patient. A comprehensive program of compensatory movements is detailed in *Glossectomee Speech Rehabilitation* by Madge Skelly (1973). Figure 18–2 demonstrates compensatory sound production for glossectomized patients.

Treatment: Surgical Options

Although complete tumor removal remains the prime objective during major head and neck cancer surgery, the emphasis today is also on immediate functional restoration through primary reconstruction. The type and extent of the surgical procedure have to be weighed against the patient's prognosis, extent of disease, and other comorbid factors influencing wound healing (e.g., history of radiation, chemotherapy, or diabetes).

The type of procedure used to reconstruct surgical defects in the oral and pharyngeal cavities may affect the strength, motion, and flexibility of the oral articulators as well as the shape of the resonating cavities. In general, the quality of life following radical surgery of the oral cavity is largely dependent on the adequacy of reconstruction (Myers, 1972). Small lesions can frequently be managed with primary closure (where structures are sutured onto themselves) or split-thickness skin grafts. In larger lesions, local or

distal flaps may be required. Secondary surgical procedures that may improve tongue mobility may also enhance the oropharyngeal resonating cavity (in the case of strictures) or improve velopharyngeal incompetence and articulation after major head and neck surgery.

Patients who have undergone reconstruction with a split-thickness skin graft typically have better speech than those reconstructed with myocutaneous or hemitongue flaps (McConnell, Teichgraeber, & Adler, 1987). Split-thickness flaps are thinner and provide less bulk. In contrast, a hemitongue flap may have reduced motion with tethering toward the defect and thus restrict articulation. Patients undergoing distal flap reconstructions may experience worse impairment in speech due to the adynamic nature of the flap and the lack of sensation and/or motor control. Speech intelligibility is influenced more by the mobility of the residual tongue than by its volume (Imai & Michi, 1992). The extent of involvement in adjacent structures may also affect the degree of speech impairment (Leonard, Goodrich, McMenamin, & Donald, 1992). In addition, bulky distal flaps may interfere with the critical range, rate, and coordination necessary for good speech and swallowing function (Pauloski et al., 1993).

Increasing experience with microvascular techniques and better patient selection have led to the increased use of free flaps as the primary choice of reconstruction for many patients (Urken, Moscoso, Lawson, & Biller, 1994). Free flaps have an advantage over traditional local or regional myocutaneous flaps by allowing sensory feedback (through sensory nerve reanastomosis) and providing more predictable tissue compatibility. The type of free flap (musculocutaneous, osseomusculocutaneous, or cutaneous) may be designed to more closely, aesthetically and functionally, reconstitute the surgically ablated area. In cases where the mandible is reconstructed, immediate placement of osteointegrated dental implants may further enhance the patient's ability to masticate and articulate more clearly. Reconstruction

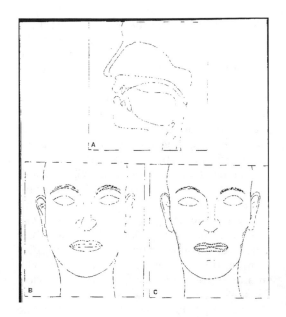

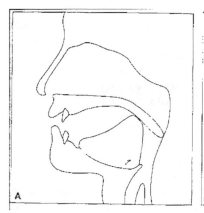

A. Normal tongue placement for [l]. The diagram does not show the lateral escape of air regarded as necessary to adequate phomeme production. B. Normal lip position for [l]. The lips can be abducted to a greater degree within phonemic limits. C. Compensatory lip and check position for [l].

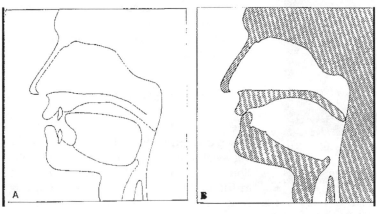

A. Normal tongue placement for [d] and [t]. B. Compensatory lip placement for [d] and [t].

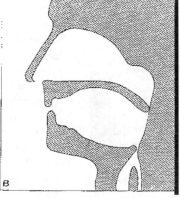

A. Normal tongue placement for [g] and [k]. B. Compensatory posterior pharyngeal bulge.

Figure 18–2. Examples of normal and compensatory sound production for /l/ (**A**), /d/ and /t/ (**B**), and /g/ and /k/ (**C**).

principles and methods are further discussed in Chapter 6.

Treatment: Prosthetic Options

Prosthetic options to assist articulatory deficits include dentures (Figure 18–3A) and palatal reshaping devices (Figure 18–3B). For example, the edentulous patient may have difficulty achieving the correct placement for interdentalized sounds. Furthermore, dentures that fit prior to surgical manipulation or irradiation may need to be adjusted due to alterations in the configuration of the oral cavity and the status of the mucosa during treatment.

Partially or totally glossectomized patients may experience difficulty making contact points between the residual tongue tissue and the palate. A palatal reshaping prosthesis lowers the palatal vault to allow the palate to contact the remaining tongue tissue and improve the articulation, including palatolingual phonemes (Colangelo et al., 1996). Rehabilitation using these devices is best accomplished through coordinated efforts between the prosthodontist and speech-language pathologist. Modifications in the shape and configuration of the palatal portion of the prosthesis frequently need to be made as the patient adjusts to the device. Specific needs are assessed by the speech-language pathologist and fabricated by the prosthodontist. Attempts have also been made to design a prosthetic tongue, although the results to date have not been especially encouraging.

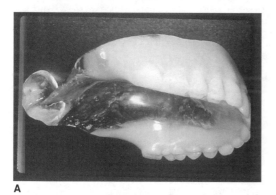

A

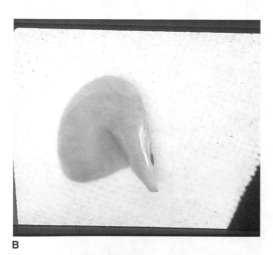

B

Figure 18–3. Prosthetic options to assist articulation production include denture prosthesis for patient post-composite resection (**A**) and palatal lowering prosthesis for partial glossectomy patient (**B**).

RESONANCE

The primary function of the soft palate is to separate the oral and nasal cavities during swallowing to prevent nasal regurgitation and to aerate and equalize pressures in the middle ear. The secondary objective of velopharyngeal closure is for speech purposes. Velopharyngeal closure is produced by sphincteric actions of the levator veli palatini and the superior pharyngeal constrictor muscles (Aronson, 1985). Closure is selective during production for all vowels and consonants except for the nasal consonants (*m, n, -ng*).

Velopharyngeal incompetence (VPI), even in small degrees, can lead to the perception of hypernasality. This may result from surgical resection of lesions extending to the palate with remaining insufficient tissue bulk, secondary scarring, and/or inadequate tissue mobility (Figure 18–4). In addition, neurological denervation (cranial nerves IX and X) may temporarily or permanently interfere with palatal motion.

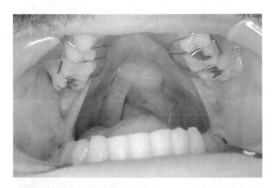

Figure 18–4. Sugical excision of a soft palate lesion with resultant hypernasality due to velopharyngeal insufficiency.

This may result from direct tumor invasion, from radiation fibrosis with compression along the nerve roots, or from necessary sacrifice during surgical resection. Velopharyngeal incompetence may also develop as part of a more centrally-based dysarthria subsequent to a primary or metastatic brain lesion or after skull base resection. In these cases, hypernasality is more often seen within the constellation of other features of a dysarthria that include respiratory, phonatory, and articulatory deficits (Aronson, 1985). Occasionally, VPI may result in nasal regurgitation.

Hyponasality is typically perceived when there is blockage of nasal airflow during production of the nasal consonants. Nasal airflow can be impeded due to a space-occupying lesion in the nasopharynx, severe obstruction of the nasal cavities, or after overcorrection of VPI.

Depending on the severity of blockage, nasal breathing may also be impaired. Treatment of hyponasality is most frequently directed to correcting the anatomic reason for obstructed nasal airflow.

Velopharyngeal closure is best assessed through videonasendoscopy in which dynamic images of the nasopharynx during production of specific speech tasks are viewed. In rare cases where nasendoscopy cannot be successfully performed, videofluoroscopic images can be obtained in lateral and basal views. Cephalometric or other static radiographs are unsatisfactory to capture the dynamic nature of sphincter closure. Completeness of closure and analysis of any gap pattern are essential to planning treatment. Small gaps with minimal bubbling of secretions may be managed with speech therapy alone. More significant VPI may require a combined approach of prosthetics, surgical reconstruction, and speech intervention.

Treatment: Speech Therapy

Speech rehabilitation is most effective in cases of mild VPI and for those that are neurologically based. Although structural defects may not improve with time or therapeutic exercise, patients may compensate for the lack of tissue bulk. Short-term therapy aimed at maximizing palatal and articulatory efforts may allow for improved velopharyngeal closure. Larger defects need either surgical reconstruction or prosthetic management.

VPI related to neurological compromise is more likely to respond to traditional speech therapy techniques aimed at increasing palatal and articulatory effort. With neurological injury, controlling the rate of speech production is also helpful. Exercises designed to force the production of velar consonants may assist in increasing strength in the soft palate musculature while also improving the accuracy of these sounds, but the benefits of palatal exercises such as blowing have not been demonstrated to have a beneficial effect on speech production.

Individuals with VPI frequently develop compensatory measures to attempt to decrease some of the nasal airflow, which may include using increased respiratory effort, articulatory techniques, or high nasal airway resistance (Warren, 1986). The use of increased vocal effort via greater respiratory support has recently received attention, particularly the Lee Silverman Voice Treatment program in its application in individuals with Parkinson's disease (Ramig, Bonitati, Lemke, & Horii, 1994). A variation on this program has been used with patients demonstrating VPI following traumatic brain injury, and increased velopharyngeal closure was observed (McHenry, 1997). Although this approach may seem appealing in its simplicity, the long-term effects of increased vocal effort on the laryngeal mechanism are not known.

Increased nasal airway resistance has also recently received attention with regard to improving VPI. Continuous positive airway pressure was designed for the management of individuals with sleep apnea. It provides a continuous flow of positive air pressure introduced into the nasal passageways via a mask and prevents collapse of the tissues of the upper respiratory system. The same technology has recently been introduced as a method of strengthening the muscles involved with velopharyngeal closure and thus reducing hypernasality (Kuehn, 1991). Positive air pressure provides a resistance for the levator muscles to work against in an isometric-like fashion to increase their strength. Increasing nasal airflow is thought to load the muscles of closure and increase resistance as opposed to unloading the muscles when pressure is increased on the oral side (Kuehn, 1997). This in turn should lead to improved velopharyngeal valving. Long-term benefits from using this technique have not been demonstrated as of yet due to its recency.

Treatment: Surgical Options

Prosthetics are still preferred as the treatment of choice for most cases of VPI after major head and neck surgery. However, primary palatal reconstruction with local, regional, or free-flaps may be indicated in select patients undergoing significant midfacial and/or palatal resections. Secondary procedures to improve VPI may also be indicated. The emphasis of flap design needs to be on reducing the abnormal nasal resonance while maintaining an adequate nasal airway. The flap design should allow for the maintenance of sufficient superior excursion of the soft palate rem-

nant (if present), and closure at the nasopharyngeal inlet level. Smaller degrees of VPI may benefit from palatopexy (surgically created adhesion of the soft palate to the posterior nasopharyngeal wall) and/or transnasal injection of autogenous materials into the nasopharyngeal wall (such as Teflon).

Treatment: Prosthetic Options

Prosthetic management of VPI includes the use of palatal obturators (Figure 18–5) and lifts. Defects in the hard palate following maxillectomy are more easily managed through obturation as the area is not dynamic and separation of the oral and nasal cavities is the only requirement. Management of VPI related to defects in the soft palate is more challenging due to the dynamic nature of posterosuperior palatal movement necessary for closure. Although the obturator may fill the surgical defect, its lack of dynamic motion may not result in complete and functional velopharyngeal closure. Typically, the obturator is individualized and designed to be larger than the original defect to allow the additional bulk to make contact with the posterior pharyngeal wall. A fine balance must be obtained to allow adequate closure while maintaining nasal breathing.

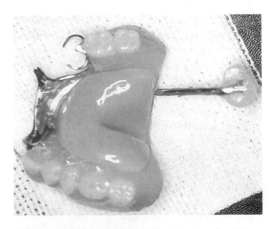

Figure 18–5. Palatal bulb obturator for management of palatal lesion surgical defect.

Overclosure may result in hyponasality. These devices may need to be altered as the patient adjusts over time with therapy. In addition, pain related to radiation treatment may inhibit optimal use of the prosthesis, and the fit may need to be adjusted following its completion (Colangelo et al., 1996).

Palatal lifts are used more often where VPI is secondary to a neurological etiology. A dental appliance is attached to the upper dentition and conforms to the shape of the hard and soft palates. An extension is then created to conform to the area of incomplete closure. In the case of a unilateral palatal paralysis, the extension would be fabricated on the affected side to permit closure when the uninvolved side actively closes. Patient tolerance is usually satisfactory, as a gag reflex is reduced or absent in many of these individuals.

VOICE

The production of normal vocal quality is dependent not only on the status of the larynx but also on the ability to control a steady stream of air that drives the vocal folds into vibration and the characteristics of the resonating tube (vocal tract). Hoarseness may not always represent an abnormality in the vocal folds. This is especially true in patients presenting with dysphonia following treatment for head and neck cancer. Persistent dysphonia may be due to vocal fold scarring, side effects from radiation or chemotherapy, maladaptive compensatory laryngeal and/or ventilatory behaviors, deterioration in general health and fitness, or emotional status (Orlikoff & Kraus, 1996).

Dysphonia may present after treatment for early glottic carcinoma. Treatment of a T1 lesion of the glottis with either radiation or surgical excision has an 85–90% 5-year cure rate (Zeitels, 1996). Treatment selection must then consider the functional result in terms of vocal quality. Prior studies have suggested better vocal quality following radiation therapy. Dysphonia is usually observed when glottic closure is incomplete because of tissue loss following surgical treatment and the resultant vocal-edge excavation (Zeitels, 1995). As the depth of the excision is increased, there may be increased subglottal pressures and flows, increased acoustic instability (jitter and shimmer), and increased patterns of supraglottal muscle strain (Zeitels, 1996). In addition, the tumor bulk of a glottic carcinoma and tissue invasion may result in a pair of vocal folds that are mismatched structurally and biomechanically (Orlikoff & Kraus, 1996). The lack of symmetrical vocal fold vibration may then lead to a perception of hoarseness. In addition, when the superficial lamina propria is excised as a component of the cancer resection, the regenerated epithelial surface may adhere to the underlying body of the vocal fold, resulting in stiffness (Zeitels, 1995). The lack of propagation of a mucosal wave in these cases is likely to result in altered vocal quality.

Changes in vocal quality may also develop following radiation therapy to the neck for either a primary laryngeal lesion or nodal disease, as the ports include the larynx and vocal tract. Radiation therapy with subsequent tumor resolution can lead to scar formation (Harrison et al., 1990). In addition, the drying effects of radiation decrease the necessary lubrication of the vocal tract and may cause the patient to require greater phonatory effort (Verdolini, Titze, & Fennell, 1994). Mucosal dryness may further alter the resonating properties of the vocal tract. Edema is another typical consequence of radiation therapy. Laryngeal edema may affect glottic closure, resulting in breathy and hoarse vocal quality. In addition, edema may alter the perception of pitch due to its mass effect. Some of the changes experienced following radiation are transient but dryness is frequently a more chronic problem.

Vocal difficulties may also develop due to unilateral or bilateral vocal fold immobility. This may be due to neurological compromise during surgery, cricoarytenoid fixation or scarring, or direct tumor involvement of the larynx or recurrent laryngeal nerve. The resultant immobility may be either temporary or permanent. A bilateral impairment in mobility may present as an emergent airway problem if the vocal folds are fixed in the midline position, despite having a near-normal voice. By contrast, if both vocal folds are fixed in a lateral position, the patient is more likely to present with a breathy, weak voice and possible aspiration when swallowing liquids. Unilateral immobility may interfere with glottic closure, resulting in glottal incompetence and a breathy and weak voice.

Weak vocal quality may develop as a result of inadequate pulmonary support or lack of overall conditioning. Primary lung lesions or pulmonary metastasis can decrease lung volumes and adversely affect the ability to control a steady airstream for phonation. Chronic obstructive pulmonary disease is a common finding in these patients exposed to chronic tobacco usage and can adversely affect respiratory support. In addition, lack of conditioning following extensive treatments may interfere with pulmonary support.

The need for a tracheostomy tube may also compromise phonatory quality. Occasionally, patients may require a temporary tracheostomy due to edema of the glottis or airway that may develop due to direct compression or obstruction by the tumor or sequelae of treatment. The location of the edema affects the patient's ability to speak with the tracheostomy tube occluded.

Trismus or decreased oral opening may adversely affect vocal quality. A small oral cavity space may act as a damping device on the vocal tone, decreasing the fullness and intensity of resonation.

Treatment: Speech Therapy

Speech rehabilitation following treatment for laryngeal lesions or vocal fold immobility focuses on two areas: vocal hygiene and directed voice therapy. Vocal hygiene must be addressed to maximize the conditioning of the entire vocal tract. The promotion of hydration and avoidance of any sub-stances that may act as a dehydrant on the vocal tract are critical to countering the drying effects of radiation and other treatments. Antireflux precautions are also important. Gastric acid may cause inflammation of the posterior portion of the larynx, resulting in edema and worsening of vocal quality (Koufman, 1991). Vocal conservation should also be emphasized. Voice rest has not been demonstrated to improve vocal quality. However, great care should be used against unnecessary overuse of the voice such as speaking over background noise.

Directed voice therapy is indicated when the patient's vocal habits interfere with his or her potential voice outcome. It has been shown that concurrent voice therapy and instruction on vocal hygiene can substantially reduce the extent of tissue damage and dysphonia associated with laryngeal radiation (Fex & Henricksson, 1970). Individuals may develop compensatory behaviors to overcome inefficiencies in their voice. The clinician's primary goal is to work with the patient toward maximizing vocal function, voice quality, and intelligibility, while expanding vocal range, flexibility, and capability (Orlikoff & Kraus, 1996). Ensuring appropriate pulmonary/abdominal support is vital for vocal intensity, endurance, and stability of tone. In addition, promotion of an appropriate pitch level, phrasing, and vocal inflection may all help to give the patient a more functional voice. Therapy is usually of short duration, with sessions aimed at monitoring the patient's status, with progression to home exercises.

Voice therapy for the dysphonia that results from a unilateral vocal fold paralysis follows the same parameters as previously discussed. However, if glottic incompetence is more significant, surgical medialization may need to be considered. Pushing exercises are no longer indicated, as they tend to promote hyperfunction of the entire laryngeal mechanism instead of the intended goal of achieving compensation past midline of the unaffected vocal fold.

Treatment: Surgical Options

The method of choice for medialization of a unilaterally paralyzed vocal fold will depend on the specific clinical situation, condition of the patient, and experience of the surgeon (McCaffrey, 1993). Terminally ill patients with a poor prognosis may benefit from vocal fold injection, on an outpatient basis, with Gelfoam, collagen, Teflon, or autogenous fat. These materials are readily available, and, in experienced hands, sufficient medialization may be achieved to address problems due to aspiration and breathy dysphonia secondary to glottal incompetence. These materials may be injected transcutaneously through the cricothyroid space or, when this is not possible, transorally through a direct laryngoscopy approach. Teflon injections have been used successfully since the early 1960s for the treatment of paralytic dysphonia (Arnold, 1964). Possible disadvantages include the potential for overinjection, with granuloma formation and airway compromise, permanent change in the vocal fold vibratory characteristics,

irreversibility, and the need for direct laryngoscopy in most circumstances, unless the physician is skilled at office-based transcutaneous (transcervical) or transoral flexible fiberoptic techniques of vocal fold injection. Disadvantages of the direct laryngoscopy approach are the increased discomfort to the patient if done under local anesthesia and the suboptimal physiological conditions to evaluate whether sufficient injection has occurred. In addition, there is an increased cost due to operating room utilization. Older patients with degenerative cervical spine disease may have limited exposure of the vocal folds due to limitation of even minor degrees of neck extension. Where general anesthesia is necessary, the precision of the technique in maximizing the medialization is much more limited. In addition, there are inherent risks to the general anesthesia.

In healthier patients with a better prognosis, laryngeal framework surgery (thyroplasty type I or medialization laryngoplasty; Figure 18–6) may be indicated over injection methods (Isshiki, Olamura, &

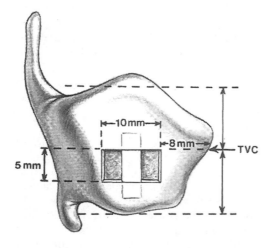

A

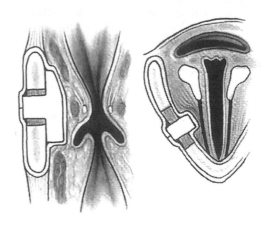

B

Figure 18–6. Thyroplasty type I or medialization laryngoplasty. **(A)** approximate measurements for thyroplasty window. **(B)** Silastic implant placement in thyroplasty window. *Source:* "Surgical Therapy for Swallowing Disorders," by G. Wisdom and A. Blitzer 1998.. From *Otolaryngologic Clinics of North America, 31*, p. 551.

Ishikawa, 1975). Advantages include its potential for reversibility, better patient tolerance, improved predictability, preservation of vocal fold vibratory characteristics, and good voice results (Koufman, 1986). Despite the fact that this is an outpatient procedure, disadvantages include the increased costs and need for an external incision with inherent potential for wound complications (i.e., infection and implant extrusion). Although laryngeal framework surgery is not absolutely contraindicated, patients with a prior history of radiation therapy to the neck may also be at risk for increased implant extrusion. Perceptually, thyroplasty type I results in increased loudness, decreased breathiness and hoarseness, and less diplophonia with longer phrasing (Lu, Casiano, Lundy, & Xue, 1996).

Surgical options for glottal incompetence secondary to vocal fold scarring after partial laryngectomy or laser cordectomy are limited by the degree of tissue loss and the degree of fibrosis. Medialization surgery does not address cases where scarring may be extensive and the linearity of the vocal fold vibrating edge is not intact. Thyroplasty for vocal fold scarring results in a poorer voice outcome than that achieved in patients with vocal fold paralysis (Isshiki et al., 1975). Vocal fold injection (with Teflon, autogenous fat, and so forth.) to augment the area is difficult due to the degree of fibrosis and the insufficient amount of compliant tissue for deposition of the injected material. Techniques using local tissue flaps designed to reconstitute the linear vocal fold edge with more compliant tissue would be better suited but may require a temporary tracheotomy during the immediate postoperative period. A discussion of vocal fold medialization and augmentation techniques also may be found in Chapter 6.

Treatment: Prosthetic Options

Prosthetic options for the patient with a voice disorder are somewhat limited. Voice amplifiers may be beneficial for those with decreased vocal intensity. In addition, the tracheotomized patient may benefit from a speaking valve if adequate ability to produce vocal fold adduction exists. Patients with nonfunctional larynges may benefit from the use of an artificial larynx on either a permanent or temporary basis, depending on their needs.

Trismus may be improved using a Therabite Jaw Motion Rehabilitation System (Rodriguez, 1995). Therabite is an appliance that gradually applies an opening pressure to the upper and lower dental arches. Increasing the oral opening can have beneficial effects not only on the resonance of the vocal tone but also on articulation, mastication, and swallowing (Figure 18–7).

Alaryngeal Speech Options

Current methods of alaryngeal speech rehabilitation include the development of esophageal speech, use of an artificial larynx, or surgical voice restoration via a tracheoesophageal puncture (TEP). Reported success rates are variable. In a comprehensive study, Gates et al. (1982) found that 55% of laryngectomees were functionally rehabilitated with either esophageal speech or use of an electrolarynx. In contrast, Ackerstaff, Hilgers, Aaronson, and Balm (1994) found that 78% of laryngectomized individuals communicated functionally with a TEP, 14% used esophageal speech, and 3% spoke with an artificial larynx. Animal studies looking at laryngeal transplantation are being evaluated. However, it is not a realistic option at this point in time.

Artificial larynges can be divided into those that are driven by pulmonary airflow and those that are electronic. The most widely used ones are the electronic devices that are placed either against the soft tissues of the neck or directly into the oral cavity via an oral adapter. Sound is transmitted into the open space of the oral cavity whereby the individual articulates the intended message. Short-term speech therapy is usually required to instruct the patient in attaining maximal sound transmission, appropriate timing between tone

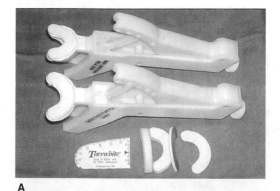

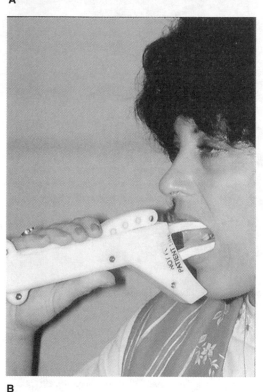

Figure 18–7. Therabite jaw mobilization appliance (**A**) and its use to prevent jaw hypomobility. (**B**).

generation and articulation, and emphasizing overarticulation. Modifications are currently underway to reduce the characteristic metallic quality of electronic larynges (Chalstrey, Bleach, Cheung, & Van Hasselt, 1994). An intraoral device is also available which has the advantage of being cosmetically unobtrusive. However, it requires a handheld switch to control the tone generator.

Surgical voice restoration using a TEP is currently the preferred method of alaryngeal speech rehabilitation in select patients (Singer & Blom, 1980). A fistula is surgically created between the posterior tracheostomal wall and the esophagus. A one-way valve is then inserted to allow pulmonary air to pass from the tracheal side through to the esophagus while preventing esophageal contents from being aspirated (Figure 18–8). A TEP can be performed as a primary procedure at the time of laryngectomy or as a secondary procedure after adequate healing. The role of the speech-language pathologist begins with the selection process to determine candidacy based on the anatomic configuration of the stoma, articulation, motivation, and air insufflation testing to rule out the possibility of cricopharyngeal spasm. The clinician then fits the patient with an appropriate-sized voice prosthesis and instructs in the coordination between respiration, stomal occlusion, phonation, and articulation. Modifications in prosthesis design and surgical technique, improvement of tracheostomal valves for independent occlusion of the stoma, refinement of the selection criteria, and assessment of the efficacy of using this type of procedure in individuals undergoing more extensive surgical procedures and reconstructions are underway (Casiano & Lundy, 1996).

Alaryngeal speech is generally considered successful if the individual is able to produce a fluent and intelligible voice for an adequate duration of time and is socially acceptable (Izdebski, Reed, Ross, & Hilsinger, 1994). Despite the evidence for superiority of speech quality with a TEP (Williams & Watson, 1985), patient choice must always be considered and respected.

CONCLUSIONS

The ultimate goals in treating patients with head and neck cancers are to maintain, promote, and/or restore their ability to enjoy an optimal quality of life. These

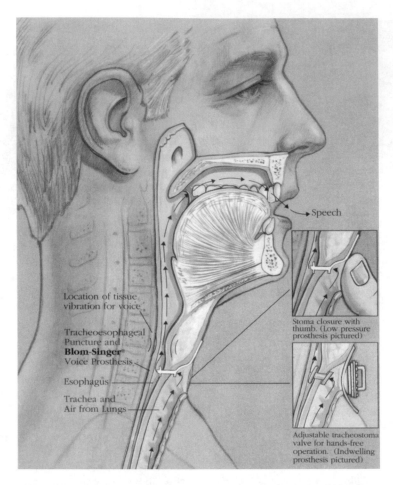

Figure 18–8. Placement of the Blom-Singer voice prosthesis and speech production using digital occlusion of the stoma and the hands-free speaking valve. Reprinted with permission of InHealth Technologies.

goals need to include concern for economy of the patient's time, energy, and expense while maintaining realistic expectations as determined by the degree of surgery and/or medical therapy. Rehabilitation efforts also need to emphasize methods that are minimally obtrusive and achieve the desired goals in the least amount of time.

REFERENCES

Ackerstaff, A. H., Hilgers, F. J. M., Aaronson, N. K., & Balm, A. J. M. (1994). Communication, functional disorders and lifestyle changes after total laryngectomy. *Clinical Otolaryngology, 19*, 295–300.

Arnold, G. E. (1964). Further experiences with intrachordal Teflon infection. *Laryngoscope, 74*, 802–815.

Aronson, A. E. (1985). *Clinical voice disorders. An interdisciplinary approach* (2nd ed.). New York: Thieme.

Atha, J. (1982). Strengthening muscle. *Exercise and Sport Sciences Reviews, 9*, 1–73.

Casiano, R. R., & Lundy, D. S. (1996). Voice and speech rehabilitation following laryngectomy. *Current Opinion in Otolaryngology, Head and Neck Surgery, 4*, 94–97.

Chalstrey, S. E., Bleach, N. R., Cheung, D., & Van Hasselt, C. A. (1994). A pneumatic artificial larynx popularized in Hong Kong. *Journal of Laryngology and Otology, 108*, 852–854.

Clark, D. H. (1973). Adaptations in strength and muscular endurance resulting from exercise. *Exercise and Sport Sciences Reviews, 1*, 73–102.

Colangelo, L. A., Pauloski, B. R., Logemann, J. A., Stein, D. W., Beery, Q. C., Heiser, M. A., & Cardinale, S. (1996). Effects of intraoral prostheses on speech in oropharyngeal cancer patients. *American Journal of Speech-Language Pathology, 5,* 43–55.

Fex, S., & Henriksson, B. (1970). Phoniatric treatment combined with radiotherapy of laryngeal cancer for the avoidance of radiation damage. *Acta Otolaryngologica, 263,* 128–129.

Fox, E. L., Kirby, T. E., & Fox, A. R. (1987). *Bases of fitness.* New York: Macmillan.

Gates, G. A., Ryan, W., Cooper, J. C., Lawlis, G. F., Cantu, E., Hayashi, T., Lauder, E., Welch, R. W., & Hearne, E. (1982). Current status of laryngectomee rehabilitation: I. Results of therapy. *American Journal of Otolaryngology, 3,* 1–7.

Harrison, L. B., Solomon, B., Miller, S., Fass, D. E., Armstrong, J., & Sessions, R. B. (1990). Prospective computer-assisted voice analysis for patients with early stage glottic cancer: A preliminary report of the functional result of laryngeal irradiation. *International Journal of Radiation Oncology, Biology, Physics, 19,* 123–127.

Heyward, V. H. (1991). *Advanced fitness assessment and exercise prescription.* Champaign, IL: Human Kinetics Books.

Imai, S., & Michi, K. (1992). Articulatory function after resection of the tongue and floor of the mouth: Palatometric and perceptual evaluation. *Journal of Speech and Hearing Research, 35,* 68–78.

Isshiki, N., Olamura, H., & Ishikawa, T. (1975). Thyroplasty type I (lateral compression) for dysphagia due to vocal cord paralysis or atrophy. *Acta Otolaryngology (Stockholm), 80,* 465–473.

Izdebski, K., Reed, C. G., Ross, J. C., & Hilsinger, R. L. (1994). Problems with tracheoesophageal fistula voice restoration in totally laryngectomized patients. *Archives of Otolaryngology—Head and Neck Surgery, 120,* 840–845.

Koufman, J. A. (1986). Laryngoplasty for vocal cord medialization: An alternative to Teflon. *Laryngoscope, 96,* 726–731.

Koufman, J. A. (1991). Otolaryngologic manifestations of gastroesophageal reflux disease (GERD): A clinical investigation of 225 patients using ambulatory 24-hr pH monitoring and an experimental investigation of the role of acid and pepsin in the development of laryngeal injury. *Laryngoscope, 101* (Suppl. 53), 1–78.

Kuehn, D. P. (1991). New therapy for treating hypernasal speech using continuous positive airway pressure (CPAP). *Plastic and Reconstructive Surgery, 88,* 959–966.

Kuehn, D. P. (1997). The development of a new technique for treating hypernasality: CPAP. *American Journal of Speech-Language Pathology, 6,* 5–8.

Leonard, R., Goodrich, S., McMenamin, P., & Donald, P. (1992). Differentiation of speakers with glossectomies by acoustic and perceptual measures. *American Journal of Speech-Language Pathology, 1,* 56–63.

Logemann, J. A., Pauloski, B. R., Rademaker, A. W., & Colangelo, L. A. (1997). Speech and swallowing rehabilitation for head and neck cancer patients. *Oncology, 11,* 651–663.

Lu, F. L., Casiano, R. R., Lundy, D. S., & Xue, J. W. (1996). Longitudinal evaluation of vocal function following thyroplasty type I in the treatment of unilateral vocal paralysis. *Laryngoscope, 106,* 573–577.

McCaffrey, T. V. (1993). Transcutaneous Teflon injection for vocal cord paralysis. *Otolaryngology—Head and Neck Surgery, 109,* 54–59.

McConnell, F., Teichgraeber, J., & Adler, R. (1987). A comparison of three methods of oral reconstruction. *Archives of Otolaryngology—Head and Neck Surgery, 113,* 496–500.

McHenry, M. A. (1997). The effect of increased vocal effort on estimated velopharyngeal orifice area. *American Journal of Speech-Language Pathology, 6,* 55–61.

Myers, E. N. (1972). Reconstruction of the oral cavity. *Otolaryngology Clinics of North America, 5,* 413–433.

Orlikoff, R. F., & Kraus, D. H. (1996). Dysphonia following nonsurgical management of advance laryngeal carcinoma. *American Journal of Speech-Language Pathology, 5,* 47–52.

Pauloski, B. R., Logemann, J. A., Rademaker, A. W., McConnel, F. M. S., Heiser, M. A., et al. (1993). Speech and swallowing function after anterior tongue and floor of mouth resection with distal flap reconstruction. *Journal of Speech and Hearing Research, 36,* 267–276.

Ramig, L. O., Bonitati, C. M., Lemke, J. H., & Horii, Y. (1994). Voice treatment for patients with Parkinson disease: Development of an approach and preliminary efficacy data. *Journal of Medical Speech-Language Pathology, 2,* 191–210.

Rodriguez, B. (1995). *Management of trismus in head and neck practice.* Presented at Society of Otorhinololaryngology and Head-Neck Nurses Nineteenth Annual Congress, New Orleans, LA.

Saxon, K. G., & Schneider, C. M. (1995). *Vocal exercise physiology.* San Diego, CA: Singular Publishing Group.

Singer, M. I., & Blom, E. D. (1980). An endoscopic technique for restoration of voice after laryngectomy. *Annals of Otology, Rhinology, and Laryngology, 89,* 529–533.

Skelly, M. (1973). *Glossectomee speech rehabilitation.* Springfield, IL: Charles C. Thomas.

Urken, M. L., Moscoso, J. F., Lawson, W., & Biller, H. F. (1994). A systematic approach to functional reconstruction of the oral cavity following partial and total glossectomy. *Archives of Otolaryngology—Head and Neck Surgery, 120,* 589–601.

Verdolini, K., Titze, I. R., & Fennell, A. (1994). Dependence of phonatory effort on hydration level. *Journal of Speech and Hearing Research, 37,* 1001–1007.

Warren, D. W. (1986). Compensatory speech behaviors in individuals with cleft palate: A regulation/control phenomenon? *Cleft Palate Journal, 23,* 250–260.

Williams, S. E., & Watson, J. B. (1985). Differences in speaking proficiencies in three laryngectomee groups. *Archives of Otolaryngology, 111,* 216–219.

Zeitels, S. M. (1995). Premalignant epithelium and microinvasive cancer of the vocal fold. The evolution of phonomicrosurgical management. *Laryngoscope, 67* (Suppl.), 1–5.

Zeitels, S. M. (1996). Phonomicrosurgical treatment of early glottic cancer and carcincoma in situ. *American Journal of Surgery, 172,* 704–709.

19

Clinical Dysphagia Intervention

Paula A. Sullivan, M.S., CCC-SLP

Dysphagia, or impaired swallowing, in cancer patients may result from the disease process or from the side effects of treatment. Oropharyngeal and esophageal dysphagia induced by localized tumor results from tumor mass, tissue fixation, neuromuscular deficits, local inflammation, and pain. Surgical intervention, radiation therapy, and chemotherapy often result in temporary or prolonged dysphagia resulting from anatomic abnormalities, including tracheotomy, fibrosis and scar, decreased saliva production, mucosal inflammation and infection, and sensory alterations. Primary brain tumors or metastatic disease with central nervous system involvement can interfere with cranial nerve function, resulting in sensory and motor deficits, thus resulting in dysphagia. The multifactorial causes of deglutition problems in cancer are discussed in Chapter 2. In addition, Chapters 3–11 detail swallowing problems related to various tumor sites and cancer treatment modalities.

Any patient presenting with dysphagia and the inability to take adequate nutrition and hydration by mouth is considered at high nutritional risk. Malnutrition is a common comorbidity in cancer patients. Untreated or poorly managed dysphagia and nutrition in this high-risk population will adversely affect quality of life, will interfere with cancer treatment, and may lead to life-threatening conditions. Although the speech-language pathologist and the dietitian work most closely and intensively with the dysphagic patient, a team approach to intervention is essential to achieving optimum clinical outcomes.

An understanding of basic dysphagia assessment and management issues by the reader is assumed. In addition, a thorough review of dysphagia and its management with various types and sites of tumors and treatment combinations is beyond the scope of this chapter. Rather, this chapter provides a framework or fundamental approach to dysphagia management that can be used by the speech-language pathologist and care team throughout the cancer care continuum. This framework provides a practical, comprehensive, and efficient approach to intervention by preventing or reducing complications of dysphagia.

PRINCIPLES OF DYSPHAGIA INTERVENTION IN ONCOLOGY

Multidisciplinary Management

Due to the complexity of medical, nutritional, swallowing, communication, and psychosocial management issues related to cancer and its treatment, multidisciplinary intervention is essential to reducing morbidity and mortality and achieving optimal functional outcomes. A team-based approach to swallowing and nutritional intervention also will ensure continuity of care throughout the cancer care continuum. Multidisciplinary team organization and requisite skills, swallowing and nutritional outcomes of care teams, and essential components of an effective multidisciplinary care team are discussed in detail in Chapter 2.

Consultative Approach

Speech-language pathologists have been prepared to deliver dysphagia services using a traditional rehabilitation approach. However, cancer patients are at risk for swallowing and nutritional problems at any point in their continuum of cancer care and require a nontraditional medically focused approach to intervention. The cancer care continuum consists of nine phases or stages in which a variety of services are provided based on the patient's distinct needs. These stages are screening and prevention, diagnosis, staging, treatment, supportive care, rehabilitation, palliative care, home care, and hospice care. Using the consultative approach described by Johnson, Valachovic, and George (1998; *evaluation/diagnosis of the swallowing disorder, intensive monitoring of clinical symptoms and intervention, and education/counseling*), a comprehensive and integrated approach to dysphagia intervention is ensured throughout the patient's course of cancer care. A schematic representation of the consultative model is presented in Figure 19–1.

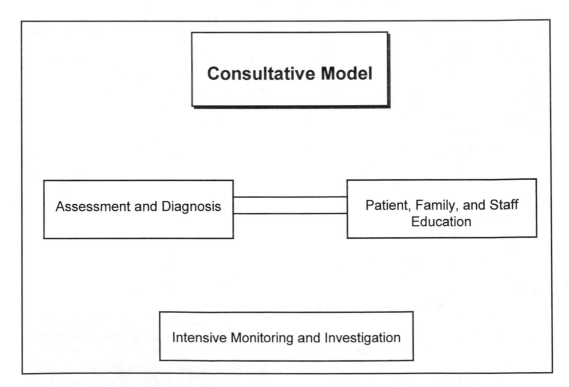

Figure 19–1. The consultative model. *Source:* Adapted from "Speech-Language Pathology Practice in the Acute Care Setting: A Consultative Approach," by A. F. Johnson, A. M. Valachovic, and K. P. George. In *Medical Speech-Language Pathology: A Practitioner's Guide*, edited by A. F. Johnson and B. H. Jacobson, 1998, New York: W.B. Saunders.

Patients most frequently are referred for dysphagia *evaluation* following cancer treatment. Rarely do patients with dysphagia secondary to malignancy initially present to the speech-language pathologist. Cancer should be suspected in patients presenting with weight loss accompanied by odynophagia. Radiographic examination also may reveal carcinoma of the head and neck or esophagus. Pretreatment swallowing evaluation often is performed to detect subtle deficits and document the effects of treatment, document the recovery, or identify complications. Decline of function during cancer treatment may reflect temporary problems due to treatment side effects or signal poor response to medical treatment. This information will assist in determining medical status and treatment plan. Following swallowing evaluation, recommendations should be written and placed in the patient's medical record and personally communicated to members of the patient's care team to ensure compliance. Critical members of this team include the patient, family, and/or other care providers. Recommendations should be concise and address pertinent issues of care, including feeding status, treatment/management issues, discharge status, and referrals to other services (Johnson et al., 1998).

Patients typically require *frequent monitoring of clinical symptoms* while undergoing cancer *treatment* to monitor clinical course, reduce or prevent treatment side effects, and modify intervention goals. The primary goals during the *treatment phase* are more medically than rehabilitationally oriented. This can be seen in the need for placement of a nasogastric feeding tube should mucositis interfere with oral intake during the patient's course of radiation therapy. Changes in swallowing function can be charted using selected monitoring tools and careful behavioral observation. Frequent patient monitoring not only will provide objective information regarding change in swallowing function but also will signal change in medical or oncologic condition.

Education and counseling by the speech-language pathologists must be focused in two major areas: (a) the patient and family and (b) the patient's cancer care team. Both the patient and his or her family must be educated and counseled at various times during the care continuum regarding basic information about the swallowing disorder and the recommended plan of care. This information also will provide the patient and family a better understanding of the course of medical and/or swallowing treatment. For example, the patient who understands that temporary placement of a nasogastric tube is necessary to ensure adequate nutrition and hydration, facilitate resolution of mucositis, and prevent interruption of radiation therapy is more likely to comply with the recommendation for its insertion. The goal of education and counseling with a terminally ill individual might be to discuss the need for eventual progression to combined or nonoral feeding methods. The priorities and goals of the patient and family must be considered and respected in all discussions about care and treatment planning. Referral to other care team members—including the social worker, psychologist, psychiatrist, clergy, and/or volunteer cancer survivor—may be necessary to assist with adjustment difficulties. The speech-language pathologist must increase care team awareness of swallowing problems, their symptoms, and referral procedures. In addition, immediate communication of dysphagia evaluation results and recommendations, whether face-to-face, by telephone, by voice mail, or by electronic mail, is critical as the participation of other team members is often required to ensure compliance.

Establishing Rehabilitation Goals

Dysphagia intervention in oncology is dynamic and ongoing and must be provided in an integrated manner through the continuum of care. Goal setting with cancer patients typically focuses on compensation as opposed to the traditional rehabilitation approach of long-term improvement in swallowing function, although more traditional approaches will be used during the *rehabilitation* phase of care.

Goals are short-term and are frequently modified as a patient progresses from one level of care to the next; they may be changed on a day-to-day basis when the patient is undergoing daily cancer treatments. In addition, a number of other patient characteristics should be considered when establishing treatment goals with the cancer patient. These include diagnosis, including type and extent of cancer treatment(s), prognosis, ability to tolerate therapy, severity of the patient's dysphagia, patient motivation and desire to eat, and respiratory function. For example, a thorough understanding of the exact extent and nature of surgical reconstruction in oral and oropharyngeal cancer patients is critical. This information will provide the speech-language pathologist critical information needed to predict or determine the nature of the swallowing problem and assist with goal setting. For patients receiving *palliative, home,* or *hospice care*, goals should accommodate a decline in swallowing function. A primary goal with a terminal patient may be to facilitate "adequate" but not "optimal" function (Twycross, 1981). For example, a patient may choose to continue oral feeding despite documented aspiration. The treatment goal for this patient is to determine and recommend food textures and compensatory strategies that minimize aspiration.

Timing of Rehabilitation Intervention

The goal of oncology treatment is to achieve cancer control or cure while minimizing functional impairment. Each cancer treatment method can result in temporary or long-term disorders in swallowing function. Optimum rehabilitation of the patient requires early and ongoing intervention by the speech-language pathologist and members of the cancer care team that begins before cancer treatment, at the time of cancer *diagnosis* and tumor *staging*. The patient and family members are integral team members and should participate in treatment selection and planning. Treatment planning ideally is discussed in a multidisciplinary tumor conference where treatment options specific to the patient

and his or her disease can be discussed. Issues to be discussed include selection of treatment and its potential effects on speech and swallowing, the prospective schedule of rehabilitation, and specific psychosocial concerns (Logemann, 1989).

Pretreatment assessment by the dietitian is critical to the identification of patients with the potential for or who are at high nutritional risk. Aggressive intervention with a goal of nutritional repletion is not always feasible prior to the initiation of treatment. A decision for the need of temporary or long-term nutritional support should be made prior to the initiation of treatment based on type of therapy, anticipated disease course, duration of treatment, and patient comfort and motivation (Robuck, 1987). Intensive clinical and nutritional monitoring by care team members should be conducted throughout the patient's cancer treatment and continuum of care. Consultation with the dentist is necessary to identify any dental disease, preserve healthy dentition, and plan for intraoral prostheses.

The patient ideally should be seen by the speech-language pathologist for pretreatment counseling. Patients considered at risk for development of posttreatment swallowing deficits should be seen for swallowing screening. The use of sensitive and standardized assessment protocols will detect subtle pretreatment deficits, document posttreatment effects, document recovery, or identify potential complications (Johnson et al., 1998). Counseling should focus on preparing the patient and his or her family for the potential of any treatment-related swallowing deficits, predict the rehabilitation course, provide patient and family reassurance, and assure them of the availability of rehabilitation support.

During the course of radiation therapy and/or chemotherapy and during the early postoperative period, the patient and family are provided *supportive* care. Often, questions are answered and patients are provided assurance regarding predictable treatment or posttreatment complications such as edema, hyposalivation, and mucositis. In surgically treated head and neck patients, swallowing intervention is initiated when the surgeon determines that suture lines have healed sufficiently to begin range of motion (ROM) exercises (developed following careful anatomic and physiological assessment of oral, laryngeal, and pharyngeal function). This typically varies from 7 to 14 days postsurgery. If patients are scheduled to undergo induction, primary, or postoperative irradiation to the head and neck, with or without chemotherapy, an appropriate home program of tongue, jaw, and pharyngeal/laryngeal ROM exercises is introduced. These may include tongue base exercises, gliding up and down the musical scale, and maintaining and improving mandibular opening using stacked tongue depressors. A noninclusive list of ROM exercises will be discussed later in this chapter (see Table 19–5). Patients are instructed to perform these exercises daily, as tolerated, throughout the course of their radiation treatment and for at least 6 weeks to reduce the formation of fibrotic tissue in the oral cavity and pharyngeal structures and thus preserve flexibility of the swallow mechanism. Pauloski, Rademaker, Logemann, and Colangelo (1998) have demonstrated that increased use of tongue ROM exercises by postsurgical oral cancer patients both during and after radiation therapy may reduce the formation of fibrotic tissue in the oral cavity and improve pharyngeal clearance by maintaining contact of the posterior tongue to the pharyngeal wall.

The *rehabilitation* phase of dysphagia intervention typically is initiated when medical treatments are completed. Rehabilitation goals often are long-term and traditionally defined and focus on optimizing functional status. The cancer care team should closely monitor for deterioration in the patient's swallowing function and nutritional status throughout the entire care continuum as well as during the *palliative*, *home*, and *hospice* phases of care. Deterioration in swallowing function may be an indication of disease recurrence. Patients also may demonstrate long-term effects to swallowing function as a result of

cancer treatments that begin at 6 months or more after treatment. Irradiated patients may exhibit significant changes in pharyngeal peristalsis secondary to increased fibrosis of the pharyngeal constrictors (Ekberg & Nylander, 1983). During the *palliative*, *home*, and *hospice* phases of care, emphasis is on consultative practice with a focus on quality-of-life issues and health needs of the patient.

DYSPHAGIA INTERVENTION THROUGHOUT THE CONTINUUM OF CANCER CARE

Dysphagia intervention is integrated and ongoing throughout all points of the patients' oncologic treatments. In this section, management principles for swallowing and nutrition problems related to cancer and its treatment are presented as they relate to the continuum of cancer care. Specifically, dysphagia intervention principles pertinent to *screening* and *prevention*, *treatment*, *rehabilitation*, and *palliative*, *home*, and *hospice* care will be highlighted, as it is at these points in the patient's cancer care where involvement by the speech-language pathologist and care team is most active. The reader is reminded that all patients do not transition through all phases of the care continuum. For example, a patient may experience a total response from his or her oncologic treatments and never require *palliative*, *home*, or *hospice* care. In addition, there typically is overlap in the phases of cancer care, as the primary focus of intervention may be *supportive* during the immediate postoperative period or during *diagnosis*, *staging*, and the *treatment* phases of care.

Prevention and Screening

Cancer *prevention* should be an integral focus of practice by speech-language pathologists and cancer care team members but frequently is overlooked. The economics of preventive interventions must be a primary focus in an increasingly capitated health care environment, as prevention of disease and disorders typically costs less than treatment. The American Speech-Language-Hearing Association's three levels of prevention activity related to communication disorders can be adapted for use with swallowing and nutrition disorders by cancer care providers (see Table 19–1). For example, head and neck cancer *prevention* and *rehabilitation* are appropriate and needed roles of speech-language pathologists in the prevention and early detection of oral cancer. Primary prevention can focus on educating teenagers about the increased risk of oral cancer associated with tobacco and alcohol use. Speech-language pathologists should be vigilant in screening high-risk individuals for signs of oral cancer and refer to appropriate medical specialists if symptoms are observed. Early detection and treatment of oral cancer is considered secondary prevention. Care providers also serve a preventive role with patients who are undergoing radiation and/or chemotherapy. An understanding of the potential treatment-induced swallowing toxicities and their prevention and therapy is needed by speech-language pathologists and other care team members. This information will make them more informed and competent health care providers and patient advocates and help prevent or reduce oral complications.

Pneumonia, particularly aspiration pneumonia, is a major cause of morbidity and mortality among the hospitalized elderly (Jones, 1993). Medical conditions that occur predominantly in the elderly and are associated with swallowing problems are considered predisposing to aspiration pneumonia, including head and neck cancer. Aspiration pneumonia is a difficult to diagnose multifactorial phenomenon that can result from both prandial and nonprandial factors. Cancer patients often have multiple risk factors for aspiration pneumonia. These risk factors include tracheostomy tubes, older age, tube feedings, poor nutritional status, immunocompromise, gastric reflux, oropharyngeal colonization of pathogenic bacteria, and multiple medications. Predicting a cancer patient's likelihood for aspiration and its prevention primary intervention goals of care teams. A prospective study by Martin et al. (1994) examined the cooccurrence of dysphagia with aspiration pneumonia in patients with pneumonia in an acute care hospital. A high incidence of dysphagia was discovered in patients with aspiration pneumonia when compared to patients with non-aspiration-related pneumonia. The modified barium swallowing evaluation is one method used to clearly delineate the pathophysiology of prandial aspiration. Although prandial aspiration is an important factor in aspiration pneumonia, it generally is not sufficient to result in pneumonia unless other risk factors are present. The best predictors of aspiration pneumonia are dependence for oral care and feeding, number of decayed teeth, tube feeding, more than one medical diagnosis,

TABLE 19–1. Prevention of Communication (*Swallowing and Nutrition*) Disorders

Primary Prevention	Elimination or inhibition of the onset and development of a communication (*swallowing and nutrition*) disorder by making behavioral modifications or personal choices that minimize risk factors associated with communication (*swallowing and nutrition*) disorders.
Secondary Prevention	Early detection and treatment of communication (*swallowing and nutrition*) disorders, which may lead to the elimination of the disorder or the retardation of the disorder's progress, thereby preventing further complications.
Tertiary Prevention	Reduction of a disability by attempting to restore effective functioning.

Source: Adapted from *Position Statement on Prevention of Communicable Disorders,* by the American Speech-Language-Hearing Association, 1998, Washington, DC: Author.

number of medications, and smoking (Langmore et al., 1998). Significant predictors of aspiration pneumonia are illustrated in Figure 19–2. These studies underscore the need for an aggressive team approach to the evaluation, prevention, and treatment of aspiration and aspiration pneumonia to reduce or prevent patient morbidity and mortality. *Prevention* measures include swallowing evaluation, swallowing therapy designed to facilitate safe and efficient bolus transit, implementation of safe feeding techniques, nonoral intake, and patient and care provider education. Nonprandial interventions also must be addressed including the promotion of oral hygiene, implementation of reflux precau-

tions, accurate placement and monitoring of feeding tubes, and interventions to aid pulmonary clearance such as regular percussion and auscultation and increasing a patient's activity.

Dysphagia screening procedures are designed to identify patients at significant risk for dysphagia but they do not define the nature of the patients' problems. Screening procedures look at symptoms of dysphagia while diagnostic procedures examine anatomy and physiology. In addition, they provide baseline information about swallowing function useful in tracking and comparing a patient's swallowing ability throughout the care continuum. Screening procedures should be relatively quick to administer, be generally noninvasive, and provide little risk to the patient. It is important that the speech-language pathologist use a system or screening tool that provides quantitative measures of swallowing function for useful indices of change. This is particularly important in oncology, as screening measures must detect swallowing changes that may signal disease recurrence or may be a result of long-term treatment effects. Currently, there are many commercially available dysphagia screening tests available to the clinician. When choosing a dysphagia screening tool for cancer patients, monitoring tools should be quick to administer, be quantifiable, and have relatively equal sensitivity and specificity. Generally, most currently available dysphagia screening tools have high sensitivity (identifies with high likelihood that a patient has dysphagia) but low specificity (overidentifies patients who do not have dysphagia). A checklist of items for dysphagia screening with fairly equal sensitivity and specificity can be found in other sources (Logemann, 1998).

Other dysphagia screening procedures may be performed to identify patients at risk for a pharyngeal phase dysphagia and who need further diagnostic workup. These include the bedside or clinical examination, cervical auscultation, blue dye test, and the fiberoptic endoscopic examination of swallowing (FEES).

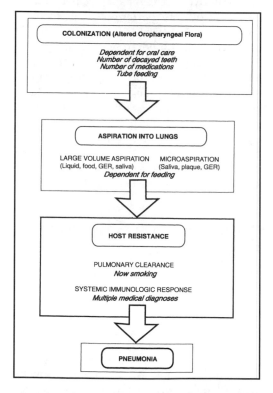

Figure 19–2. *Significant predictors of aspiration pneumonia positioned in the model.* (*Source:* From "Predictors of Aspiration Pneumonia: How Important is Dysphagia?" by S. E. Langmore, M. S. Terpenning, A. Schork, Y. Chen, J. E. Murray, D. Lopatin, and W. J. Loesche, 1998, *Dysphagia, 13,* pp. 69–81. Copyright 1998 by Springer-Verlag. Reprinted with permission.)

Bedside or Clinical Examination

The bedside or clinical examination of dysphagia is a screening test for the pharyngeal phase of swallowing. However, it can be used as an oral phase diagnostic test for head and neck cancer patients. The examination is intended to provide the speech-language pathologist and care team members information critical for use in dysphagia diagnosis and management. The examination is conducted by the speech-language pathologist in conjunction with various team members, such as the dietitian, physician, and neurologists, as no one discipline can comprehensively assess all phases of swallowing. The bedside or clinical examination often is divided into (a) the preparatory examination with no bolus swallows and (b) the initial swallowing examination when trial food swallows are attempted. Logemann (1998) reports that the bedside or clinical examination should provide the clinician the following information about the patient:

1. current medical diagnosis, medical history, and history of the swallowing disorder, including the patient's awareness of the swallowing disorder and indications of the localization and nature of the swallowing disorder;
2. medical status including nutritional and respiratory status;
3. oral anatomy;
4. respiratory function and its relationship to the swallow;
5. labial control;
6. lingual control;
7. palatal function;
8. pharyngeal wall contraction;
9. laryngeal control;
10. the patient's ability to follow directions and monitor and control behavior;
11. reaction to oral sensory stimulation, including taste, temperature, and texture; and
12. reactions and symptoms during attempts to swallow.

Cervical Auscultation

Cervical auscultation is a procedure used to detect the sounds of swallow and respiration via a stethoscope placed on the patient's larynx (Bosma, 1992). The clinician can detect the inspiratory and expiratory phases of the respiratory cycle and define the phase of respiration during which the patient swallows. Cervical auscultation is an imprecise clinical method for evaluating aspiration, and currently there are no data to support the correlation of acoustic sounds with swallowing events (Zenner, Losinski, & Mills, 1995).

Blue Dye Test

The blue dye test consists of placement of blue food dye on the tongue or in foods of a patient with a tracheostomy. The patient is suctioned immediately and at regular intervals over a 1-hr period, and the presence of any dye in the tracheal secretions is noted. The test has been found to have both positive and negative error rate. Results should be interpreted conservatively and interpreted in the context of the complete clinical examination. However, it can provide the clinician an indication of gross airway competence (Dikeman & Kazandjian, 1995).

Flexible Endoscopic Examination of Swallowing

FEES uses a fiberoptic nasopharyngoscope to directly visualize the pharynx before and after the swallow (Langmore, Schatz, & Olsen, 1988). FEES is considered a screening procedure, as the actual swallow itself cannot be visualized. Therefore, the exact nature of the patient's physiological swallow disorder can only be inferred based on postswallow food residual. FEES is particularly useful with head and neck cancer patients, as it can provide information about anatomic changes in the pharynx and how these changes relate to swallowing. The videoendoscopic procedure can also provide biofeedback for training patients in airway closure maneuvers. Using FEES technology, the severity of oropharyngeal secretions in the laryngeal vestibule can be directly visualized and assessed using a four-level rating scale. Murray, Langmore, Ginsberg, and Dostie (1996) found that the accumulation of visible oropharyngeal secretions in the laryngeal vestibule was highly predictive of prandial aspiration. The rating scale for determining severity of accumulated oropharyngeal secretions can be found in Table 19–2.

Treatment and Supportive Care

While undergoing cancer *treatment*, whether recovering from surgery or undergoing radiation therapy with or without chemotherapy, the patient often is unable to tolerate traditional rehabilition interventions. Goals primarily are consultative and *supportive* in nature. Supportive care is provided during ongoing cancer treatments with emphasis on reducing cancer-related disability through rehabilitation interventions. The primary emphasis is to prepare the patient and family for the rehabilitation phase of care that will begin when oncologic treatments are completed. Activities of preparing the patient for rehabil-

itation, as described for the acute hospital stay by Johnson et al. (1998), are applicable to cancer patients in the treatment phase of care. These include (a) differential diagnosis of the swallowing problem, (b) assessment of severity as the patient's condition improves or worsens, (c) aggressive communication with members of the care team, (d) manipulation of the environment to facilitate immediate swallowing and health needs of the patient, (e) patient and family education about the swallowing disorder including the prognosis and anticipated follow-up, (f) development of discharge and follow-up plans, (g) short-term treatment to facilitate swallowing in the immediate environment, and (h) participation in the overall care of the patient.

Consultative and *supportive* roles of the speech-language pathologist, dietitian, and other care team members most frequently are provided to patients receiving radiation therapy, with or without chemotherapy, for malignancies to the upper aerodigestive tract. Patients are counseled about predictable oral complications, which may include mucositis, pain, xerostomia, and loss of or altered taste. To prevent or reduce fibrosis of soft tissues and prevent trismus, patients are encouraged to perform oral ROM exercises on a daily basis, as tolerated. Oral supplementation or temporary

TABLE 19–2. Four-Level Scale for Determining Severity of Accumulated Oropharyngeal Secretions

Rating	Description
0	Normal rating. No visible secretions anywhere in the hypopharynx or some transient bubbles visible in the valleculae and pyriform sinuses. Secretions are not bilateral or deeply pooled.
1	Any secretions evident upon entry or following a dry swallow that were bilaterally represented or deeply pooled. This rating would include cases where there is a transition in the accumulation of secretions during the period of observation.
2	Any secretions that changed from a "1" rating to a "3" during the period of observation
3	Most severe rating. Any secretions seen in the area defined as the laryngeal vestibule. Pulmonary secretions are included if they are not cleared by swallowing or coughing.

Source: Adapted from "The Significance of Accumulated Oropharyngeal Secretions and Swallowing Fequency in Predicting Aspiration," by J. Murray, S. E. Langmore, S. Ginsberg, and A. Dostie, 1998, *Dysphagia, 11,* pp. 99–103.

placement of a nasogastric tube may be recommended if weight loss or decline in swallowing function is observed. Head and neck postsurgical patients may be encouraged to dry swallow or assisted with tracheostomy decannulation when medical clearance is obtained. Insufficient or excessive saliva and secretion production can have a deleterious effect on swallowing function and interfere with airway protection. Care team members can play a role in saliva and secretion management in patient's undergoing cancer treatments using a number of intervention approaches, including pharmacological, behavioral, surgical, or lifestyle.

Rehabilitation

The goals of swallowing rehabilitation are multiple and include reestablishment of oral intake, eliminating aspiration, reducing the risk of pneumonia and other pulmonary complications, and improving hydration and nutritional status. Management of dysphagia is possible only after oropharyngeal swallow anatomy and physiology have been thoroughly assessed using an appropriate instrumental procedure.

Swallowing Assessment

The instrumental procedure selected by the speech-language pathologist should be based on the information needed specific to each patient. The two most commonly used instrumental swallowing assessment procedures are the modified barium swallow and FEES and will be discussed in greater detail. Other instrumental techniques that will not be discussed include ultrasound (Shawker, Sonies, Hall, & Baum, 1984), scintigraphy (Muz, Hamlet, Mathog, & Farris, 1994), surface electromyography (Perlman, 1993), and manometry (Ergun, Kahrilas, & Logemann, 1993). In addition, a number of these instrumental techniques have been used concurrently, such as videofluoroscopy and manometry (Kahrilas, Logemann, Lin, & Ergun, 1992).

MODIFIED BARIUM SWALLOW. The most frequently used and comprehensive method for assessing the oral and pharyngeal phases and cervical esophageal region is the modified barium swallow. It has been referred to by a variety of names including *cookie swallow* and *videofluoroscopic swallow study*. The videofluoroscopic evaluation of oral and pharyngeal swallowing function typically is performed colloboratively by the speech-language pathologist, who is interested in swallow function, and the radiologist, whose focus is structural abnormalities.

The presence of a radiologist during the modified barium swallow is critical with cancer patients, as the procedure alone is not adequate for assessment of structural abnormalities and mucosal abnormalities. Additional techniques to assess structural abnormalities and mucosal lesion of the pharynx may be necessary including rapid sequence with x-ray spot film and double contrast pharyngography. The purposes of the modified barium swallow procedure should be identification of (a) the anatomic and/or physiological oropharyngeal swallow dysfuctions, (b) the relationship of swallow physiology to the patient's symptoms, (c) treatment strategies to improve the pharyngeal swallow and the conditions under which the patient can eat safely, (d) the need for any nonoral intake if aspiration cannot be eliminated, (e) the type of swallowing therapy required, and (f) the need for and timing of swallowing reassessment (Logemann, 1998). The procedure for the modified barium swallow will not be discussed, as it is well detailed in other sources (Logemann, 1993). However, the added use of an objective numerical rating tool will provide objective and sensitive monitoring of patient change in function and provide valuable material for future research and clinical applications. One such tool is the Duke University Medical Center Rating of Radiologic Swallowing Abnormalities (Horner, Riski, Ovelmen-Levitt, & Nashold, 1992). A four-level scale ranks critical components of the oropharyngeal swallow including: oral preparatory phase, reflex initiation phase, pharyngeal phase, pharyngeal appearance in anterior-posterior projection, aspiration, and pharyngeal-esophageal phase screening. Another valuable standardized videfluoroscopic rating tool is the Penetration-Aspiration Scale (Rosenbek, Robbins, Roecker, Coyle, & Wood, 1996), which is presented in Figure 19–3. The Penetration-Aspiration Scale is particularly useful with cancer patients, as

Penetration-Aspiration Scale		
Category	Score	Descriptions
No Penetration or Aspiration	1	Contrast Does Not Enter the Airway
P E N E T R A T I O N	2	Contrast Enters the Airway, Remains Above the Vocal Folds, No Residue
	3	Contrast Remains Above Vocal Folds, Visible Residue Remains
	4	Contrast Contacts Vocal Folds, No Residue
	5	Contrast Contacts Vocal Folds, Visible Residue Remains
A S P I R A T I O N	6	Contrast Passes Glottis, No Sub-Glottic Residue Visible
	7	Contrast Passes Glottis, Visible Sub-Glottic Residue Despite Participant's Response
	8	Contrast Passes Glottis, Visible Sub-Glottic Residue, Absent Participant Response

Figure 19–3. Schematic representation of the 8-Point Penetration Scale. *Source*: From "Differentiation of Normal and Abnormal Airway Protection During Swallowing Using the Penetration-Aspiration Scale," J. A. Robbins, J. Coyle, J. C. Rosenbek, E. Roecker, & J. Wood, submitted for publication. Adapted with permission.

it provides clinical information regarding amount of aspiration, depth of passage of aspirate into the airway, and the patient's ability to expel the aspirate. This information is critical in the management of high-risk populations such as patients with lung cancer who may be placed at significant risk for further pulmonary complications from even small amounts of aspiration.

FLEXIBLE ENDOSCOPIC EXAMINATION OF SWALLOWING. Videoendoscopic examination of pharyngeal dysphagia is being used with increased frequency. Diagnostic limitations previously have been addressed in this chapter. The endoscopic procedure is particularly useful in understanding altered pharyngeal anatomy and its impact on swallowing in patients with anatomic alteration due to surgical excision of the head and neck or base of skull. FEES also is a valuable diagnostic tool for use in examining patients with lung cancer presenting with severe pulmonary disease or in patients who are severely debilitated from cancer and its treatment. Clinical usefulness of FEES in cancer populations can be found in Table 19–3. The endoscopic procedure for examining swallowing function can be found in other sources (Karnell & Langmore, 1998).

FUNCTIONAL MEASUREMENTS TOOLS. Speech-language pathologists and care teams may use or develop functional swallowing measures specific to patient populations served. The Performance Status Scale for Head and Neck Cancer (List et al., 1996) provides ratings of normalcy of diet and public eating, which are represented in Table 19–4.

Swallowing Management

Approaches to management of a swallowing problem can be either medical, prosthetic, or behavioral, or a combination of methods. *Medical* intervention can be categorized according as surgical or pharmacological. Pharmacological interventions are discussed in Chapter 14. Examples of surgical interventions include vocal fold augmentation and medialization, laryngeal suspension, dilation of scar tissue in the pharynx, and cricopharyngeal myotomy. Surgical procedures also are used for management of unremitting aspiration including tracheostomy, glottic and supraglottic laryngeal closure, laryngeal diversion, and total laryngectomy (Blitzer, Krespi, Oppenheimer, & Levine, 1988). *Prosthetic* management includes a maxillary intraoral prosthetic to restore resected portions of the oral cavity and provide improved tongue-to-palate contact for swallowing. A palate-lowering or augmentation device typically is required if the surgical resection has compromised 50% of more of the tongue or if remaining tongue mobility is significantly reduced either vertically or laterally. The speech-language pathologist provides the maxillofacial prosthodontist information about the patient's tongue structure and ROM to

TABLE 19–3. Clinical Usefulness of FEES in Oncology

Postsurgery to the larynx and pharynx
Pharyngeal mucosal appearance after chemotherapy and/or radiation therapy
Concern about excess radiation exposure
Severely dehibilated patients
Assess impact of accumulated secretions and mucus in the laryngopharynx
Biofeedback, to teach airway closure maneuvers
Assess effects of tracheostomy placement
Evaluation of patients with severe pulmonary disease, such as lung cancer
Cranial neuropathies

TABLE 19–4. Performance Status Scale for Head and Neck Cancer: Normalcy of Diet and Public Eating Subscales

Normalcy of Diet	Public Eating
100 Full diet (no restrictions)	100 No restriction of place, food, or companion
90 Full diet (liquid assist)	75 No restriction of place, but restricts diet when in public
80 All meat	50 Eats only in presence of selected persons and in selected places
70 Raw carrots, celery	25 Eats only at home in presence of selected persons
60 Dry bread and crackers	0 Always eats alone
50 Soft chewable foods	
40 Soft foods requiring no chewing	
30 Pureed foods	
20 Warm liquids	
10 Cold liquids	
0 Nonoral feeding	

Source: Adapted from "The Performance Status Scale for Head and Neck Cancer and the Functional Assessment of Cancer Therapy-Head and Neck Scale," by M. A. List, L. L. D'Antonio, D. F. Cella, A. Siston, P. Mumby, D. Haraf, and E. Vokes, 1996, *Cancer, 77*, 2294–2301.

assist with prosthesis design. The majority of postsurgical oral and oropharyngeal cancer patients fitted with intraoral prostheses experience either unchanged swallowing function or mixed results (Pauloski et al., 1996). This highlights the need for patient evaluation and selection for prosthetics based on the extent of resection, nature of reconstruction, and function of remaining oral structures. Research has demonstrated that swallowing rehabilitation can facilitate a return to oral intake in greater than 80% of patients with oropharyngeal dysphagia (Rademaker et al., 1993). As *behavioral* intervention methods are used to rehabilitate the majority of patients with oropharyngeal dysphagia by the speech-language pathologist, this discussion will focus on swallowing therapy. Behavioral methods typically are less costly, lower risk, and more effective in the treatment of oropharyngeal swallowing problems due to cancer and its treatment.

As previously mentioned, a comprehensive discussion of swallowing management strategies specific to each tumor site or cancer treatment modality is beyond the scope of this chapter. General manage-

ment principles have been addressed in preceding chapters, and principles of dysphagia intervention in oncology were highlighted earlier in this chapter. Rather, an approach to swallowing therapy based on pathophysiology of the swallow will be emphasized.

Swallowing procedures are either compensatory or rehabilitative in nature. The effectiveness of *compensatory* treatment procedures typically is assessed during the assessment procedure, and these procedures are designed to control food flow and eliminate the patient's symptoms. Compensatory strategies include (a) postural changes, (b) increasing sensory input, (c) modifying volume and speed of food presentation, (d) changing food consistency or viscosity, and (e) intraoral prosthetics (Logemann, 1998b). *Rehabilitative* therapy procedures are designed to change swallow physiology and are categorized as indirect or direct. *Indirect* therapy procedures are used with patients who are deemed unsafe for any oral intake. No food or liquid is used and therapy involves exercises and swallows of saliva. *Direct* therapy procedures involve actual food or liquid swallows using specified swallowing sequences. Commonly used indirect and direct management techniques and their physiological effect on swallowing are listed in Table 19–5.

Although space prohibits discussion of each of the swallowing treatment strategies presented in Table 19–5, their application is demonstrated in this profile of a patient with head and neck cancer presenting to our care team. *F. A., a 46-year-old male of Cuban descent, presented to our head and neck team for second opinion of recurrent Stage III, T3 N0 M0 squamous cell carcinoma of the tongue that involved most of the right side of the tongue and some of the tongue base. Six months prior to presentation, the patient underwent right partial glossectomy. The plan of care subsequently discussed at the multidisciplinary tumor board included right hemiglossectomy and right modified neck dissection with postoperative radiation therapy. The patient and his family agreed with this plan of care and decided to receive treatments at our cancer center. Pretreatment intervention by the speech-language pathologist included patient and family consultation and baseline swallowing assessment. Clinical assessment revealed hypersalivation and odynophagia. Diet was limited to soft chewable foods. The patient was limiting his public eating due to pain and diet constraints. This resulted in significant lifestyle and vocational disturbances, as Mr. A. reported that entertaining was an important and necessary part of his job. Modified barium swallow revealed a safe and functional swallow, but postswallow coating was observed on the tongue base. Laryngeal penetration also was exhibited by the patient and assigned a rating of 5 on the Penetration-Aspiration Scale. Psycho-oncology referral was made to address psychosocial concerns voiced by the patient and family due to rapid disease recurrence. Mr. A.'s postoperative status was monitored during his 5-day hospitalization. Consultation also was requested and provided to the patient's adult daughter regarding her father's functional speech and swallowing prognosis. Three days fol-* *lowing his discharge home, Mr. A. was seen at the time of his return postoperative medical appointment. Hyperfractioned (twice daily) radiation therapy with concurrent chemotherapy was recommended to the patient by his surgeon, as the surgical pathology report showed close margins with perineural spread. Supportive care was provided to the patient and his wife, as concerns were voiced about the recommendation for additional aggressive medical treatment. The patient's tracheostomy tube was removed but medical clearance was not received to initiate direct or indirect swallowing therapy. The patient returned a week later and an oromotor exercise program was initiated, as the patient's surgeon determined that postoperative healing was complete. Tongue ROM exercises included tongue tip and tongue base elevation, tongue protrusion, and tongue lateralization. Yawning, gargling, and tongue retraction movements were encouraged to improve tongue base retraction. Mandibular mobilization using tongue depressors was initiated and a Therabite Jaw Motion Rehabilitation System was ordered for the patient. Mr. A. was encouraged to try to manage his saliva using the effortful swallow maneuver and the suck-swallow exercise. He was instructed to perform these exercises 5 to 10 times a day for 2 to 3 min each time. Mr. A. was seen in follow-up at the time of his otolaryngology appointment approximately 4 days later. Medical clearance to initiate oral intake was received, as the tracheostomy site was completely healed and the patient was managing his saliva. Modified barium swallow was conducted and revealed the following: premature bolus loss, residue on the tongue and tongue base, mild delay in the initiation of the pharyngeal response, and mild-moderate vallecular residue resulting in aspiration that was assigned a rating of 6 on the Penetration-Aspiration Scale. A safe and efficient swallow was observed when the following compensatory strategies and swallow maneuvers were implemented: head tilt to the left, bolus placement on the left, sensory enhanced sour bolus, and effortful swallow. The patient's nasogastric*

TABLE 19–5. Common Direct and Indirect Therapy Procedures for Dysphagia

Category	Techniques	Physiological Effect
Postural techniques	Chin down; chin-up; heat rotation to damaged side; head tilted to stronger side; side-lying	Redirect bolus flow and change pharyngeal dimensions (Logemann et al., 1994; Rasley et al., 1993)
Combined postures and swallow maneuvers	Evaluated separately then in combination during MBS based on pathophysiology of the swallow	Attain safe and efficient swallow
Lip ROM exercises	Stretch lips in /i/ position; pucker lips tightly; press lips together	Improve labial closure
Tongue ROM exercises	Tongue tip elevation; tongue base elevation; tongue protrusion; tongue lateralization	Improve tongue ROM and oropharyngeal swallow efficiency (Logemann et al., 1997)
Tongue resistance exercises	Provide resistance to the tongue against a tongue depressor, spoon, or clinician's finger in the following directions: tongue up, to the side, and forward	Improve tongue ROM and strength (Jordan, 1979)
Bolus control exercises	Provide patient progressively smaller objects, controlled by the clinician, to manipulate in the mouth with eventual control by the patient; patient progresses to holding both liquid and paste boluses in a cohesive manner	Improve lingual control of the bolus
Bolus propulsion exercises	Patient pushes upward and backward on a liquid-soaked gauze; gauze thickness is reduced with accompanying improvement in tongue ROM	Improve anterior-posterior movement of the bolus
Jaw ROM exercises	Unassisted mandibular opening; mechanically assisted mandibular mobilization with stacked tongue depressors; Therabite Jaw Motion Rehabilitation System	Prevents jaw hypomobility (Buchbinder et al., 1993)
Chewing exercises	Patient chews on gauze, gum, or food	Improve jaw ROM and tongue control for chewing
Tongue base exercises	Patient pulls tongue back and holds; patient pretends to gargle and releases; patient pretends to yawn; effortful swallow maneuver; super-supraglottic swallow	Improve tongue base ROM
Suck-swallow exercise	Patient uses increased vertical tongue-jaw sucking movements with lips closed	Facilitates triggering of the pharyngeal response and improves saliva control

continued

TABLE 19–5. *continued*

Category	Techniques	Physiological Effect
Sensory-motor integration techniques	Thermal-tactile stimulation; cold bolus; textured bolus; larger bolus	Sensitizes and improves triggering of the pharyngeal response (Lazzara et al., 1986); improves initiation of the pharyngeal swallow (Bisch et al., 1994)
Vocal fold adduction exercises	Patient holds breath while pushing or pulling; patient lifts or pushes with simultaneous voicing; patient lifts or pushes while prolonging phonation; easy breath-hold; effortful breath-hold	Improve vocal fold and arytenoid movement
Laryngeal ROM exercises	Patient glides up the scale then prolongs; patient glides down the scale then prolongs	Improve laryngeal elevation
Swallow maneuvers	Dry or repeated swallows; washing food through the pharynx; effortful swallow; Mendelsohn maneuver; tongue-hold maneuver	Improve bolus clearance
Swallow maneuver	Tongue-hold maneuver	Improve tongue base to pharyngeal wall contact and exercise the glossopharyngeus muscle (Fujiiu & Logemann, 1996)
Swallow maneuver	Effortful swallow	Improve tongue base retraction and improve pressure generation (Pouderoux & Kahrilas, 1995)
Swallow maneuver	Supraglottic swallow	Closes vocal folds before and during the swallow (Martin et al., 1993)
Swallow maneuver	Super-supraglottic swallow	Increase anterior tilting of the arytenoid and retraction of the tongue base for airway entrance closure (Ohmae et al., 1995)
Swallow maneuver	Mendelsohn maneuver	Accentuate and prolong laryngeal elevation and anterior movement to improve laryngeal elevation and increase extent and duration of cricopharyngeal opening (Kahrilas et al., 1988); improve coordination of pharyngeal swallow (Lazarus et al., 1993)

Note: MBS = modified barium swallow.

tube subsequently was removed and he began oral intake of soft foods and sensory enhanced liquids using the compensatory strategies and swallow maneuvers deemed effective during videofluroscopic swallowing examination. A program of tongue resistance exercises was introduced for strengthening. The tongue-hold and effortful swallow maneuvers also were provided to improve tongue base retraction and pressure generation. In addition, consultation with the medical oncologist and radiation oncologist for postsurgery cancer treatment planning was arranged. The patient's progress was periodically monitored when he returned for postoperative follow-up in head and neck clinic and throughout his course of concurrent chemotherapy and radiation therapy. Intervention provided at these points during the patient's cancer care included review of daily food diary, gradual progression to a regular diet, weight monitoring, and increased duration and frequency of exercise to extend muscle function. The patient was encouraged to perform his speech and swallowing exercises daily, as tolerated, throughout radiation and for at least 6 weeks after irradiation to prevent fibrosis. At the completion of his 2nd week of therapy, the patient's speech and swallowing were assessed to be well within normal limits but he complained of uncomfortable, dry mouth. Pilocarpine hydrochloride (Salagen) was prescribed and other dietary and hydration recommendations were provided to lessen the effects of xerostomia. During week 3 of the patient's 6-week course of chemoradiation therapy, he demonstrated a 5-lb weight loss and ability to tolerate only liquids due to moderate mucositis. Nutritional consultation was obtained and an aggressive program of oral supplementation was initiated. A prescription of "magic mix" was provided to the patient to lessen the oral impact of treatment. Weight stabilized during the next 7 to 10 days. However, a nasogastric tube was placed during the 5th week of postoperative treatment due to the development of additional combined treatment toxicities. Feeding tube placement provided adequate nutrition, hydration, and patient comfort, which allowed Mr. A. to complete his cancer treatment without interruption. Resolution of all treatment side effects was observed approximately 2 weeks posttreatment completion, and the patient reinitiated his daily speech and swallowing exercise program.

He gradually resumed full oral intake of a regular diet, with liquid assist, over the subsequent 2-week period. Repeat modified barium swallow was performed to assess improvement and assist with nasogastric tube removal. Mr. A. subsequently was seen for follow-up 3 months and 6 months posttreatment completion. Clinical dysphagia assessment revealed scores of 100 on the normalcy of diet, public eating, and understandability of speech subscales on the Performance Status Scale for Head and Neck Cancer. The patient has returned to work on a full-time basis and has resumed his former lifestyle.

Other Swallowing Treatment Considerations

Biofeedback

Instrumental procedures can be used to provide patients biofeedback while they learn swallowing maneuvers and exercises. Biofeedback procedures include surface electromyography, ultrasound, videoendoscopy, and videoflurosopy. The Kay Swallowing Workstation also contains a number of biofeedback applications, including combined surface electromyography and respiratory phase signal to improve coordination between swallowing and respiration and intraoral tongue array with multiple sensors for tongue-strengthening exercises (Figure 19–4).

Functional Dysphagia

Dysphagic cancer patients also may present with accompanying psychological components to their oropharyngeal swallowing disturbance, particularly in oral phase deficits. Psychological distress, particularly anxiety (Barofsky & Fontaine, 1998), related to their disease, dysphagia, or fear of swallowing can be common etiologies. Patients undergoing chemotherapy and radiation therapy typically develop loss of appetite or anorexia. Other contributing factors may include altered oropharyngeal sensation and biomechanics secondary to cancer and its treatments. For

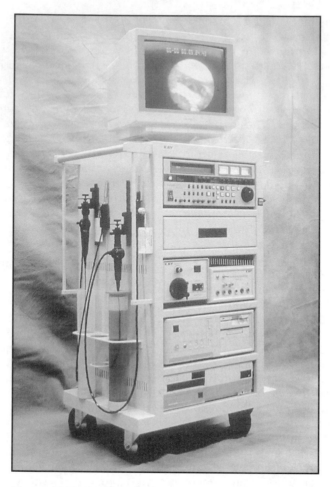

Figure 19–4. Kay Swallowing Workstation provides clinicians multiple biofeedback applications.

example, patients may exhibit difficulty with swallow initiation associated with previous oral pain from mucositis during radiation therapy. Careful swallowing assessment is required to determine psychological accompaniments to the patient's oropharyngeal dysphagia.

Cultural and Religious Differences

With the rapidly changing racial and ethnic composition of the American population, the care team needs to be aware of and sensitive to the religious and cultural practices of patients. For example, many religions such as Catholicism and Judaism have specific regulations regarding food. The Catholic faith has four delineations for the feeding of dying patients. Patients from lower socioeconomic levels and or with little education may rely on folk remedies and beliefs rather than comply with medical recommendations for oral intake. Likewise, clinicians need to be familiar with common ethnic foods when providing food consistency recommendations. For example, picadillo is a common food puree texture that can be recommended to Hispanic patients. Issues should be identified and honored in therapy, as they will affect compliance to treatment recommendations.

Palliative, Home, and Hospice Care

For patients with terminal cancer, intervention principles are modeled after those used with patients with degenerative neurological disease. Palliative goals are directed at improving or maintaining the comfort and independence of patients, allowing them to be least dependent. Regular swallowing assessment is essential so that decline in function can be compensated for, aspiration and pulmonary risks are minimized, and optimum nutrition and hydration are maintained by initiation of partial or total nonoral feeding methods when needed (Logemann, 1998b). Dysphagia intervention involves (a) progressively changing strategies, (b) modifying and restricting the nature of the diet, and (c) recommending combined feeding with eventual transition to nonoral feeding (Logemann, 1998a). Considerations in goal setting with terminally ill patients are discussed in Chapter 20, "Caring for Patients at the End of Life." Counseling, education, and supportive care of patients and families are an essential component of service delivery by care team members. It serves to provide these individuals a better understanding of the anticipated clinical course and intervention goals. An informed patient and family will be better able to realistically assess the risks and benefits of clinical intervention. Most importantly, the decision-making right of the patient must be respected.

CONCLUSIONS

Dysphagia in cancer is multifactorial and complex and often is intensified by the disease process and its treatment. Early prevention as well as ongoing monitoring and treatment throughout the continuum of care provided by a multidisciplinary team approach are required to prevent and reduce morbidity and mortality and achieve optimum clinical outcomes. The speech-language pathologist is a critical team member and plays a key role in dysphagia intervention at every stage in the care continuum. In this chapter, we have attempted to outline general intervention approaches and activities of the clinician at each of these care stages. In order to effectively manage cancer patients with dysphagia, speech-language pathologists require a sound knowledge of dysphagia treatment goals and procedures. In addition, a thorough understanding of cancer and its treatment and the potential impact on swallowing function and nutrition is essential. This knowledge will make care providers more effective and competent team members and ensure a systematic, integrated approach to dysphagia intervention. Although this chapter has not described all dysphagia evaluation and treatment approaches, it does aspire to provide a starting place for individuals and teams interested in addressing the unique challenges provided by cancer patients.

REFERENCES

Barofsky, I., & Fontaine, K. R. (1998). Do psychogenic dysphagia patients have eating disorders? *Dysphagia, 13*, 24–27.

Bastian, R. W. (1991). Videoendoscopic evaluation of patients with dysphagia: An adjunct to the modified barium swallow. *Otolaryngology—Head and Neck Surgery, 104*, 339–350.

Bisch, E. M., Logemann, J. A., Rademaker, A. W., Kahrilas, P. J., & Lazarus, C. L. (1994). Pharyngeal effects of bolus volume, viscosity and temperature in patients with dysphagia resulting from neurologic impairment and in normal subjects. *Journal of Speech and Hearing Research, 37*, 1041–1049.

Blitzer, A., Krespi, Y. P., Oppenheimer, R. W., & Levine, T. M. (1988). Surgical management of aspiration. *Otolaryngologic Clinics of North America, 21*, 743–750.

Bosma, J. F. (1992). Development and impairments of feeding in infancy and childhood. In M. Groher (Ed.), *Dysphagia diagnosis and management* (2nd ed., pp. 107–141). Stoneham, MA: Butterworth-Heinemann.

Buchbinder, D., Currivan, R. B., Kaplan, A. J., & Urken, M. L. (1993). Mobilization regimens for the prevention of jaw hypomobility in the radiated patient: A comparison of three techniques. *Journal of Oral and Maxillofacial Surgery, 51*, 863–867.

Dikeman, K. J., & Kazandjian, M. S. (1995). *Communication and swallowing management of tracheostomized and ventilator-dependent adults.* San Diego, CA: Singular Publishing Group.

Ekberg, O., & Nylander, G. (1983). Pharyngeal dysfunction after treatment for pharyngeal cancer with surgery and radiotherapy. *Gastrointestinal Radiology, 8,* 97–104.

Ergun, G. A., Kahrilas, P. J., & Logemann, J. A. (1993). Interpretation of pharyngeal manometric recording. Limitations and variability. *Diseases of the Esophagus, 6,* 11–16.

Fujiu, M., & Logemann, J. A., (1996). Effect of a tongue holding maneuver on posterior pharyngeal wall movement during deglutition. *American Journal of Speech-Language Pathology, 5,* 23–30.

Horner, J., Riski, J. E., Ovelmen-Levitt, J., & Nashold, B. S. (1992). Swallowing in torticollis before and after rhizotomy. *Dysphagia, 7,* 117–125.

Johnson, A. F., Valachovic, A. M., & George, K. P. (1998). Speech-language pathology practice in the acute care setting: A consultative approach. In A. F. Johnson & B. H. Jacobson (Eds.), *Medical speech-language pathology: A practitioner's guide* (pp. 96–130). New York: Thieme.

Jones, J. (1993). Risk and outcome of aspiration pneumonia in a city hospital. *National Medical Association Journal, 85,* 533–536.

Jordan, K. (1979). Rehabilitation of the patients with dysphagia. *Ear, Nose and Throat Journal, 58,* 86–87.

Kahrilas, P., Dodds, W. W., Dent, J., Logemann, J., & Shaker, R. (1988). Upper esophageal sphincter function during deglutition. *Gastroenterology, 95,* 52–62.

Kahrilas, P. J., Logemann, J. A., Lin, S., & Ergun, G. A. (1992). Pharyngeal clearance during swallow: A combined manometric and videofluoroscopic study. *Gastroenterology, 103,* 128–136.

Karnell, M. P., & Langmore, S. (1998). Videoendoscopy in speech and swallowing for the speech-language pathologist. In A. F. Johnson & B. H. Jacobson (Eds.), *Medical speech-language pathology: A practitioner's guide* (pp. 563–584). New York: Thieme.

Langmore, S. E., Schatz, K., & Olsen, N. (1988). Fiberoptic endoscopic examination of swallowing safety: A new procedure. *Dysphagia, 2,* 216–219.

Langmore, S. E., Terpenning, M. S., Schork, A., Chen, Y., Murray, J. T., Lopatin, D., & Loesche, W. J. (1998). Predictors of aspiration pneumonia: How important is dysphagia? *Dysphagia, 13,* 69–81.

Lazarus, C., Logemann, J. A., & Gibbons, P. (1993). Effects of maneuvers on swallow function in a dysphagic oral cancer patient. *Head and Neck, 15,* 419–424.

Lazzara, G., Lazarus, C., & Logemann, J. A. (1986). Impact of thermal stimulation on the triggering of the swallowing reflex. *Dysphagia, 1,* 37–77.

List, M. A., D'Antonio, L. L., Cella, D. F., Siston, A., Mumby, P., Haraf, D., & Vokes, E., (1996). The Performance Status Scale for Head and Neck Cancer and the Functional Assessment of Cancer Therapy-Head and Neck Scale. *Cancer, 77,* 2294–2301.

Logemann, J. A. (1983). *Evaluation and treatment of swallowing disorders.* Austin, TX: Pro-Ed.

Logemann, J. A. (1989). Speech and swallowing rehabilitation for head and neck tumor patients. In E. N. Myers & J. Y. Stuen (Eds.), *Cancer of the head and neck* (2nd ed., pp. 1021–1043). New York: Churchill Livingstone.

Logemann, J. A. (1993). *Manual for the videofluorographic study of swallowing* (2nd ed.). Austin, TX: Pro-Ed.

Logemann, J. A. (1998a). Dysphagia: Basic assessment and management issues. In A. F. Johnson & B. H. Jacobson (Eds.), *Medical speech-language pathology: A practitioner's guide* (pp. 17–37). New York: Thieme.

Logemann, J. A. (1998b). *Evaluation and treatment of swallowing disorders* (2nd ed.). Austin, TX: Pro-Ed.

Logemann, J. A., Kahrilas, P. J., Kobara, M., & Vakil, N. B. (1989). The benefit of head rotation on pharyngoesophageal dysphagia. *Archives of Physical Medicine and Rehabilitation, 70,* 767–771.

Logemann, J. A., Pauloski, B. R., Rademaker, A. W., & Colangelo, L. (1997). Speech and swallowing rehabilitation in head and neck cancer patients. *Oncology, 11,* 651–659.

Logemann, J. A., Rademaker, A. W., Pauloski, B. R., & Kahrilas, P. J. (1994). Effects of postural change on aspiration in head and neck surgical patients. *Otolaryngology—Head and Neck Surgery, 110,* 222–227.

Martin, B. J. W., Corlew, M. M., Wood, H., Olson, D., Golopol, L. A., Wingo, M., & Kirmani, N. (1994). The association of swallowing dysfunction and aspiration pneumonia. *Dysphagia, 9,* 1–6.

Martin, B. J. W., Logemann, J. A., Shaker, R., & Dodds, W. J. (1993). Normal laryngeal valving patterns during three breath-hold maneuvers: A pilot investigation. *Dysphagia, 8,* 11–20.

Murray, J., Langmore, S. E., Ginsberg, S., & Dostie, A. (1996). The significance of accumulated oropharyngeal secretions and swallowing frequency in predicting aspiration. *Dysphagia, 11,* 99–103.

Muz, J., Hamlet, S., Mathog, R., & Farris, R. (1994). Scintigraphic assessment of aspiration in head and neck cancer patients with tracheostomy. *Head and Neck, 16,* 17–20.

Ohmae, Y., Logemann, J. A., Kaiser, P., Hanson, D. G., & Kahrilas, P. J. (1995). Timing of glottic closure during normal swallow. *Head and Neck, 17,* 394–402.

Pauloski, B. R., Logemann, J. A., Colangelo, L. A., Stein, D., Beery, Q., Heiser, M. A., & Cardinale, S.

(1996). Effect of intraoral prostheses on swallowing function in postsurgical oral and oropharyngeal cancer patients. *American Journal of Speech-Language Pathology, 5,* 31–46.

Pauloski, B. R., Rademaker, A. W., Logemann, J. A., & Colangelo, T. A. (1998). Speech and swallowing in irradiated and nonirradiated postsurgical oral cancer patients. *Otolaryngology—Head and Neck Surgery, 118,* 616–624.

Perlman, A. L. (1993). Electromyography and the study of the oropharyngeal swallowing. *Dysphagia, 8,* 351–355.

Perlman, A. L., Lu, C., & Jones, B. (1997). Radiographic contrast examination of the mouth, pharynx, and esophagus. In A.L. Perlman & K. Schulze-Delrieu (Eds.), *Deglutition and its disorders* (pp.153–199). San Diego, CA: Singular Publishing Group.

Pouderoux, P., & Kahrilas, P. J. (1995). Deglutitive tongue force modulation by volition, volume and viscosity. *Gastroenterology, 108,* 1418–1426.

Rademaker, A. W., Logemann, J. A., Pauloski, B. R., Bowman, J., Lazarus, C., Sisson, G., Milianti, F., Graner, D., Cook, B., Collins, S., Stein, D., Berry, Q., Johnson, J., & Baker, T. (1993). Recovery of postoperative swallowing in patients undergoing partial laryngectomy. *Head and Neck, 15,* 325–334.

Rasley, A., Logemann, J. A., Kahrilas, P. J., Rademaker, A. W., Pauloski, B. R., & Dodds, W. J. (1993). Prevention of barium aspiration during videofluoroscopic swallowing studies: Value of change in posture. *American Journal of Roentgenology, 160,* 1005–1009.

Robuck, J. T., & Fleetwood, J. B. (1992). Nutrition support of the patient with cancer. *Focus on Critical Care, 19,* 129–130, 132–134, 136–138.

Rosenbek, J. C., Robbins, J. A., Roecker, E. B., Coyle, J. L., & Wood, J. L. (1996). A penetration-aspiration scale. *Dysphagia, 11,* 93–98.

Shawker, T., Sonies, B., Hall, T., & Baum, G., (1984). Ultrasound analysis of tongue hyoid and laryngeal activity during swallowing. *Investigative Radiology, 19,* 82–86.

Twycross, R. G. (1981). Rehabilitation in terminal cancer patients. *International Rehabilitation Medicine, 3,* 135–144.

Zenner, P. M., Losinski, D. S., & Mills, R. H. (1995). Using cervical auscultation in the clinical dysphagia examination in long-term care. *Dysphagia, 10,* 27–31.

Caring for Patients at the End of Life

Helen M. Sharp, M.S., and S. Kirk Payne, M.D.

Recent cancer mortality statistics suggest that life expectancy and cure rates for some forms of cancer have improved; however, new cancer treatments have not made a significant impact on overall survival rates (Bailar & Gornik, 1997; Ries et al., 1997). Despite earlier detection and new therapies, many patients with cancer develop progressive disease that requires a shift from curative to palliative goals of care. The World Health Organization (1990) defines palliative care as:

> The active total care of patients whose disease is not responsive to curative treatment. Control of pain, of other symptoms, and of psychological, social and spiritual problems is paramount. The goal of palliative care is achievement of the best quality of life for patients and their families. Many aspects of palliative care are also applicable earlier in the course of the illness in conjunction with anticancer treatment (p. 11).

In this chapter we discuss the treatment of a patient with laryngeal cancer as she moves through a continuum of care: from diagnosis, to disease-specific therapy, to palliative care at the end of her life. This case illustrates the challenges that face patients who are terminally ill and high-

lights opportunities for clinicians to respond to these challenges.

Mrs. Johnson is a 52-year-old widow with a 4-month history of progressive hoarseness and difficulty swallowing. An otolaryngologist diagnoses locally advanced squamous cell carcinoma of the larynx. Members of the head and neck oncology team (medical oncologist, radiation oncologist, otolaryngologist, nurse, social worker, and speech-language pathologist) evaluate Mrs. Johnson. The team members provide her with information about the risks and benefits of therapeutic interventions and the rehabilitation options associated with surgery with postoperative radiation therapy versus induction chemotherapy with definitive radiation therapy. After much reflection and several discussions with Mrs. Smythe, a close friend, Mrs. Johnson selects concomitant radiation and chemotherapy, because she wishes to preserve her larynx and voice. Her desire to keep her voice is largely driven by her wish to continue working as a real estate sales agent.

Mrs. Johnson's treatment is complicated by pain, fatigue, nausea, and dysphagia. Her swallowing is significantly impaired and a gastrostomy tube is recommended for nutritional support. Following completion of chemoradiation therapy, aggressive dysphagia therapy allows her to transition to primarily oral feeding with subsequent removal of the gastrostomy tube.

Following an 18-month remission, Mrs. Johnson returns to the clinic for follow-up and reports difficulty swallowing. Examination shows a suspicious lesion and a biopsy confirms the diagnosis of recurrent squamous cell carcinoma. Radiographic imaging shows that the tumor is unresectable.

The head and neck oncology team offers Mrs. Johnson the following treatment options for the recurrent disease: radiation therapy, salvage chemotherapy, or enrollment in a Phase II experimental trial (a study to determine if a new treatment is safe and shows signs of efficacy in patients with a given disease). After careful consideration of the risks and benefits of each option, and of the small chance that any intervention would significantly prolong her survival, Mrs. Johnson declines further treatment for her cancer.

WHEN PATIENTS REFUSE TREATMENT

Patients frequently choose to receive aggressive treatments for malignant diseases, and clinicians may be surprised when a patient elects to forgo cancer treatments. A patient's right to refuse treatment, even when the treatment is potentially life saving, has been discussed extensively in the legal, medical, and ethics literature (see Weir, 1989). This right to make health care decisions for oneself is increasingly recognized as an important ethical principle in patient care. This emphasis on patient self-determination has evolved as public perceptions of physicians' roles have changed and as medical technologies have proliferated. Many of these technologies offer doctors the opportunity to alter the trajectory of the dying process, giving rise to increasingly complex ethical dilemmas in medicine, many of which have been discussed in the growing field of clinical medical ethics (Beauchamp & Childress, 1989; Jonsen, Siegler, & Winslade, 1998).

A frequently cited example of a patient's decision and right to forgo life-sustaining treatment is the refusal of blood transfu-

sion. Some members of the Jehovah's Witnesses faith believe that receiving blood is a sin. Even though a blood transfusion may be a life-saving therapy, the courts and the majority of scholars in bioethics recognize that an adult with **decision-making capacity** (DMC) has a right to refuse blood transfusions as well as other life-saving treatments (*Melideo*, 1976; *Schloendorff v. Society of New York Hospitals*, 1914). Recognizing a patient's right to self-determination (also referred to as respect for a patient's **autonomy**) is widely recognized as an important ethical principle. The principle of autonomy is frequently invoked to support a competent patient's right to accept or refuse any medical assessments or interventions (*Cruzan v. Director, Missouri Department of Health*, 1990; President's Commission for the Study of Ethical Problems in Medicine and Biomedical and Behavioral Research, 1982).

Respecting a patient's decision to forgo a potentially life-saving therapy may be difficult for clinicians, especially when the proposed treatment presents few risks and is likely to benefit the patient. Occasionally, clinicians are morally opposed to a patient's decision to forgo medically beneficial treatment. In such situations, clinicians may recognize that they can no longer participate in a therapeutic relationship with the patient and should arrange to transfer the clinical responsibility for the patient's care to another qualified clinician who is more comfortable with the patient's decision (Jonsen et al., 1998). Clinicians should avoid threatening to abandon or discontinue care for patients when they choose to forgo recommended treatments. Although continuing to care for the patient may be emotionally difficult for the clinician, most patients value the continuity of care. Preserving the clinician-patient relationship may strengthen the patient's trust in the clinician. With ongoing discussions clinicians may gain a clearer understanding of the patient's goals and wishes about treatment and give patients an opportunity to reexamine their decision to refuse treatment.

Few circumstances justify overriding a patient's informed decision to refuse treatment (Wear & Brahams, 1991). However, when a patient refuses treatment, clinicians must determine whether or not the patient has the cognitive capacity to make decisions about his or her health care (Appelbaum & Grisso, 1988). Decisions to override a patient's refusal and provide treatment usually only occur when the physician or health care team determines that the patient lacks DMC or when the decision to forgo treatment places other people (staff, family members, or other patients) at risk. For example, a patient who refuses treatment for tuberculosis presents a significant health risk to family members, the public, health care workers, and other patients. Many states have laws that mandate treatment for such communicable diseases, even if the patient has DMC and refuses treatment (Gostin, 1993). In such clinical situations, society's interest in protecting the health of third parties takes priority over a patient's right to informed refusal of treatment (Gostin, 1986; Merritt, 1986). However, most treatment refusals involve only the patient. Therefore, when a patient refuses treatment, the primary objective should be to determine if the patient has DMC.

Determining a Patient's Decision-Making Capacity

Clinicians should assess a patient's capacity to participate in decision making for most nonemergent clinical decisions. A patient's decision to forgo treatment often raises specific questions about his or her ability to make informed decisions. When a patient refuses treatment, the team should evaluate the patient to determine if he or she possesses the cognitive capacity to make such a refusal. This evaluation ensures that the health care team does not honor a refusal for treatment from a patient who is unable to comprehend the consequences of making this refusal.

Clinicians often use the terms *competent* and *incompetent* in the context of patients' cognitive capacities. *Competence* is a legal term that refers to patients' ability to live and conduct their affairs in the communi-

ty (Appelbaum, Lidz, & Meisel, 1987). Adults are considered to be competent, unless proved otherwise in a court proceeding (Lo, 1995). If a person is declared "incompetent" he or she is judged to be unable to manage finances, vote in elections, or consent to marriage (Boyle, 1995). Clinicians do not typically focus on patients' competence, but rather on patients' capacity to understand the specific treatment decision and the consequences of giving or refusing consent for that treatment. In Mrs. Johnson's case, the team focuses on her ability to make an informed choice about whether or not she wants further treatment for her cancer. Thus, the team members caring for Mrs. Johnson focus on assessing her DMC rather than her competence. In order to demonstrate that she has DMC, Mrs. Johnson must demonstrate that she can (a) understand her current condition, (b) understand the treatment options available, (c) use a rational thought process in making choices, (d) understand the consequences of her decision, and (e) express a choice (Appelbaum & Grisso, 1988).

The attending physician, a team of clinicians, or consultants can assess DMC. The presence of depression, a cognitive impairment, or a communication disorder may complicate this assessment. True clinical depression can be difficult to distinguish from appropriate sadness about facing death (Mussie & Holland, 1990). In some cases medical personnel may incorrectly assume that a patient is depressed because he or she openly discusses a readiness to die. When the clinical team identifies concerns about depression, a psychiatrist, psychologist, or other mental health professional may be asked to determine if clinical depression impairs the patient's DMC (Sullivan & Youngner, 1994). For patients with cognitive and/or communication disorders, speech-language pathologists may facilitate the assessment of DMC by providing compensatory strategies for cognitive impairments (e.g., memory or attention problems), augmentative communication systems, assistance with speech or voice impairments, or suggestions for enhancing comprehension. Speech-language pathologists may serve a unique role in facilitating the assessment of DMC among patients with communication disorders because the criteria for demonstrating DMC rely heavily on the patient's language comprehension and expression skills. A speech-language pathologist may assist the patient and the team by identifying strategies to maximize the patient's comprehension or ways to facilitate verbal or nonverbal expression using therapeutic strategies or augmentative devices. Furthermore, a speech-language pathologist may be the first team member to identify the patient's capacity to communicate and is thus able to advocate for the patient's participation in decision making. In addition to these specialists, many hospitals, nursing homes, and rehabilitation centers also have clinical ethics consultants who are trained to assist in determining patients' decision-making abilities.

It is important to note that DMC is not an "all or none" phenomenon. A patient may have the ability to make some decisions, such as what to eat or whether to accept a flu shot, but lack the capacity to weigh the risks and benefits of major surgery (Elliot, 1991; Faden & Beauchamp, 1988). For some patients, DMC fluctuates from day to day, so it may be important to periodically reevaluate the patient's capacity to participate in decision making, especially when the patient's cognitive and/or language status is expected to improve (Lo, 1995).

Mrs. Johnson demonstrates that she has DMC through her clear understanding of her medical condition and the ability to discuss the consequences of her decisions. Through her discussions with the team it is clear that she has read about laryngeal cancer and is aware that further treatment would be palliative and unlikely curative. Initially, she chooses to decline further treatment based on her experience with the side effects of treatment and her knowledge of the limited potential for benefit given her current disease state. However, after several weeks of ongoing discussions with the team, Mrs. Johnson elects to receive palliative radiation treatment, with the goals of

potentially decreasing her pain and improving her swallowing. She explicitly states that she does not want another gastrostomy tube.

Following 2 weeks of palliative radiation therapy, a clinical examination and a computed tomography scan show continued growth of the recurrent tumor. In consultation with the team, Mrs. Johnson decides to discontinue further radiation therapy. The team offers experimental therapy, which Mrs. Johnson also declines. She retires from work and plans a trip to visit her daughter and new grandson in California. She enjoys spending time with her neighbor, Mrs. Smythe, who often accompanies her to follow-up appointments. Mrs. Johnson continues to eat a modified diet at home and requires only intermittent pain medication to control her symptoms.

Three weeks later, Mrs. Smythe brings Mrs. Johnson to the emergency room for evaluation of fever, shortness of breath, and lethargy. Mrs. Johnson has become increasingly lethargic over the past few days. Clinical assessment shows that Mrs. Johnson is dehydrated, is malnourished, and has aspiration pneumonia. The emergency room physician intubates her for impending respiratory failure and admits her to the intensive care unit. Mrs. Smythe explains to the physician that Mrs. Johnson has repeatedly stated that she does not want to be "hooked up to machines."

When a Patient Loses Decision-Making Capacity

When health care providers determine that patients are unable to make decisions about their medical treatment, difficult questions arise. Has the patient previously expressed a preference about the treatments he or she wishes to receive? If so, how should these wishes be interpreted within the context of the patient's current status? If not, who should the team look to as the appropriate **surrogate decision maker** or person to speak on behalf of the patient?

When a patient lacks DMC, the team should determine whether the patient has previously expressed any treatment preferences that could guide current decisions (Patient Self-Determination Act [PSDA], 1990). Empirical research suggests that it is preferable to obtain a patient's wishes directly rather than relying on a surrogate decision maker because surrogates accurately predict the decisions the patient would make for themselves only slightly more often than the odds of chance (guessing) predict (Seckler, Meier, Mulvihill, & Cammer Paris, 1991). Physicians' predictions about patients' preferences were even less accurate than those of patient-designated surrogates (Seckler et al., 1991; Uhlmann, Pearlman, & Cain, 1988; Zweibel & Cassel, 1989). The data suggest that, although surrogates do not always predict the patients' preferences, they tend to provide more accurate reflections of the patients' values than do clinicians. The relatively poor ability of clinicians and surrogates to predict patients' preferences underscores the importance of encouraging patients to document their treatment preferences, in written directives and through discussions with family members, caregivers, and clinicians.

Most states have passed legislation that recognizes both living wills and durable powers of attorney for health care, although the specific application of these documents may vary slightly from state to state. In general, a **living will** is a written request to forgo specific treatments or procedures in the event of a terminal or irreversible illness (Miles, Koepp, & Weber, 1996; PSDA, 1990). The definition of *terminal illness* varies between states, and interpreting the applicability of living wills to nonterminal events can be difficult. A **durable power of attorney for health care** is a document that allows the patient to designate a person to make health-related decisions on the patient's behalf should he or she lose the capacity to make such decisions (PSDA, 1990; Miles et al., 1996). A durable power of attorney for health care is especially useful because it allows the health care team to discuss the risks and benefits of treatment options with a person who is chosen by the patient and who is usually familiar with the patient's ideas and preferences.

Clinicians should ask patients and families about written **advance directives**, such as living wills or durable powers of attorney for health care, and should request copies of these documents so they can be placed in the medical record. Advance directives should be interpreted carefully to ensure that the patient's preferences for medical care guide the decisions of surrogates and clinicians.

Although most Americans express support for written advance directives (Burg, McCarty, Allen, & Denslow, 1995; Edinger & Smucker, 1992), it is estimated that only 15–25% of adults complete these documents (Burg et al., 1995; Gallup & Newport, 1991; Gilligan & Jensen, 1995). Many people, like Mrs. Johnson, have verbally expressed preferences about specific treatments to family, friends, or clinicians, but do not complete written advance directives. Verbal statements, though often not as clear as written directives, should be given serious consideration (Sachs & Siegler, 1991). In this case, Mrs. Johnson has stated on several occasions that she does not want a gastrostomy tube in order to sustain her nutritional status if she is unable to eat by mouth. Furthermore, her neighbor reports to the team that Mrs. Johnson has stated on many occasions that she does not want to be "hooked up to machines." Although these statements appear definitive, it is unclear whether she might agree to the temporary use of "machines" (e.g., mechanical ventilation or tube feeding) to treat a potentially reversible disease process. The goal of short-term treatment might be to improve her clinical and cognitive status, thereby allowing her to return home and resume independent living.

The decision whether to provide or to withhold life-saving therapies is especially challenging when there is uncertainty about the patient's prognosis and about what the patient would choose. Many patients use advance directives to request that treatments, such as a feeding tube or mechanical ventilation, be withheld to avoid long-term life support that merely prolongs the dying process. It is difficult to know whether such refusals apply to the short-term use of these technologies in potentially reversible situations. In discussions with her neighbor, Mrs. Johnson explicitly stated her preference not to be "hooked up to machines". Therefore, one could argue against continuing mechanical ventilation, even for a short time. On the other hand, Mrs. Johnson did not specify her preference for the short-term use of technological support, in the event that her condition is potentially reversible. In Mrs. Johnson's case, the team believes that her aspiration pneumonia is treatable and probably reversible with ventilatory support and antibiotics. One may also consider that, because there is some uncertainty about her preferences in this circumstance, it would be best to treat Mrs. Johnson aggressively with the goal of restoring her ability to decide for herself.

In cases where clinical uncertainty is coupled with uncertainty about the patient's preferences, a time-limited trial may be a helpful strategy (President's Commission for the Study of Ethical Problems in Medicine and Biomedical Research, 1983). A time-limited trial is a treatment plan designed to increase clinical certainty about prognosis and to determine how well the patient will tolerate the treatment over a specific time interval. The goal of a time-limited trial is to answer questions about the potential to treat the disease and/or to restore the patient's DMC. In Mrs. Johnson's case, a time-limited trial of mechanical ventilation would provide more clinical information about her prognosis and potentially restore her DMC. This therapy would be conducted with the understanding that the outcome of treatment will be evaluated after a specific time period and that further decisions about continuing or stopping treatment will be addressed at that time with the benefit of the information gained during the trial.

Clinicians and patients often raise questions about the legal and ethical implications of stopping a treatment once it has been started. Legal and ethical analyses draw little distinction between a decision to withdraw ongoing treatment and the decision to withhold treatment (Jonsen, Siegler, & Winslade, 1992; President's Commission for the Study of Ethical Problems in Medicine and Biomedical Research, 1983). If the patient continues to deteriorate during a time-limited trial, the decision to discontinue treatment may be made with greater clinical certainty about the patient's prognosis. However, when withdrawing a treatment is determined to be an ethically acceptable option, it may present a significant psychological burden for the staff who care for the patient. The temporal relationship between treatment termination and the patient's death increases the psychological and emotional pressures for clinicians. However, staff education and team-based decisions about the goals of time-limited trials often help staff understand the rationale and ethical basis for such trials and ease the emotional burdens.

Mrs. Johnson's case presents three options: (a) withdraw mechanical ventilation, (b) continue mechanical ventilation, or (c) continue mechanical ventilation for a limited time period. Although each of these options may be ethically acceptable, Mrs. Johnson cannot participate in the decision making, so who should make the decision?

Mrs. Johnson has given the team permission to discuss her care with Mrs. Smythe, who is often present during clinic visits. The two women have had many conversations about treatments and personal preferences as Mrs. Johnson's disease progressed. However, the social worker raises a concern about the legality of turning to Mrs. Smythe because Mrs. Johnson has not executed an advance directive naming her as a durable power of attorney for health care. The social worker reminds the team that Mrs. Johnson has a daughter who lives in California. Although the team shares her concern, they have never met the patient's daughter because she lives 700 miles away and she has been unable to visit. According to Mrs. Smythe, the daughter calls regularly for updates on her mother's condition, but she rarely calls the hospital directly. She has not been available to participate in her mother's care. Nevertheless, the social worker and other team members remain concerned about who the appropriate decision maker should be in this case.

Identifying an Appropriate Surrogate Decision Maker

When clinicians are uncertain about a patient's preferences for treatment, the patient's proxy or surrogate decision maker may provide helpful guidance. Although empirical studies document relatively poor agreement between the preferences of competent patients and their chosen surrogates' beliefs about the patient's preferences, family members are more accurate in identifying patient's preferences than are physicians (Seckler et al., 1991; Uhlmann et al., 1988). Therefore, if the patient does not have a legal guardian and has not named a proxy decision maker, clinicians may request the assistance of family members to participate in a process of shared decision making. The process of identifying a decision maker may be achieved through discussions with available family members or friends. For end-of-life decision making, some states have developed a list prioritizing who can make decisions about end-of-life care on behalf of a patient who lacks DMC. For example, the Illinois Health Care Surrogate Act (Illinois Public Act 87-749, 1991) suggests the following hierarchy for selecting a proxy decision maker: legal guardian, spouse, adult child, parent, adult sibling, adult grandchild, close friend, guardian of the estate. Such legislation facilitates the identification of an appropriate decision maker to speak on behalf of a patient who is terminally ill and lacks DMC, without going to court. However, these laws do not necessarily allow the team to select who the decision maker should be when someone without a strong legal relationship has a strong personal relationship with the patient. As in the case of Mrs. Johnson, a friend who has no legally recognized relationship to the patient may be in the best position to provide information about the patient's preferences. Although Mrs. Johnson has a daughter, her unrelated, closely involved friend

may be willing to participate as a decision maker. Similar situations arise among patients who are HIV positive and have a domestic partner; the patient's partner may have the best understanding of what the patient would want. However, under a strict reading of the legal guidelines for decision makers for dying patients, a "friend" would rank lower in priority as the appropriate decision maker than an estranged parent (Illinois Public Act 87-749, 1991). Such circumstances may lead the clinician to identify a legally appropriate decision maker who is not necessarily the most ethically appropriate choice. In addition, legislation may not provide guidance when disagreements occur within families (Menikoff, Sachs, & Siegler, 1992). When disagreements arise about who should speak for the patient, it may be helpful to encourage the decision makers to use substituted judgment. **Substituted judgment** requires that the decision maker approach decisions from the perspective of what the patient would want in this circumstance, rather than what the decision maker wants for the patient. Conflict mediation may also be a preferable alternative to using the potentially costly and time-consuming legal system to resolve disagreements about difficult clinical decisions. In rare circumstances, it may be necessary to go to court to appoint a legal **guardian**. However, in most cases it is possible to arrive at mutually agreeable solutions in a more timely way, through discussions about mutual interests in the patient's overall welfare.

A conference involving Mrs. Smythe, Mrs. Johnson' daughter (on a speakerphone), and the health care team is convened to identify a decision maker for Mrs. Johnson. Mrs. Johnson's daughter expresses concern about her mother and is tearful at the prospect of her imminent death. She states that her mother has discussed her desire not to have her suffering prolonged, but is unsure how her mother would view a time-limited trial of mechanical ventilation for pneumonia, which may respond to treatment. The patient's daughter makes arrangements to travel to the hospital as soon as possible. The team is concerned that the daughter's wish for aggressive interventions may reflect her own preferences rather than those of Mrs. Johnson. However, a time-limited trial of mechanical ventilation is arranged, and agreed on by all parties.

Mrs. Johnson's pneumonia responds to treatment with antibiotics and she is easily weaned from the ventilator. Her mental status returns to normal. The clinicians explain the reason for the trial of therapy and Mrs. Johnson agrees they made the best decision possible. She worries, however, that she will die a prolonged and painful death. Mrs. Johnson, her daughter, and Mrs. Smythe meet with the team to discuss plans for further treatment. During the discussion, the team encourages Mrs. Johnson to complete advance directives. After extensive discussions with her neighbor (Mrs. Smythe) and daughter, Mrs. Johnson completes a living will and a durable power of attorney for health care naming Mrs. Smythe as her surrogate decision maker. Her daughter agrees that Mrs. Smythe is the best person to articulate her mother's wishes because she is nearby, has a close relationship with her mother, and is comfortable with the responsibility. The daughter requests that Mrs. Smythe and the team keep her informed of changes in her mother's condition.

Mrs. Johnson's clinical status improves and she decides to resume oral feeding. The care team is concerned, however, about possible deterioration of her swallowing function and questions whether her compromised swallowing caused her aspiration pneumonia. A consultation by a speech-language pathologist is requested. A case manager from Mrs. Johnson's insurance carrier requests justification for the referral for this rehabilitative service, based on documentation in the medical record that Mrs. Johnson is terminally ill.

SETTING REHABILITATION GOALS WITH A PATIENT WHO IS TERMINALLY ILL

Rehabilitation clinicians, such as speech-language pathologists, often work with patients who are expected to make long-term improvements in their functional abilities. Therapists who work with patients who are terminally ill must formulate different rehabilitation goals. Rather than striving for optimal function, the dying patient's goal may be adequate function with minimal intervention (Twycross, 1981). For patients with progressive terminal diseases, rehabilitation goals should have the flexibility to accommodate a potential decline in function rather than traditionally defined goals that focus on improved functional status. For example, a goal of intervention might be to familiarize the patient with a variety of communication tools in anticipation that he or she will need to select an augmentative system in the future. Although such an intervention may be emotionally difficult for the patient, it offers the patient an opportunity to ask questions and discuss the benefits and burdens of various devices. The patient's personal goals and priorities should guide the therapist and the treatment plan for rehabilitation.

Mrs. Johnson is an appropriate candidate for an initial screening of her swallowing function. She expresses her desire to continue oral nutritional support for as long as possible, even though she has experienced a case of aspiration pneumonia. The speech-language pathologist often needs to justify the expense of an assessment by clarifying that it will contribute to managing the patient in two ways: first, by identifying the physiological oral and/or pharyngeal factors that contribute to the patient's swallowing dysfunction and, second, by determining the effectiveness of intervention strategies designed to maximize the patient's efficiency in swallowing and minimize the risk of aspiration. For many patients with cancer of the head and neck, compensatory strategies are easily learned and are helpful (Logemann, 1994). The outcome of a swallowing evaluation may include recommendations for "safer" food consistencies, together with the compensatory strategies, such as postural changes, most appropriate for the patient.

For patients with degenerative diseases that influence swallowing, it can be tempting to anticipate a decline in function and make recommendations for food textures or a modified diet that will be safest for the patient, even following some deterioration. However, some patients may prefer to eat a diet that is slightly higher risk for as long as possible, rather than eat a pureed diet or drink thickened liquids in anticipation that they will need the additional safety in the future. The goal for patients, such as Mrs. Johnson, is to allow continued oral feeding while minimizing the risk of complications. The care team and Mrs. Johnson expect her swallowing function to decline as her tumor increases in size. Thus, her immediate goal is adequate (but perhaps not optimal) nutrition with adequate (but perhaps not optimal) safety. If a patient is unable to swallow safely or is unlikely to be able to sustain adequate intake to meet nutritional needs, the speech-language pathologist and other team members should revisit the discussion of the benefits and burdens of tube feedings with the patient. There are questions about the appropriate role of the speech-language pathologist in facilitating oral feeding in a patient known to aspirate (Segel & Smith, 1995; Sharp & Genesen, 1996). However, the refusal of a feeding tube and/or recommendations for diet modification can usually be handled in a similar way to other refusals of treatment (Sharp & Genesen, 1996; see also the section "When Patients Refuse Treatment").

Mrs. Johnson returns to her home with home health nursing support. Two weeks later she returns to the clinic complaining of severe pain at the disease site. Her physician had prescribed morphine elixir as needed for pain; however, she reports that she takes only half the prescribed dose because she fears she is "taking too much pain medication and will become addicted to morphine." The team admits Mrs. Johnson to the hospital for management of uncontrolled pain. Intravenous morphine is started and carefully titrated to relieve her symptoms. Within 2 hr of initiating treatment, her pain has resolved and she is able to sleep for the first time in several days.

BARRIERS TO EFFECTIVE PAIN MANAGEMENT

The World Health Organization estimates that between 75% and 90% of patients with advanced cancer experience pain (in Bonica, 1990). Forbes (1997) studied 38 patients with head and neck cancer who were admitted to hospice and found that 79% reported pain related to their disease. Although 75% to 85% of cancer pain can be controlled using oral, rectal, or transdermal medication (Management of Cancer Pain Guideline Panel, 1994), studies show that only about half of the patients with cancer receive adequate analgesia (Cleeland et al., 1994). Barriers to achieving adequate pain control occur at the level of the physician and the patient.

Mrs. Johnson's case illustrates how patients' misconceptions about pain management may interfere with treatment. Surveys of attitudes toward pain show that many patients believe "good" patients do not complain about pain (Ward et al., 1993). In addition to underreporting pain, patients are often reluctant to take medication as prescribed because of fear of addiction. This fear persists despite the finding that drug addiction is extremely rare among cancer patients treated with opioids (Porter & Jick, 1980; Ward et al, 1993). Patients also report a fear that they will develop tolerance to pain medications and will suffer with unrelieved pain in the future if they "overuse" prescribed pain medications (Hill, 1993). However, increased pain among patients with cancer is rarely due to tolerance to medications and usually represents progression of the cancer (Gonzales, Elliot, Portenoy, & Foley, 1991). Finally, many patients dislike the sedative side effects of analgesics. When pain medications are properly prescribed and titrated, side effects such as sedation and constipation can usually be managed successfully. It is important for clinicians to be aware of patients' perceptions so they can educate and reassure patients about their concerns.

Physicians may also present barriers to effective pain control. Physicians frequently cite concerns about the potential for patients to become addicted to narcotics and the legality of prescribing what they perceive to be high doses of morphine (Weissman, 1993). Because there is no specific opioid dose that will provide relief for all patients, providing an appropriate dose of pain medication may prove especially challenging. However, the treatment of pain should be similar to the treatment of other medical conditions. Just as doses of insulin are increased to control elevated blood sugar in some patients with diabetes or doses of antihypertension medications are increased to treat high blood pressure, the amount of pain medication necessary to treat cancer pain should be increased to the amount required to eliminate the patient's pain (Levy, 1994). If doses of pain medication are carefully and responsibly titrated to achieve the relief of symptoms, life-threatening side effects such as profound respiratory depression are rarely encountered. In fact, morphine has been reported to be effective and safe for treating shortness of breath associated with cancer (Bruera, MacEachern, Ripamonti, & Hanson, 1993).

Mrs. Johnson experiences difficulty taking adequate oral pain medication secondary to problems with swallowing; therefore the team discusses the use of an intravenous patient-controlled analgesia pump that will allow her to titrate the dose of opioid necessary to relieve her pain. Patient-controlled analgesia pumps allow patients to self-administer a prescribed subcutaneous or intravenous dose of pain medication; a lock-out mechanism prevents patients from delivering too much medication and the pump records medication use.

Mrs. Johnson is given a continuous infusion of opioid with a patient-controlled analgesia pump and she learns to administer additional doses to control her pain. When her pain is well controlled, the dose of opioid used is calculated and converted to a drug that can be delivered using a transdermal delivery system. The transdermal opioid "patch" system proves effective and Mrs. Johnson is discharged to her home with nursing care. Her physician speaks with her 3 days after discharge, and she reports that her pain is well controlled.

Seventeen days later Mrs. Johnson returns to the clinic complaining of increased pain and somnolence. A physical examination shows severe dehydration. Her home care needs have greatly increased, and her neighbor is no longer able to provide the level of care that she needs, even with assistance from home health nurses. Mrs. Johnson's oral intake is now limited to small sips of juice, and she is clearly unable to achieve adequate nutrition or hydration using oral feeding alone. Once again she discusses with her doctor her wish not to have her life prolonged with artificial nutrition and hydration. Although she has repeatedly made this preference clear to her neighbor, family, and health care team, several team members and Mrs. Smythe express concern that they are allowing Mrs. Johnson to "starve to death."

WHEN PATIENTS REFUSE FOOD AND WATER

Clinicians may be uncomfortable supporting a patient's decision to forgo **artificially administered nutrition and hydration**. Food and water are considered a basic human need and the withholding of nutrition may be regarded as cruel behavior (Anscombe, 1981; Callahan, 1983). Most patients agree to accept nutritional support when they lose the ability to swallow. The artificial provision of food and fluids is often considered standard care for patients when there is any chance of a benefit, particularly when the patient's wishes are unknown (Beauchamp & Childress, 1989). However, some patients, like Mrs. Johnson, decide not to prolong their own lives with this technology. As previously discussed, patients have a right to refuse treatment, even if the treatment is potentially life sustaining. The artificial administration of nutrition and hydration is considered a medical treatment as are mechanical ventilation, antibiotic therapy, chemotherapy, and surgery (*Bowvia v. Superior Court*, 1986; *Cruzan v. Director, Missouri Department of Health*, 1990; Lynn & Childress, 1983).

When a patient refuses nutritional support, the refusal should first be considered indicative of a potential medical problem. For example, among patients who have received radiation therapy, the refusal to eat may be secondary to pain associated with radiation-induced mucositis (mucosal irritation) rather than a refusal of nutritional support. Similarly, some cancer patients refuse oral feeding because of recurrent nausea. Although medications are available to treat symptoms of nausea and anorexia associated with treatment, cachexia and anorexia are recognized as a normal part of the dying process (Ashby & Stoffell, 1995).

A patient's informed decision to refuse supplemental nutrition or hydration should be respected. A recent study of cancer patients who made this decision involved interviews with patients and family members throughout the process of dying by starvation (McCann, Hall, & Groth-Juncker, 1994). Careful monitoring of these patients revealed that, although they were consistently offered food and fluids, their intake gradually decreased. Most patients reported that as long as good oral care with oral moisture was maintained, they did not feel pain or experience discomfort during the dying process. Family members were also interviewed and typically reported that they perceived the patient was comfortable. Surprisingly, patients who elected to continue hydration were more likely to report pain than those for whom both hydration and nutrition were stopped (McCann et al., 1994).

Many patients who are terminally ill elect to continue supportive nutrition. Several studies have been conducted to quantify the relative benefits and burdens of sustaining nutritional support throughout the dying process. Some authors argue that continued feeding promotes wound healing and improves quality of life (Ottery, 1995). Others conclude that clinical studies fail to demonstrate that tube feeding extends days of life or improves patient comfort when a patient is terminally ill (Lynn & Childress, 1983; Quill, 1989; Vigano, Watanabe, & Bruera, 1994). The potential burdens of tube feedings include complications such as diarrhea, pain, nausea, vomiting, dyspnea, or aspiration pneumonia (Ciocon, Silverstone, Graver, & Foley, 1988) and the use of chemical and mechanical restraints (Quill, 1989).

Discontinuing food and fluids is likely to remain a controversial issue. Interpreting the research and opinions regarding nutritional support for patients who are in the terminal stages of disease is fraught with subjectivity and uncertainty. For example, it is critical to consider that the patients who participated in the study by McCann et al. (1994) *elected* to discontinue nutritional support. For many patients, such an option would be abhorrent and their reports of the process of dying without food or water could be considerably different. Because feeding carries so many social and emotional overtones, decisions to continue feeding, despite risks of prolonging a potentially painful dying process, or to withdraw nutrition, despite risks of potentially shortening one's life, remain intensely personal and individual. When surrogate decision makers are asked to decide about continuing or discontinuing feeding, it is important to question whether artificially administered feeding meets the patient's goals or is continued for the benefit of the family. Despite the importance of considering the artificial provision of nutrition and hydration on an individual basis, the recent data challenge clinicians and patients to rethink the goals of artificial nutrition and hydration as a standard part of "comfort care" in the dying patient (Billings, 1985; McCann et al., 1994).

The day after admission, Mrs. Smythe and the care team (including a dietitian) meet with Mrs. Johnson to discuss her goals of care and treatment. They reach an agreement that continuing to provide artificial nutrition and hydration would be of minimal benefit, given Mrs. Johnson's poor prognosis. During the discussion the team clarifies that without food or fluids Mrs. Johnson is likely to die within 4 to 14 days. Maximizing pain control and patient comfort are clearly identified as the goals of treatment. These goals appear to be consistent with the philosophy of hospice care and Mrs. Johnson agrees to an evaluation by the palliative care team. A plan of treatment involving a return to home with nursing and home care support, the support of her neighbor, and a plan for her daughter to return home for a few weeks is agreed on by everyone. Mrs. Johnson is discharged home the next day. She remains comfortable with occasional lucid periods, and dies in her sleep on day 5 following discharge. Mrs. Smythe and the daughter each write letters of thanks to the team and report that Mrs. Johnson appeared comfortable and that her death happened in a manner consistent with her wishes.

REFERENCES

Anscombe, G. E. M. (1981). Ethical problems in the management of some severely handicapped children: Commentary 2. *Journal of Medical Ethics, 7,* 122–123.

Appelbaum, P. S., & Grisso, T. (1988). Assessing patient's capacities to consent to treatment. *New England Journal Medicine, 319,* 1635–1638.

Appelbaum, P. S., Lidz, C. W., & Meisel, A. (1987). *Informed consent: Legal theory and clinical practice.* New York: Oxford University Press.

Ashby, M., & Stoffell, B. (1995). Artificial hydration and alimentation at the end of life: A reply to Craig. *Journal of Medical Ethics, 21,* 135–140.

Bailar, J. C., III, & Gornik, H. L. (1997). Cancer undefeated. *New England Journal of Medicine, 336,* 1569–1574.

Beauchamp, T. L., & Childress, J. F. (1989). *Principles of biomedical ethics* (3rd ed, pp. 163–169). New York: Oxford University Press.

Billings, J. A. (1985). Comfort measures for the terminally ill: Is dehydration painful? *Journal of the American Geriatrics Society, 33,* 808–810.

Bonica, J. J. (1990). Cancer pain. In J. J. Bonica (Ed.), *The management of pain* (2nd ed., Vol. 1, pp. 400–460). Philadelphia: Lea & Febiger.

Bouvia v. Superior Court, No. B019134 (Cal. App. 2d Dist. April 16, 1986).

Boyle, R. J. (1995). Determining patients' capacity to share in decision making. In J. C. Fletcher, C. A. Hite, P. A. Lombardo, & M. F. Marshall (Eds.), *Introduction to clinical ethics* (p. 66). Frederick, MD: University Publishing Group.

Bruera, E., MacEachern, T., Ripamonti, C., & Hanson, J. (1993). Subcutaneous morphine for dyspnea in cancer patients. *Annals of Internal Medicine, 119,* 906–907.

Burg, M. A., McCarty, C., Allen, W. L., & Denslow, D. (1995). Advance directives: Population prevalence and demand in Florida. *Journal of the Florida Medical Association, 82,* 811–814.

Callahan, D. (1983). On feeding the dying. *Hastings Center Report, 13,* 22.

Ciocon, J. O., Silverstone, F. A., Graver, L. M., & Foley, C. J. (1988). Tube feedings in elderly patients. *Archives of Internal Medicine, 148,* 429–433.

Cleeland, C. S., Gonin, R., Hatfield, A. K., Edmonson, J. H., Blum, R. H., Stewart, J. A., & Pandya, K. J. (1994). Pain and its treatment in outpatients with metastatic cancer. *New England Journal of Medicine, 330,* 592–596.

Cruzan v. Director, Missouri Department of Health, 497 U.S. 261, 110 S. Ct. 2841 (1990).

Edinger, W., & Smucker, D. R. (1992). Outpatient's attitudes regarding advance directives. *Journal of Family Practice, 35,* 650–653.

Elliot, C. (1991). Competence as accountability. *Journal of Clinical Ethics, 2,* 167–171.

Faden, R., & Beauchamp, T. (1988). *A history and theory of informed consent.* New York: Oxford University Press.

Forbes, K. (1997). Palliative care in patients with cancer of the head and neck. *Clinical Otolaryngology, 22,* 117–122.

Gallup, G., & Newport, F. (1991). Mirror of America: Fear of dying. *Gallup News Service, 55,* 1–6.

Gilligan, M. A., & Jensen, N. (1995). Use of advance directives: A survey in three clinics. *Wisconsin Medical Journal, 94,* 239–243.

Gonzales, G. R., Elliot, K. J., Portenoy, R. K., & Foley, K. M. (1991). The impact of a comprehensive evaluation in the management of cancer pain. *Pain, 47,* 141–143.

Gostin, L. (1986). The future of communicable disease control: Toward a new concept in public health. *Milbank Quarterly, 64* (Suppl. 1), 79–96.

Gostin, L. O. (1993). Controlling the resurgent tuberculosis epidemic: A 50-state survey of TB statutes and proposals for reform. *JAMA, 269,* 255–261.

Hill, C. S. (1993). The barriers to adequate pain management with opioid analgesics. *Seminars in Oncology, 20* (Suppl. 1), 1–5.

Illinois Pub. Act 87–749, H.B. 2334, 87th Gen. Assembly, 91st Sess. (1991).

Jonsen, A. R., Siegler, M., & Winslade, W. J. (1992). *Clinical ethics* (3rd ed.). New York: McGraw-Hill.

Jonsen, A. R., Siegler, M., & Winslade, W. J. (1998). *Clinical ethics* (4th ed.). New York: McGraw-Hill.

Levy, M. H. (1994). Pharmacologic management of cancer pain. *Seminars in Oncology, 21,* 718–739.

Lo, B. (1995). *Resolving ethical dilemmas: A guide for clinicians* (pp. 82–89). Baltimore: Williams & Wilkins.

Logemann, J. A. (1994). Rehabilitation of the head and neck cancer patient. *Seminars in Oncology, 21,* 359–365.

Lynn, J., & Childress, J. F. (1983). Must patients always be given food and water? *Hastings Center Report, 13,* 17–21.

Management of Cancer Pain Guideline Panel. (1994). *Management of cancer pain: Clinical practice guideline* (AHCPR Publication 94–0592). Rockville, MD: U.S. Public Health Service, Agency for Health Care Policy and Research.

McCann, R. M., Hall, W. J., & Groth-Juncker, A. (1994). Comfort care for terminally ill patients: The appropriate use of nutrition and hydration. *JAMA, 272,* 1263–1266.

Melideo 88 Misc. 2d 974, 390 N.Y.S. 2d 523 (1976).

Menikoff, J. A., Sachs, G. A., & Siegler, M. (1992). Beyond advance directives—Health care surrogate laws. *New England Journal of Medicine, 327,* 1165–1169.

Merritt, D. J. (1986). The constitutional balance between health and liberty. *Hastings Center Report, 16* (Suppl.), 2–10.

Miles, S. H., Koepp, R., & Weber, E. P. (1996). Advance end-of-life treatment planning: A research review. *Archives of Internal Medicine, 156,* 1062–1068.

Mussie, M. J., & Holland, J. C. (1990). Depression and the cancer patient. *Journal of Clinical Psychiatry, 51,* 12–17.

Ottery, F. D. (1995). Supportive nutrition to prevent cachexia and improve quality of life. *Seminars in Oncology, 22* (Suppl. 3), 98–111.

Patient Self-Determination Act. In Omnibus Budget Reconciliation Act of 1990. Pub. L. No. 101–508 4206, 4751 (1990).

Porter, J., & Jick, H. (1980). Addiction rare in patients treated with narcotics. *New England Journal of Medicine, 302,* 123.

President's Commission for the Study of Ethical Problems in Medicine and Biomedical and Behavioral Research (1982). Washington, DC: U.S. Government Printing Office.

President's Commission for the Study of Ethical Problems in Medicine and Biomedical and Behavioral Research. (1983). *Deciding to forego life-sustaining treatment* (pp. 82–83). Washington, DC: U.S. Government Printing Office.

Quill, T. E. (1989). Utilization of nasogastric feeding tubes in a group of chronically ill, elderly patients in a community hospital. *Archives of Internal Medicine, 149,* 1937–1941.

Ries, L. A. G., Kosary, C. L., Hankey, B. F., Miller, B. A., Harras, A., & Edwards, B. K. (Eds.). (1997). *SEER cancer statistics review, 1973–1994, National Cancer Institute* (NIH Publication No. 97–2789). Bethesda, MD.

Sachs, G. A., & Siegler, M. (1991). Guidelines for decision making when the patient is incompetent. *Journal of Critical Illness, 6,* 348–359.

Schloendorff v. Society of New York Hospitals, 211 NY 125, 129, 105 N.E. 92, 93 (1914).

Seckler, A. B., Meier, D. E., Mulvihill, M., & Cammer Paris, B. E. (1991). Substituted judgment: How accurate are proxy predictions? *Annals of Internal Medicine, 115,* 92–98.

Segel, H. A., & Smith M. L. (1995). To feed or not to feed. *American Journal of Speech-Language Pathology, 4,* 11–14.

Sharp, H. M., & Genesen, L. B. (1996). Ethical decision-making in dysphagia management. *American Journal of Speech-Language Pathology, 5,* 15–22.

Sullivan, M. D., & Youngner, S. J. (1994). Depression, competence, and the right to refuse lifesaving medical treatment. *American Journal of Psychiatry, 151,* 971–978.

Twycross, R. G. (1981). Rehabilitation in terminal cancer patients. *International Rehabilitation Medicine, 3,* 135–144.

Uhlmann, R. F., Pearlman, R. A., & Cain, K. C. (1988). Physicians' and spouses' predictions of elderly patients' resuscitation preferences. *Journal of Gerontology, 43,* M115–121.

Vigano, A., Watanabe, S., & Bruera, E. (1994). Anorexia and cachexia in advanced cancer patients. *Cancer Surveys, 21,* 99–115.

Ward, S. E., Goldberg, N., Miller-McCauley, V., Mueller, C., Nolan, A., Pawlik-Plank, D., Robbins, A., Stormoen, D., & Weissman, D. E. (1993). Patient-related barriers to management of cancer pain. *Pain, 52,* 319–324.

Wear, A. N., & Brahams, D. (1991). To treat or not to treat: The legal, ethical, and therapeutic implications of treatment refusal. *Journal of Medical Ethics, 17,* 131–135.

Weir, R. F. (1989). *Abating treatment with critically ill patients: Ethical and legal limits to the medical prolongation of life* (pp. 65–105). New York: Oxford University Press.

Weissman, D. E. (1993). Doctors, opioids, and the law: The effect of controlled substances on cancer pain management. *Seminars in Oncology, 20* (Suppl. 1), 53–58.

World Health Organization (1990). *Cancer pain relief and palliative care.* (Tech. Rep. Series 804). Geneva, Switzerland: Author.

Zweibel, N. R., & Cassel, C. K. (1989). Treatment choices at the end of life: A comparison of decisions by older patients and their physician-selected proxies. *Gerontologist, 29,* 615–621.

GLOSSARY

Advance directive—A statement through which an individual expresses preferences about health care in order to direct his or her physician and other members of the health care team. Most states recognize two forms of written advance directives: the living will and the durable power of attorney for health care.

Artificially administered nutrition and hydration—Any nonoral method of delivering nutrition and hydration to a person; it includes, but is not limited to, total parenteral nutrition (TPN), intravenous (IV) fluids, nasogastric (NG) tube, oral-gastric tube, gastrostomy (G) tube, jejunostomy (J) tube. Alternative means of nutritional support does not include assisted or adaptive feeding techniques such as spoon or bottle feeding.

Autonomy—A patient's right to self-determination.

Decision Making Capacity (DMC)—An individual's ability to understand the information being given, use a rational thought process to manipulate the information, and express a choice. DMC is task-specific, so a patient may have DMC for one decision, but lack DMC for another (see Appelbaum & Grisso, 1988).

Durable power of attorney for health care (DPAHC)—A signed, witnessed document completed by an individual 18 years of age or older that designates a person to act as an agent to make health care decisions on his or her behalf, at any time that the individual is unable to make decisions for him- or herself. An agent appointed as a DPAHC has the power to consent to or refuse any medical treatment, including life-sustaining treatment. A DPAHC is not authorized to make financial or other non-health-related decisions.

Guardian—A person appointed through a legal proceeding and authorized by the courts to make health care, financial, and all other decisions on behalf of a person who has been evaluated and found to be legally incompetent.

Living will—A signed, witnessed document completed by an individual 18 years of age or older that instructs the health care team about the individual's treatment preferences. The living will usually applies only to decisions to withhold or withdraw life-sustaining treatments in the event that the individual both is unable to make decisions for him- or herself and is judged to be terminally ill and that treatment would only prolong the dying process.

Surrogate decision maker—An individual identified to make decisions on behalf of a patient, when the patient lacks the capacity to make his or her own decisions. A surrogate decision maker may be identified by the patient (e.g., durable power of attorney for health care or named verbally), by the courts (i.e., legal guardian), or by the physician (or care team) when the patient is unable to name a person to make decisions on his or her behalf.

Substituted judgment—A decision made by a surrogate decision maker that reflects as nearly as possible the decision the patient would make under specific circumstances. Substituted judgment is the preferred standard for decision making by a surrogate decision maker when the patient lacks decision-making capacity or is unable to express his or her wishes

21

Shaping the Future

Albert B. Einstein, Jr., M.D.

Rehabilitation of the patient who has experienced disability due to destructive cancer treatment or the disease itself is obviously important for the quality of the patient's life as well as returning the patient to a useful functional role in society (Dietz, 1981). The economic costs of the rehabilitation efforts can be measured, but the economic and human costs of not rehabilitating the patient are more difficult to estimate.

The evolution of health care in the 1990s has created the need to evaluate, standardize, and justify, in terms of both clinical and economic outcomes, the clinical practices that we previously have taken for granted. Cancer rehabilitation strategies need to be incorporated into disease management guidelines to ensure that they are appropriately considered and used. Clinical pathways that describe optimal cost-efficient rehabilitation therapy with definable outcome measures relating to functional improvement, patient satisfaction, and cost need to be developed to justify the procedures in today's cost-driven managed care environment.

HEALTH CARE REFORM IN THE 1990S

Prior to 1993, most Americans' health care benefits were provided through corporate-sponsored commercial indemnity insurance or government benefit programs such as Medicare or Medicaid. Health care providers, including rehabilitation specialists, were reimbursed on a fee-for-service basis. The charges for procedures and services had little or no relationship to the actual cost in providing the service. Providers had no incentive to consider or account for costs of the care they provided to be reimbursed (Einstein, 1996).

In the 1970s the federal government first recognized a rapid increase in health care costs under the fee-for-service system and attempted, but failed, to control the rise by requiring a certificate of need for hospitals considering major capital investments (Einstein, 1996). In 1985, Congress took the step of creating a prospective payment system to limit the Medicare hospital costs (Igelhart, 1992). The diagnosis-related groups (DRGs) were created to provide a fixed payment for a hospital admission based on the principal diagnosis, regardless of the length of stay or the services provided (Einstein, 1996). The subsequent impact has been tighter management of hospital stays, decreased bed use, shorter length of stays, and a shift in services from the inpatient to the outpatient environment (Einstein, 1996). Medicare physician fee reimbursement became regulated in 1991 with the Resource Based Relative

343

Value System (Dernberg, 1992; Igelhart, 1993; Xistris & Houlihan, 1994). Physician office and hospital evaluation and management fees were based on the physician's work, practice costs, and malpractice expense. In the next couple of years, Medicare plans to introduce a second prospective payment system for outpatient hospital procedures.

Meanwhile, in the commercial health care industry, health maintenance organizations (HMOs) established by the HMO Act of 1973 showed significant growth in the 1980s. Most major HMOs were either cooperatives or not-for-profit staff model organizations such as Group Health Cooperative of Puget Sound and the Kaiser Foundation Health Plan (Einstein, 1996). By the 1990s, for-profit managed care organizations began to emerge, particularly in California and Minnesota, as the predominant HMO model. They would contract with selected hospitals and physicians for the care of populations of patients at significantly discounted reimbursement rates. They began to introduce other models of provider organizations such as preferred provider organizations and other reimbursement strategies such as case rates and capitation to reduce the cost of physician and hospital care. New provider organizations, such as independent physician associations (IPAs) and physician hospital organizations (PHOs), formed to facilitate competing for and acquiring managed care contracts (Campbell, 1995; Einstein, 1996).

In 1993, the cost of health care accounted for 13% of the gross national product, a level perceived by many as being intolerable and significantly higher than in other Western industrialized countries. Corporations found it harder to produce a profit for their shareholders in part because of the uncontrolled rise in health care costs. Federal and state governments had fewer budgetary dollars available for other competing services such as education and social welfare services.

In 1992, Bill Clinton was elected president of the United States on a platform that promised health care reform to cor-

rect its uncontrolled growth. Despite concerted effort by the executive branch, however, the Congress failed in 1993 to adopt an overall sweeping reform plan (Annas, 1995; Blumenthal, 1995; Heclo, 1995; Skocpol, 1995). Meanwhile, several states—including Washington, Minnesota, Florida, and Oregon—adopted health care reform measures (Brown, 1993; Crittenden, 1993; Igelhart, 1994; Rogal & Helm, 1993). Many of the state initiatives, however, were reversed by the 1994 elections when the Republican Party captured power in many of the state legislatures. Despite these political activities, the underlying pressures demanding cost reduction in health care did not disappear.

Into the void created by the federal government's inaction has stepped the for-profit managed care industry. It has rapidly penetrated many of the major health care markets, offering corporations and government a means to control their health care costs. Managed care organizations now control over 50% of care in some major metropolitan areas, with a corresponding reduction in traditional indemnity insurance. Managed care plans are now being implemented for both Medicare and Medicaid beneficiaries. Some large corporations have adopted the principles of managed care in operating their self-insurance plans. For all payers, their overt mission in the 1990s has been to reduce their cost of health care.

For the health care provider, the impact of managed care and the emphasis on cost control have created major changes. Both hospitals and physicians have experienced marked reductions in reimbursement, decreased revenues, and increased competition for patients. Hospital admissions and lengths of stays have decreased as care has shifted from the inpatient setting to the less expensive ambulatory care setting. All hospitals have had to reduce costs in an attempt to maintain a profit margin. Some unprofitable hospitals have closed; others have been forced to merge or affiliate with other hospitals in their communities (Einstein, 1996). Specialized services, such as cancer and rehabilitation, have in some communities been centralized in designated hospitals within a health care system rather than each facility's duplicating the services.

Physicians have experienced loss of control over their practices and increased administrative overhead. Managed care gatekeepers and case managers may determine what services are to be provided and by whom. Physician access to patients is now determined by the managed care plan. Physicians are being forced to abandon solo or small group independent practice in favor of networks, practice management arrangements, and group practice to be competitive for managed care contracts (Berger, 1995; Campbell, 1995; Einstein, 1996). To what degree managed care will dominate an individual market may vary, but currently it remains the major force for cost containment by the payers.

Although most managed care contracts are currently based on discounted fee-for-service reimbursement, risk-sharing contracts are beginning to emerge in the form of case rates for an episode of care, global fees bundling both physician and hospital reimbursement, and capitation, where the provider is paid a set reimbursement for defined services on a per patient per month basis, regardless of utilization. Providers are rewarded not for delivery of services but for the appropriate utilization of services. In the risk-sharing arrangements, profitability depends on the provider's ability to control utilization and costs of services. The fewer the resources expended, the greater the reward for the providers. The cost of care and the utilization of services of individual physicians or hospitals can now be measured and compared to peers (Einstein, 1996). Some argue that risk sharing represents a perverse incentive for the provider to not deliver appropriate services; others argue that providers need to be appropriately incentivized to control costs and utilization. Necessary and appropriate services such as rehabilitation services for cancer can no longer be taken for granted and need to be continuously justified on the basis of outcomes.

THE CONTINUUM OF CANCER CARE AND ITS MANAGEMENT

The cancer care management model has also evolved as health care in general has shifted from the fee-for-service reimbursement system to the managed-care methodology. Cancer care consists of a continuum of cancer services that includes screening and prevention, diagnosis, staging, treatment, supportive care, rehabilitation, palliative care, home care, and hospice care. In the ideal model all of these services are managed in a seamless fashion for the benefit of the patient and his or her family. Traditionally, the cancer care model has been the multidisciplinary hospital-based cancer program as defined by the American College of Surgeons and the Association of Community Cancer Centers. This model included a screening program, an inpatient oncology unit, a tumor board, a cancer committee, a tumor registry, as well as hospital-based patient support and rehabilitation services. The oncologists would provide inpatient treatment usually on a dedicated inpatient oncology nursing unit and outpatient treatment either in their private offices or the hospital outpatient clinic. Most, if not all, oncology services were centralized and provided by a single hospital. Fee-for-service reimbursement allowed both the physician and the hospital to get paid independently for their services without the need for cost management (Einstein, 1996).

With the increased penetration of managed care and particularly capitated or risk-sharing contracts, the traditional cancer care paradigm has evolved from a hospital-based cancer program to a cancer delivery system that is capable of managing, not just providing, cancer care over a geographically defined marketplace. The providers are now being forced to control costs if they are to successfully compete for managed-care contracts or share risk. Provider networks with the potential of managing cancer care are assuming a variety of forms: physician only, hospital systems and physicians, practice management companies and physicians, and care management companies and providers. These networks or alliances typically provide care over a geographic area defined by the managed-care marketplace. They may be single specialty, multispecialty, hospital only or physician only, or a combination of physicians and hospitals. They may consist of disease-specific, specialty-specific, or multispecialty, multiple-disease providers. To successfully manage cancer care, they must have a medical support organization that case manages, preferably using multidisciplinary provider derived clinical guidelines; information systems that support case management; as well as the typical practice administrative support systems (Campbell, 1995; Einstein, 1996).

Managing cancer care primarily requires control of clinical costs and utilization of services, but appropriate quality of care and patient satisfaction remain important outcomes. To achieve these outcomes, physicians and institutions must be willing and incentivized to standardize care, control utilization of services, and reduce individual provider variability. Standardization of care is best achieved by clinical guidelines and critical pathways. Clinical guidelines define what to do and pathways define how to do it (Einstein, 1996; Field & Lohr, 1990).

Cancer-related clinical guidelines are currently being developed by multiple national, regional, and local organizations. They are best defined by a multidisciplinary team based on the best scientific data available as well as the consensus of expert opinion when the scientific data are not definitive. They should be used by practitioners to guide, not dictate, the care in the majority of cases and should be routinely reviewed and updated (Einstein, 1996; Field & Lohr, 1990). Local physician participation in the development, adoption, review, and updating of the guidelines is essential to achieve physician buy-in to the process.

Compared to guidelines, clinical pathways or protocols define in detail the necessary events and services surrounding a

particular clinical intervention. Pathways are constructed to provide consistent, highly cost-efficient quality care. In contrast to guidelines, which describe what to do, they prescribe how to perform an intervention. The combination of guidelines and pathways provides the basis for a system to manage clinical care.

The new cancer management paradigm requires the alignment of individual provider incentives with cost containment and quality. In risk-sharing contractual arrangements, the physicians are reimbursed by controlling costs. Risk-sharing pools are established and allocated based on control of costs. Quality is defined by and maintained by the guidelines and pathways. Physician variation from guidelines, although allowed when appropriate, is discouraged by this reimbursement system.

THE ROLE OF REHABILITATION IN THE MANAGEMENT OF CANCER-RELATED SWALLOWING AND SPEECH DISORDERS

Cancers of the head and neck region and their treatment can result in major changes in the anatomy and, subsequently, the swallowing and speech functions of the patient (Dietz, 1981). Maintenance or restoration of these important functions is essential for the patient's nutritional status, quality of life, and ability to be restored as a productive, useful member of society. Evaluation of individual rehabilitation potential, goal setting, therapy planning, and outcomes measurement are important for each patient.

According to Logemann, Pauloski, and Rademaker (1992), treatment selection is the first line of rehabilitation. There is no treatment procedure for head and neck cancer that does not have some effect on speech and/or swallowing function. The importance of treatment selection cannot be overemphasized. Preferably, rehabilitation planning should begin at the time of diagnosis, and treatment planning and rehabilitation are evaluated concurrently. Speech and swallowing problems can be predicted by the oncologists and the patient can be prepared for the necessary restorative measures in advance. Successful rehabilitation requires that the oncologist work closely with the rehabilitation specialists in a collaborative fashion from the beginning of treatment planning. The restorative goals need to be realistic, planned by a multidisciplinary team, and communicated effectively to the patient.

Posttreatment evaluation of speech and swallowing defects should be performed by a speech-language pathologist and by a dentist or maxillofacial orthodontist when indicated. Disability may be short lived, associated with a particular modality of therapy, or involve long-term, potentially permanent changes to the lifestyle (Dietz, 1981).

Clinical guidelines for the management of the variety of head and neck cancers have been written by many organizations. Although the guidelines primarily address treatment modalities based on cancer site and stage, they should also clearly indicate the type and optimal timing of rehabilitation interventions in order to be complete and truly multidisciplinary. Rehabilitation specialists should be part of the multidisciplinary team's writing, reviewing, and adopting of guidelines for the management of head and neck cancers. Once the guidelines are established, the rehabilitation specialists should define clinical pathways for the significant rehabilitation interventions, taking into consideration current research findings, cost-effectiveness, patient satisfaction, and functional outcomes. Once established, these pathways should be carefully followed and compliance by rehabilitation specialists should be measured. Pertinent clinical, economic, and patient satisfaction outcomes should be identified and measured. Outcomes results can subsequently be evaluated for the defined patient population and compared with benchmark data, when available, or with historical data to assess relative performance and improvement.

Protocols for many rehabilitation interventions, including nutritional, exist in most, if not all, hospitals and rehabilitation units. More sophisticated managed care rehabilitation guidelines, pathways, and outcomes measurement systems are currently being defined, published, and used. However, the vast majority of rehabilitation-specific clinical pathways address patients with primary neurological disorders or orthopedic problems, not cancer-specific issues. Currently published guidelines, pathways, and outcomes specific or pertinent to swallowing and speech disorders associated with head and neck cancers have been relatively few.

Dietz (1981), in his monograph, *Rehabilitation Oncology*, provides an excellent discussion of the importance of rehabilitation in the restorative efforts of cancer patients and discusses the management of specific problems. Ridley (1996), in presenting the clinical practice guidelines for malignancies of the head and neck (larynx, oropharynx, and oral cavity), recommends that patients be evaluated before and after treatment for functional impairments in speech and swallowing. He proposes that an attempt be made to rehabilitate speech in all patients who undergo total laryngectomy and that a nasogastric tube be used to manage the nutritional status until the swallowing mechanism has been healed or sufficiently rehabilitated. Physical therapy related to increasing the range of motion of the neck may also be helpful. The National Comprehensive Cancer Network has published guidelines for the treatment of head and neck cancers, but they do not include rehabilitation considerations. Logemann, Pauloski, and Rademaker (1997) recently published a critical pathway for rehabilitation after supraglottic laryngectomy, and commented that critical pathways for rehabilitation are needed. Unfortunately, at present we do not have the data needed to develop such pathways for all treated patient types.

Objective clinical outcomes regarding speech and swallowing function as well as nutritional status need to be defined, measured, and reported. Logemann et al. (1997) evaluated and discussed the relevancy of bedside examination of swallowing physiology versus videofluoroscopy and the ability of head and neck cancer patients to tolerate some aspiration without developing aspiration pneumonia. Langmore (1995) addresses the definition of dysphagia program outcomes and emphasizes the importance of functional outcome measures in efficacy studies rather than just physiological measurements of swallowing. Studies such as these will help define the most appropriate clinical outcomes and enable rehabilitation specialists to begin to compare their results.

Although quality cancer care management needs to be an integrated system, the forces of managed care are tending to disrupt the established working relationships of the specialists involved in the care. Hospital lengths of stay are shorter and more care is being given in the ambulatory care setting, in many cases by non-hospital-based providers. Some specialties are being carved out and contracted for separately, sometimes on a risk-sharing basis. Specialists are finding that they need to coordinate services and work with specialists that they may not have worked with previously, possibly in different health care organizations. Speech therapy and other rehabilitation services may be provided by for-profit rehabilitation service providers not associated with the hospital in which the patient receives the cancer treatment. This potential chaos makes the planning of patients' treatment and rehabilitation more difficult.

The oncologists are beginning to react to this disruption by forming oncology-specific networks that have the capacity to contract for and manage the full continuum of cancer care on a risk-sharing basis. When the network does not provide the specific service, it would contract with the appropriate provider for the service, but continue to manage the overall care. Case managers and social workers will need to help manage patients' care among the various providers on the established clinical guidelines. Rehabilitation care will need to be provided by or contracted for by oncology networks to guarantee the coordinated planning and provision of care necessary for the optimal clinical outcomes.

In the new world of care management, coordinating cancer care and demonstrating the value of appropriate rehabilitation interventions in terms of functional outcomes, cost benefit, and patient satisfaction are considerable challenges. Participating in the new health care delivery systems and being able to present outcomes data will help rehabilitation specialists compete for managed-care contracts and be appropriately reimbursed for their services.

REFERENCES

Annas, G. J. (1995). Reframing the debate on health care reform by replacing our metaphors. *New England Journal of Medicine, 332,* 744-747.

Berger, E. L. (1995, July/August). Specialty physician networks in managed care. *Health Care Innovations,* 16-18, 37-38.

Blumenthal, D. (1995). Health care reform—Past and future. *New England Journal of Medicine, 332,* 465-468.

Brown, L. D. (1993). Commissions, clubs, and consensus: Reform in Florida. *Health Affairs, 2,* 7-26.

Campbell, B. (1995). Oncology networks: Genesis. *Oncology Issues, 10,* 22-25.

Crittenden, R. A. (1993). Managed competition and premium caps in Washington state. *Health Affairs, 12,* 82-88.

Dernberg, J. (1992). The RBRVS for oncology services. *Oncology Issues, 7,* 9-19.

Dietz, J. H. (1981). *Rehabilitation oncology.* New York: John Wiley & Sons.

Einstein, A. B. (1996). The impact of health care reform on cancer care. In V. T. Devita, S. Hellman, & S. A. Rosenberg (Eds.), *Cancer principles and practice of oncology* (5th ed., pp. 2957-2966). Philadelphia: Lippincott-Raven.

Field, M. J., & Lohr, K. N. (Eds.) (1990). *Clinical practice guidelines: Directions for a new program. Institute of Medicine, Committee on Clinical Practice Guidelines.* Washington, DC: National Academy Press.

Heclo, H. (1995). The Clinton health plan: Historical perspective. *Health Affairs, 14,* 86-98.

Igelhart, J. K. (1992). The American health care system: Medicare. *New England Journal of Medicine, 327,* 1467-1472.

Iglehart, J. K. (1993). The American health care system: Medicaid. *New England Journal of Medicine, 328,* 896-900.

Iglehart, J. K. (1994). Health care reform: The states. *New England Journal of Medicine, 330,* 75-79.

Langmore, S. E. (1995). Efficacy of behavioral treatment for oropharyngeal dysphagia. *Dysphagia, 10,* 259-262.

Logemann, J. A., Pauloski, B. R., & Rademaker, A. (1992). Impact of the diagnostic procedure on outcome measures of swallowing rehabilitation in head and neck cancer patients. *Dysphagia, 7,* 179-186.

Logemann, J. A., Pauloski, B. R., & Rademaker, A. W. (1997). Speech and swallowing rehabilitation for head and neck patients. *Oncology, 11,* 651-656.

Ridley, M. B. (1996). Clinical practice guidelines for malignancies for the head and neck: larynx, oropharynx, and oral cavity. *Cancer Control: Journal of the Moffitt Cancer Center, 3,* 442-447.

Rogal, D. L., & Helm, W. D. (1993). State models: tracking states' efforts to reform their health systems. *Health Affairs, 12,* 27-30.

Skocpol, T. (1995). The rise and resounding demise of the Clinton plan. *Health Affairs, 14,* 66-85.

Xistris, D. M., & Houlihan, N. G. (1994). Impact of reimbursement and health care reform on the ambulatory oncology setting. *Seminars in Oncology Nursing, 10,* 281-287.

I

Index

A

Abitbol, Andre A., chapter author, 47–63
Abulia, 65
Acalculia, 66
Acanthosis, 166
Acetaminophen, 58, 157
Achalasia, 100
Acidosis, 35
Acinetobacter, 233
Acoustic Neuroma Association, 74
Actinomycin, 34
Acyclovir, 145, 155, 169, 229, 230
Adenocarcinoma. *See under* Carcinoma
Adrenocortical cancer, 31
Adriamycin, 34
African-Americans, cancer incidence, 14
Ageusia, 15
Aglutition, 198
Agnosia, finger, 66
Agraphia, 66
AIDS (acquired immunodeficiency
    syndrome). See also HIV (human
    immunodeficiency virus)
  anorexia, 163
  cytomegalovirus (CMV), 169–170
  dysphagia, 163
  Epstein-Barr virus (EBV), 170
  leukoplakia, oral hairy, 170
  non-Hodgkin's lymphoma, 175
  odynophagia/oral lesions, 163
  wasting syndrome, 163, 171
Alcohol abuse, 55, 78, 86, 88, 100, 103,
    125
  psychological care, 249–250
Alexia, 67
Alkaloids, vinca, 33, 34, 175
Alkylamines, 241

Alkylsufonates, 28
Allen, Kathryn, chapter author, 195–226
Allopurinol, 231
Alopecia, 8
Alprazolam, 252
American Botanical Council, 225
American Brain Tumor Association, 73
Amifostine, 61–62
Aminogluthethimide, 31
Amphotericin, 167, 168, 230
    amphotericin B, 239
Anastrozole, 31
Androgen, 5, 31, 35
Anemia, 8, 122–125, 137, 166, 167
  aplastic, 150
  Fanconi's, 150
Anesthesia, local, 81–82, 145
Angiogenesis, 3
Angiomatosis, bacillary, HIV (human
        immunodeficiency virus), 164
Anorexia, 15, 117, 122–125, 156, 168,
        196, 199, 201, 205
  AIDS (acquired immunodeficiency
        syndrome), 163
Antacids, 214
Antibiotics, 30, 32, 129, 144, 155, 165,
        166, 171, 260
Anticachectic therapies, 124
Anticholinergics, 241
Antidepressants, 113
  tricyclic, 166, 242
Antifungals, 144, 163, 165, 166, 171
Antihistamines, 124, 241–242
Antihypertensives, 242
Antimetabolites, 29
Antineoplastic. *See* Chemotherapy
Anxiety, psychological care, 250–254

malabsorption, intervention, 215
malnutrition
    achlorhydria, 15, 200
    dumping syndrome, 15, 198, 200, 202
    etiology, 197–205
    in hospital, 195 106
    implications of, 195–196
    incidence, 129
    lung cancer, 129–132
    prevalence, 196
    treatment effect contributions, 19i
mucositis, 157
odynophagia, intervention, 214
outcome measures, 212
outcomes, 18–19, 20
parenteral/enteral debate, 131–132
pharyngitis, intervention, 214
prosthesis, esophageal, 201
radiation therapy, 58, 201–205, 204–205
reflux, intervention, 214
satiety, early, 15, 122–125, 198
    intervention, 213
stomatitis, intervention, 214
surgery, 200–201, 202
    diabetes, 202
    hyperprothrombinemia, 202
    hypoalbuminia, 202
    oral cavity, 202
    vitamin B-12 deficiency, 201, 202
treatment effects, 191, 199–100
trismus, intervention, 213
tumor effects, localized, 197–199
xerostomia, intervention, 214
Nystatin, 129, 145, 166, 167, 171, 230, 235, 239

O

Odynophagia, 15, 101, 127, 157, 183, 198, 205
    AIDS (acquired immunodeficiency syndrome), 163
Office of Alternative Medicine, National Institutes of Health, 225
ONS (Oncology Nursing Society), rehabilitation definition, 17
Orabase, 231
Oral lesions, AIDS (acquired immunodeficiency syndrome), 163
Oratect, 231

Osteoradionecrosis, 60, 142
Otalgia, 86
Otitis media, 260, 275
Ototoxicity, 44, 229–230, 242, 258, 273–276
    ASHA (American Speech-Language Hearing Association) monitoring guidelines, 276
Ovarian cancer, 28, 39, 150
Oxycodone, 58
Oxygen therapy, hyperbaric, 60

P

Paclitaxel, 30, 61
Pain management, 337–338
Panendoscopy, 79, 80
Papillomavirus, human (HPV), 100
    HIV (human immunodeficiency virus), 164, 170
Parakeratosis, 166
Paralysis, 67
    vocal fold, 168
        bilateral, 95–96
        unilateral, 93–95
Paresis, 67
Parotitis, 173
Paroxetine, 252, 253
Payne, S. Kirk, chapter author, 329–342
PCA (patient-controlled administration), medication, 157, 338
Pediatrics. *See* Children
Pentamidine, 166
Pentoxifylline, 236
Peplomycin, 231
Performance Status Scale for Head and Neck Cancer (PSS), 248
Performance Status Scale for Head and Neck Cancer (PSS-HN), 17
Periodontal disease, HIV (human immunodeficiency virus), 164
Peroxide, hydrogen, 235
Pharmacology. *See also* Chemotherapy; Drugs; individual medications
    candidiasis, oral, 233, 235
    capsaicin, 232
    chamomile, 232–233
    combination products, 239
    cryotherapy, 239–240
    drugs

Scarring, 15
Seizure, 65, 67
Serotonin receptor blockers, 32
Serratia, 143
Sertraline, 252, 253
Sezary syndrome, 136
Sharp, Helen M., chapter author, 329–342
Sialoadenitis, 51
    HIV (human immunodeficiency virus),
        173–174
Sialogogues, 125, 240, 241
Sialor 7, 241
Sialorrhea, 101
Sickle cell disease, 150
Signal transduction, cell, 2–3
Silver nitrate, 237
Sinusitis, HIV (human immunodeficiency
        virus), 164
Sjögren'syndrome, 173
Sodium alginate, 237
Sodium chloride, 156
Speech disorders, lymphoma/leukemia,
        incidence, 138–139
Speech rehabilitation
    exercise, resonance, 297
    Lee Silverman Voice Treatment Program,
        297–298
    management, 346–348
    prostheses, 296, 298–299, 302
        Blom-Singer voice prosthesis, 304
    therapy
        articulation, 292–294
            directed, 293
        compensatory techniques, 293–294,
            295
        exercises, oral facilitative, 292–293
        resonance, 296–299
        voice, 300
    treatment, surgery, 301–302
        articulation, 294, 296
        resonance, 298
    voice, overview, 299–300
Spirochetes, HIV (human
        immunodeficiency virus), 164
Splenomegaly, 136
Staging, 80, 81, 82, 86, 88–89, 92–93, 104
    head and neck cancer, 80, 81, 82, 86,
        88–89, 92–93, 104
    lung cancer, 118, 119, 120
    and ultrasound, endoscopic, 104
Staphylococci, 233

Stem cell transplantation. *See* High dose
        therapy/stem cell transplantation
Steptozocin, 28
Stereognosis, 66
Steroids, 33, 34, 44, 122, 124, 158, 167,
        173
    neutral, 31
    psychosis, 44
Stomatitis, 8, 15, 44, 151, 158, 198, 203
    laser treatment, 240
    prevention, 230–240
    symptoms, 227–228, 228
    treatment, 230–240
Streptococcus faecalis, 233
Streptozocin, 206
Sucralfate, 112, 126–127, 230, 237–238
Suicide, 252–254
Sullivan, Paula A., chapter author, 13–26,
        307–327
Support groups, 249
Surgery
    anesthesia, local, 81–82
    brain tumors, 68–69
    chemotherapy
        postsurgical, 41, 42–44
        preoperative, 40–41
    effects, 15
    electrocorticography, 69
    esophageal carcinoma, 110–111
    head and neck cancer, 77–96
        arytenoidectomy, 96
        esophageal, 104
        Gelfoam injection, vocal fold paralysis,
            94–95, 301
        glottis, 90–91
        hemiglossectomy, 85–86
        hypopharynx, 92–93
        larynx, 88–92
        oral cavity, 84–86
        oropharyngeal wall, 88
        oropharynx, 86
        overview, 77–78
        soft palate, 86
        squamous cell, 104
        subglottis, 91
        supraglottis, 88–90
        tongue base, 86–87
        tonsils, 87–88
        tracheoesophageal puncture (TEP), 92
        vocal fold paralysis, 94–95, 96
    and immunosuppression, 6
    intraoperative cortical mapping, 69